Regenerative Endodontics

Guest Editors

SAMI M.A. CHOGLE, BDS, DMD, MSD
HAROLD E. GOODIS, DDS

DENTAL CLINICS OF NORTH AMERICA

www.dental.theclinics.com

July 2012 • Volume 56 • Number 3

SAUNDERS an imprint of ELSEVIER, Inc.

W.B. SAUNDERS COMPANY
A Division of Elsevier Inc.

1600 John F. Kennedy Boulevard • Suite 1800 • Philadelphia, Pennsylvania 19103-2899

http://www.dental.theclinics.com

DENTAL CLINICS OF NORTH AMERICA Volume 56, Number 3
July 2012 ISSN 0011-8532, ISBN 978-1-4557-3850-2

Editor: Yonah Korngold; y.korngold@elsevier.com

Dental Clinics of North America (ISSN 0011-8532) is published quarterly by Elsevier Inc., 360 Park Avenue South, New York, NY 10010-1710. Months of issue are January, April, July, and October. Business and Editorial Offices: 1600 John F. Kennedy Boulevard, Suite 1800, Philadelphia, PA 19103-2899. Periodicals postage paid at New York, NY and additional mailing offices. Subscription prices are $259.00 per year (domestic individuals), $447.00 per year (domestic institutions), $122.00 per year (domestic students/residents), $310.00 per year (Canadian individuals), $563.00 per year (Canadian institutions), $375.00 per year (international individuals), $563.00 per year (international institutions), and $184.00 per year (international and Canadian students/residents). International air speed delivery is included in all *Clinics* subscription prices. All prices are subject to change without notice. **POSTMASTER:** Send address changes to *Dental Clinics of North America*, Elsevier Health Sciences Division, Subscription Customer Service, 3251 Riverport Lane, Maryland Heights, MO 63043. **Customer Service (orders, claims, online, change of address): Elsevier Health Sciences Division, Subscription Customer Service, 3251 Riverport Lane, Maryland Heights, MO 63043. Tel: 1-800-654-2452 (U.S. and Canada). Fax: 314-447-8029. E-mail: journalscustomer service-usa@elsevier.com (for print support); journalsonlinesupport-usa@elsevier.com (for online support).**

Reprints. For copies of 100 or more, of articles in this publication, please contact the Commercial Reprints Department, Elsevier Inc., 360 Park Avenue South, New York, NY 10010-1710. Tel.: 212-633-3812; Fax: 212-462-1935, E-mail: reprints@elsevier.com.

The *Dental Clinics of North America* is covered in *MEDLINE/PubMed (Index Medicus), Current Contents/Clinical Medicine, ISI/BIOMED* and *Clinahl*.

Printed in the United States of America.

Contributors

GUEST EDITORS

SAMI M.A. CHOGLE, BDS, DMD, MSD
Associate Professor, Program Director, Postgraduate Program in Endodontics, Endodontics Department, The Boston University Institute for Dental Research and Education, Dubai, United Arab Emirates; Adjunct Associate Professor, Department of Endodontics, The Goldman School of Dental Medicine, Boston University, Boston, Massachusetts; Adjunct Associate Professor, Department of Endodontics, Case School of Dental Medicine, Cleveland, Ohio

HAROLD E. GOODIS, DDS
Professor, Chief Academic Officer, The Boston University Institute for Dental Research and Education, Dubai, United Arab Emirates; Adjunct Professor, Department of Endodontics, The Goldman School of Dental Medicine, Boston University, Boston, Massachusetts; Professor Emeritus, Department of Endodontics, The University of California School of Dentistry, San Francisco, California

AUTHORS

TATIANA M. BOTERO, DDS, MS
Clinical Associate Professor, Cariology, Restorative Soicnces and Endodontics, School of Dentistry, University of Michigan, Ann Arbor, Michigan

MIQUELLA G. CHAVEZ, PhD
Postdoctoral Fellow, Department of Bioengineering and Therapeutic Sciences; Department of Orofacial Sciences, University of California, San Francisco, San Francisco, California

MO CHEN, PhD
Center for Craniofacial Regeneration, Columbia University, New York, New York

SHOKO CHO, MD, PhD
Center for Craniofacial Regeneration, Columbia University, New York, New York

SAMI M.A. CHOGLE, BDS, DMD, MSD
Associate Professor, Program Director, Postgraduate Program in Endodontics, Endodontics Department, The Boston University Institute for Dental Research and Education, Dubai, United Arab Emirates; Adjunct Associate Professor, Department of Endodontics, The Goldman School of Dental Medicine, Boston University, Boston, Massachusetts; Adjunct Associate Professor, Department of Endodontics, Case School of Dental Medicine, Cleveland, Ohio

PAUL R. COOPER, PhD
School of Dentistry, University of Birmingham, Birmingham, United Kingdom

TEJAL DESAI, PhD
Professor, Department of Bioengineering and Therapeutic Sciences; Department of Physiology, University of California, San Francisco, San Francisco, California

SUSAN Y. FU, MD, PhD
Center for Craniofacial Regeneration, Columbia University, New York, New York

TODD M. GEISLER, DDS
Member of American Association of Endodontists; Member of American Association of Endodontists Regenerative Committee; Member of Journal of Endodontics Scientific Advisory Board; President and Co-founder, BioMatRx, LLC, Minneapolis, Minnesota

HAROLD E. GOODIS, DDS
Professor, Chief Academic Officer, The Boston University Institute for Dental Research and Education, Dubai, United Arab Emirates; Adjunct Professor, Department of Endodontics, The Goldman School of Dental Medicine, Boston University, Boston, Massachusetts; Professor Emeritus, Department of Endodontics, The University of California School of Dentistry, San Francisco, California

ORAPIN V. HORST, DDS, PhD
Assistant Clinical Professor, Division of Endodontics, Department of Preventive and Restorative Dental Sciences, University of California, San Francisco, San Francisco, California

ANDREW H. JHEON, DDS, PhD
Assistant Adjunct Professor, Department of Orofacial Sciences, University of California, San Francisco, San Francisco, California

NAN JIANG, DDS
Center for Craniofacial Regeneration, Columbia University, New York, New York

MO K. KANG, DDS, PhD
Professor, Jack Weichman Endowed Chair, Section of Endodontics, Division of Associated Clinical Specialty, University of California Los Angeles School of Dentistry, Los Angeles, California

REUBEN H. KIM, DDS, PhD
Assistant Professor, Division of Restorative Dentistry; Section of Oral Biology & Medicine, University of California Los Angeles School of Dentistry, Los Angeles, California

SAHNG G. KIM, DDS, MS
Center for Craniofacial Regeneration; Assistant Professor of Clinical Dental Medicine, Division of Endodontics, College of Dental Medicine, Columbia University, New York, New York

ATHEEL M. KINAIA, DDS
Clinical Assistant Professor, Advanced Education in General Dentistry Program, The European University, Dubai, United Arab Emirates

BASSAM MICHAEL KINAIA, DDS, MS
Assistant Professor, Program Director, Postgraduate Periodontology Program, Periodontology Department, The Boston University Institute for Dental Research and Education, Dubai, United Arab Emirates; Adjunct Assistant Professor, Department of Periodontology and Oral Biology, The Goldman School of Dental Medicine, Boston University, Boston, Massachusetts; Adjunct Faculty, University of Detroit Mercy - School of Dentistry, Detroit, Michigan

OPHIR D. KLEIN, MD, PhD
Associate Professor, Department of Orofacial Sciences; Department of Pediatrics, University of California, San Francisco, San Francisco, California

ALAN S. LAW, DDS, PhD
Diplomate, American Board of Endodontics; Private Practice, The Dental Specialists, Lake Elmo, Minnesota

JEREMY J. MAO, DDS, PhD
Professor and Zegarelli Endowed Chair, Co-Director, Center for Craniofacial Regeneration, Columbia University, New York, New York

SHEBLI MEHRAZARIN, DDS
PhD Candidate, Section of Oral Biology & Medicine, University of California Los Angeles School of Dentistry, Los Angeles, California

PETER E. MURRAY, PhD
Professor, Department of Endodontics, College of Dental Medicine, Nova Southeastern University, Fort Lauderdale, Florida

CHRISTINE M. SEDGLEY, MDS, MDSc, FRACDS, MRACDS(ENDO), PhD
Associate Professor and Chair, Department of Endodontology, School of Dentistry, Oregon Health and Science University, Portland, Oregon

RICHARD M. SHELTON, BDS, PhD
School of Dentistry, University of Birmingham, Birmingham, United Kingdom

ANTHONY J. SMITH, PhD
School of Dentistry, University of Birmingham, Birmingham, United Kingdom

JAMES G. SMITH, BMedSc
School of Dentistry, University of Birmingham, Birmingham, United Kingdom

CHARLES SOLOMON, DDS
Clinical Professor of Dental Medicine, Division of Endodontics, College of Dental Medicine, Columbia University, New York, New York

SONGHEE SONG, DDS
Center for Craniofacial Regeneration, Columbia University, New York, New York

TAKAHIRO SUZUKI, DDS, PhD
Center for Craniofacial Regeneration, Columbia University, New York, New York

RUJING YANG, MD
Center for Craniofacial Regeneration, Columbia University, New York, New York

LING YE, DDS, PhD
Department of Endodontics, West China School of Stomatology, Sichuan University, Chengdu, Sichuan, China

YING ZHENG, DDS, PhD
Center for Craniofacial Regeneration, Columbia University, New York, New York

JIAN ZHOU, DDS, PhD
Center for Craniofacial Regeneration, Columbia University, New York, New York

XUEDONG ZHOU, DDS, PhD
Department of Endodontics, West China School of Stomatology, Sichuan University, Chengdu, Sichuan, China

Contents

> The search for more accessible mesenchymal stem cells than those found in bone marrow has propelled interest in dental tissues. Human dental stem/progenitor cells (collectively termed dental stem cells [DSCs]) that have been isolated and characterized include dental pulp stem cells, stem cells from exfoliated deciduous teeth, stem cells from apical papilla, periodontal ligament stem cells, and dental follicle progenitor cells. Common characteristics of these cell populations are the capacity for self-renewal and the ability to differentiate into multiple lineages. In vitro and animal studies have shown that DSCs can differentiate into osseous, odontogenic, adipose, endothelial, and neural-like tissues.

> The primary goal of regenerative endodontics is to restore the vitality and functions of the dentin-pulp complex, as opposed to filing of the root canal with bioinert materials. A myriad of growth factors regulates multiple cellular functions including migration, proliferation, differentiation, and apoptosis of several cell types intimately involved in dentin-pulp regeneration. Recent work showing that growth factor delivery, without cell transplantation, can yield pulp-dentin–like tissues in vivo provides one of the tangible pathways for regenerative endodontics. This review synthesizes knowledge on many growth factors that are known or anticipated to be efficacious in dental pulp–dentin regeneration.

> Dental tissue injury and regeneration affects the daily lives of almost everyone. Tissue engineering is emerging as a promising therapy to regenerate missing teeth and dental tissues. The aim of regenerative dental therapies is to restore patients to full oral health. This means restoring normal function to missing or damaged tissue. Regeneration approaches use a combination of scaffolds, stem cells, growth factors, tissue engineering, organ tissue culture, transplantation, and tissue grafting. There are 8 key elements to create and use tissue constructs for tissue regeneration. These will be described in detail in this article.

> Biological solutions for the repair and regeneration of the dental tissues offer significant potential for improved clinical treatment outcomes. Translation of dental tissue-engineering approaches to the clinic will make considerable contributions to these outcomes in the future, but exploiting the natural regenerative potential of dentin-pulp to enhance wound-healing responses offers solutions for maintaining pulp vitality now. Strategies to harness the natural regenerative potential of the pulp must be based on a sound biological understanding of the cellular and molecular events

taking place, and require careful consideration of the interplay of infection, inflammation, and regeneration.

The management of a tooth with incomplete root maturation and a necrotic pulp is an endodontic and a restorative challenge. Apexification procedures alone leave the tooth in a weakened state and at risk for reinfection. Regenerative endodontic procedures potentially offer advantages, including the possibility of hard tissue deposition and continued root development. Case studies have reported regeneration of human pulplike tissues in vivo, but there is no protocol that reliably regenerates pulplike tissue. This article summarizes historical, current, and future regenerative treatment approaches.

The use of regenerative endodontic techniques holds great promise for the treatment of immature teeth with necrotic pulp tissue. Several published case reports and case series have demonstrated radiographic evidence of apical bone healing, increases in root length, and root wall thickness. Although histologic changes have been demonstrated in animal models, histology in human teeth is lacking. A summary of these outcomes is discussed in this article.

Regenerative endodontics has encountered substantial challenges toward clinical translation. The adoption by the American Dental Association of evoked pulp bleeding in immature permanent teeth is an important step for regenerative endodontics. However, there is no regenerative therapy for most endodontic diseases. Simple recapitulation of cell therapy and tissue engineering strategies that are under development for other organ systems has not led to clinical translation in regeneration endodontics. Recent work using novel biomaterial scaffolds and growth factors that orchestrate the homing of host endogenous cells represents a departure from traditional cell transplantation approaches and may accelerate clinical translation.

Mesenchymal stem cells (MSCs) are adult stem cells whose self-renewal, multipotency, and immunosuppressive functions have been investigated for therapeutic applications. MSCs have used for various systemic organ regenerative therapies, allowing rescue of tissue function in damaged or failing organs. This article reviews the regenerative and immunomodulatory functions of MSCs and their applications in dental, orofacial, and systemic tissue regeneration and treatment of inflammatory disorders. It also addresses challenges to MSC-mediated therapeutics arising from tissue and MSC aging and host immune response against allogenic MSC transplantation, and discusses alternative sources of MSCs aimed at overcoming these limitations.

The work performed by researchers in regenerative endodontics and tissue engineering over the last decades has been superb; however, many questions remain to be answered. The basic biologic mechanisms must be elucidated that will allow the development of dental pulp and dentin in situ. Stress must be placed on the many questions that will lead to the design of effective, safe treatment options and therapies. This article discusses those questions, the answers to which may become the future of regenerative endodontics. The future remains bright, but proper support and patience are required.

DENTAL CLINICS OF NORTH AMERICA

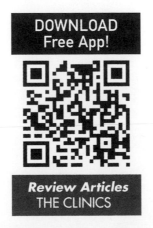

Preface

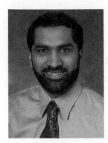
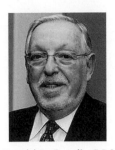

Sami M.A. Chogle, BDS, DMD, MSD   Harold E. Goodis, DDS
Guest Editors

The profession of Dentistry has evolved greatly in every major specialty and treatment area over the last fifty years. The evolution of the profession as a whole clinically has allowed dentists the ability to retain, restore, and replace teeth and other oral tissues. A large part of the process includes research pertinent to several dental specialties, including basic, translational, and clinical sciences. In endodontics, biologic solutions to healing of the dental tissues through repair and regeneration will lead to improved outcomes clinically. Retention or regeneration of the dental pulp in a vital, healthy state will occur through tissue engineering and lead to the preservation of both hard and soft tissues. The early use of direct and indirect pulp capping methods has led to an area once thought to be impossible to produce, hence, Regenerative Endodontics. As the readers will appreciate, Regenerative Endodontics is a complex, difficult area to understand in that not only retention of the original dental pulp can occur but also the generation of new pulp-dentin-enamel-like tissue can be duplicated in form and function in a manner similar to the original tissue.

Leading authors have contributed to a well-rounded review of the field of regenerative endodontics. This edition of *Dental Clinics of North America* preludes with an overview of regenerative medicine and tissue engineering and then delves into the current dental regenerative research. The tri-factor combination of dental stem cells, constructs/scaffolds, and signaling mechanisms/growth factors, integral to repair and regeneration, is discussed together as well as independently. Although a clear clinical translation is still in process, prototypical guidelines, strategies, and initial treatment outcomes are discussed in detail. With this issue the editors and authors aim to review the most current understanding of this therapy-changing field and also provide important factors for future directions. Further understanding of the ability of injured pulpal tissue to heal and repair, coupled with continued research into the processes

Dent Clin N Am 56 (2012) xiii–xiv
doi:10.1016/j.cden.2012.05.013
0011-8532/12/$ – see front matter © 2012 Elsevier Inc. All rights reserved.

necessary to create pulp-like tissues, may yield everyday regenerative therapies in the not-so-distant future.

Sami M.A. Chogle, BDS, DMD, MSD
Postgraduate Program in Endodontics
Endodontics Department
The Boston University Institute for Dental Research and Education
PO Box 505097, Dubai Healthcare City
Dubai, United Arab Emirates

Harold E. Goodis, DDS
The Boston University Institute for Dental Research and Education
PO Box 505097, Dubai Healthcare City
Dubai, United Arab Emirates

E-mail addresses:
sxc89@case.edu (S.M.A. Chogle)
harold.goodis@ucsf.edu (H.E. Goodis)

Stem Cell and Biomaterials Research in Dental Tissue Engineering and Regeneration

Orapin V. Horst, DDS, PhD[a], Miquella G. Chavez, PhD[b,c],
Andrew H. Jheon, DDS, PhD[c], Tejal Desai, PhD[b,d],
Ophir D. Klein, MD, PhD[c,e],*

KEYWORDS

- Tissue engineering • Regenerative medicine • Dental tissues • Scaffold

KEY POINTS

- Dental caries and periodontal disease are the most common diseases resulting in tissue loss. To replace or regenerate new tissues, various types of stem cells have been identified, including embryonic, somatic/adult, and induced pluripotent stem cells. Somatic and induced pluripotent stem cells can be obtained from teeth and periodontium.
- Endothelial cells and their paracrine factors mediate the formation of vasculature into engineered tissues or organs.
- Growth factors and bioactive molecules dictate various aspects of tooth morphogenesis and maturation and thus can be used to guide the formation of engineered tooth tissues in the manner recapitulating development.
- Various biomaterials can be chosen when designing a scaffold, including synthetic, natural, degradable and non-degradable materials.
- Advances in biomaterial sciences including microfabrication, self-assembled biomimetic peptides, and three-dimensional printing hold great promise for whole organ or partial tissue regeneration to replace teeth and periodontium.

Funding: The authors are supported by the NIH/NIDCR.
[a] Division of Endodontics, Department of Preventive and Restorative Dental Sciences, University of California, San Francisco, Box 0758, 521 Parnassus Avenue, Clinical Science Building 627, San Francisco, CA 94143-0758, USA; [b] Department of Bioengineering and Therapeutic Sciences, University of California, San Francisco, Box 2330, 1700 4th Street, San Francisco, CA 94158-2330, USA; [c] Department of Orofacial Sciences, University of California, San Francisco, Box 0442, 513 Parnassus Avenue, San Francisco, CA 94143-0442, USA; [d] Department of Physiology, University of California, San Francisco, Byers Hall Room 203C, MC 2520, 1700 4th Street, San Francisco, CA 94158-2330, USA; [e] Department of Pediatrics, University of California, San Francisco, Box 0442, 513 Parnassus Avenue, San Francisco, CA 94143-0442, USA
* Corresponding author. Department of Orofacial Sciences, University of California, San Francisco, Box 0442, 513 Parnassus Avenue, San Francisco, CA 94143-0442.
E-mail address: Ophir.Klein@ucsf.edu

Dent Clin N Am 56 (2012) 495–520
doi:10.1016/j.cden.2012.05.009
0011-8532/12/$ – see front matter © 2012 Elsevier Inc. All rights reserved.

INTRODUCTION

The ultimate goal for tissue engineering and regenerative medicine is to develop therapies to restore lost, damaged, or aging tissues using engineered or regenerated products derived from either donor or autologous cells. Various approaches have been considered in tissue engineering and regenerative medicine, but currently the most common is to use a biodegradable scaffold in the shape of the new tissue that is seeded with either stem cells or autologous cells from biopsies of damaged tissues.[1,2] The scaffold provides an environment that allows the implanted cells to proliferate, differentiate, and form the desired tissue or organ. Several biomimetic scaffold materials have been used for this purpose, including naturally occurring macromolecules such as collagen, alginate, agarose, hyaluronic acid derivatives, chitosan, and fibrin,[3] and man-made polymers such as polyglycolic acid (PGA), polylactic acid (PLA), poly(caprolactone) (PCL), poly(dioxanone), poly(methyl methacrylate) (PMMA), and poly(glycerol-sebacate).[4–8]

The approach of combining adult stem cells with biomimetic scaffolds and bioactive molecules is in varying stages of development for the treatment of disorders such as diabetes, arthritis, Parkinson disease, Alzheimer disease, atherosclerosis, cancer, and heart disease. This article focuses on dental diseases such as caries and periodontitis, which are pandemic, cause a permanent loss of tissues and functions, and affect the health of populations in all age groups worldwide.

PAST AND PRESENT APPROACHES IN TISSUE REGENERATION

Over the past few decades, new technologies in tissue engineering such as microfabrication, self-assembled biomimetic peptides, and 3-dimensional (3D) printing have rapidly developed. These technologies have enabled the building of simple tissues such as skin epithelium and production of composite tissues such as bone, kidney, and bladder.[9–14]

Regeneration of Nondental Tissues

The first tissue-based therapies for skin grafting were developed in India around 3000 BCE, but the synthesis of substitute materials for skin and various grafting techniques (eg, autologous and allografts) were not developed until the eighteenth century.[15] The first engineered skin tissues were generated by Howard Green and colleagues in 1975.[16,17] This product, which contained only a few layers of cells and did not contain dermis, led to the development of the first commercial skin product, named Epicel (Genzyme, Cambridge, MA, USA), which contains sheets of autologous keratinocytes. Another engineered product for skin was generated using bovine type I collagen and shark chondroitin 6-sulfate.[18,19] These compounds were crosslinked and packed into a porous matrix with a silicone sheet attached onto one side as a temporary epidermis-like barrier. A composite product of reconstituted dermis and epidermis has led to the development of a commercial skin graft product called Apligraf (Organogenesis, Canton, MA, USA).[20,21] The strategy of combining cells and extracellular matrix in skin-graft products was also used to successfully produce cartilage-graft materials. Cell-based cartilage repair techniques were first described in 1994.[22] This technology led to the development of the first commercial product for cartilage grafts, called Carticel (Genzyme). Since 2008, significant advances in tissue engineering have been made for other tissues such as bone, kidney, bladder, blood vessels, and liver.[9–14,23–26]

Unlike other tissues, the skin and cartilage do not require an extensive vascular supply.[23] An important challenge in organ regeneration is the acquisition of a functional vascular supply for the engineered organ. Endothelial cells and the paracrine factors that regulate them, such as vascular endothelial growth factor, were shown to induce angiogenesis and facilitate the integration of transplanted tissues/organs into the host. This finding led to a new treatment strategy in regenerative medicine by using peripheral blood-derived or bone marrow–derived endothelial progenitor cells to induce de novo vessel formation in regenerated organs.[27–29] Vascular endothelial cells can also be generated from human embryonic stem (ES) cells. These cells can integrate into the host and form chimeric vasculature.[30] Vascular endothelial cells can facilitate the differentiation of ES cells into various cell types such as pancreatic insulin-producing cells,[31] cardiomyocytes,[32] neurons, and glial cells.[33] 3D cardiac tissues with endothelial cell networks have been created and implanted onto infarcted rat hearts, which regain function after the surgery. The improvement of cardiac function was dependent on the endothelial cell densities within the engineered cardiac tissues. The number of capillaries in the transplanted tissues with the endothelial cell network is also greater than those without the endothelial cells.[34]

Regeneration of Dental Tissues and Supporting Structures

The regeneration of periodontium was the first tissue-engineering technology in dentistry, and was invented by Nyman and colleagues[35] in 1982. This procedure, termed guided tissue regeneration (GTR), involves inserting a barrier membrane under the periodontal tissue flap to prevent the ingrowth of gingival epithelium and connective tissue, while creating a space on the root surface for progenitor cells from the periodontal ligament including cementoblasts, fibroblasts, and osteoblasts to migrate in and form new periodontal structures including cementum, periodontal ligament, and alveolar bone. Various types of bone-graft materials such as autogenous grafts, allografts, alloplasts, or xenografts have been placed in the space above root surfaces to facilitate bone formation.[36–38]

There are 2 main types of barrier membranes, resorbable and nonresorbable. The nonresorbable membranes require a second surgical procedure to remove the membranes at 4 to 6 weeks after the initial surgery. Two types of commonly used nonresorbable GTR barrier membranes include expanded polytetrafluoroethylene (ePTFE), also known as Gore-Tex, and nonexpanded polytetrafluoroethylene (nPTFE). The resorbable barrier materials were more recently developed and are available in 2 formats, synthetic polymers and natural barrier materials. The synthetic polymer GTR materials consist of a lactide/glycolide copolymer or PLA blended with a citric acid ester. The natural barrier membranes include those made from collagen, calcium sulfate, or enamel matrix proteins.[38–40]

The regeneration of periodontium with these products requires the presence of at least one bony wall at the treatment site, most likely to provide progenitor cells and vascular supply, allowing the repair and regeneration of the periodontal tissues. To improve on the limited level of success, strategies using exogenous growth factors and stem cells have been studied and await translational application to clinical practice. Potential growth factors for periodontal regeneration include bone morphogenetic proteins, platelet-derived growth factor, amelogenin proteins, and fibroblast growth factors.[38,41–46]

Current therapeutic approaches involve replacing the missing tooth structure with artificial materials as the capacity of adult human dental tissues to regenerate is virtually nonexistent, particularly for enamel, due to the absence of ameloblasts in formed teeth. The regeneration and repair of inner-tooth dentin can be obtained only if the healthy dental pulp tissue is still present and if bacterial contamination is completely removed.[47,48] Typically, mechanical removal of decayed enamel and dentin is completed and artificial materials are used to fill in the prepared cavity, to prevent bacterial contamination and induce the formation of reparative dentin onto the dentinal floor of the cavity.

The regeneration of dentin is usually not possible in necrotic teeth. However, in children with incompletely formed teeth with wide-open root apices, pulp tissue can be regenerated through the opened root apices. Findings from prior revascularization studies of traumatized teeth showed that the success of pulp-tissue regeneration in replanted avulsed teeth depends on the diameter of the opening of root apices.[49–51] A diameter of 1 mm (1000 μm) of the opening of root apices has been suggested as a minimum requirement to allow new tissues with neural and vascular structures to regrow into the tooth.[49] Because diameters of the neural, vascular, and cellular structures are less than 100 μm (ie, 10–30-μm diameters for eukaryotic animal and human cells; 0.2–20-μm diameters for nerve fibers; and <100-μm diameters for most arteries in the dental pulp),[52–54] theoretically the regeneration of pulp tissues may not need as much as a 1000-μm–diameter opening. However, the positive correlation of clinical success in revascularization of the replanted teeth and a 1-mm minimum apical opening requirement may be due to the existence of stem cells or progenitor cells in the apical area. Further studies are needed to test this notion.

Several case series showing clinical success of pulp-tissue regeneration in immature necrotic teeth led to the growing recognition of the regenerative potential of tissues at the apical end of these immature teeth.[55–61] The recent identification of adult mesenchymal stem cells in these tissues also suggests that this cell population regrows into the tooth and regenerates the dentin-pulp complex of such immature necrotic teeth. However, the exact mechanisms by which such precursor cells contribute to clinical outcomes remain unknown.

USES OF STEM CELLS IN TISSUE REGENERATION

Cell-based therapies are the most common approaches in regenerative medicine. Challenges in applying this approach clinically are to acquire the appropriate source of cells, to identify methodologies to induce cell proliferation and differentiation, to maintain cell survival, and to remove unwanted cells.

As stem cells possess a remarkable potential to proliferate and develop into many different cell types to form the desired organ, these cells hold great promise for regenerative therapy. The progeny of stem cells may remain as unspecialized progenitors to serve as an internal source of repair and replenishment, or may differentiate into specialized cells to form the desired tissue. The most commonly used and studied stem cells are (1) ES cells, (2) somatic or adult stem cells, and (3) induced pluripotent stem cells.

Embryonic Stem Cells

ES cells are derived from the inner cell mass of early embryos, called blastocysts. ES cells were first isolated from mouse embryos in 1981.[62,63] The success of this work led to the derivation of human ES cells from in vitro fertilized human blastocysts in 1998.[64] ES cells are capable of dividing and renewing themselves for long periods without differentiating, whereas most somatic or adult stem cells cannot. In the appropriate environment, these cells can acquire epigenetic marks in their DNA to modulate their gene expression, allowing them to differentiate into any specialized cells. Various types of specialized cells derived from ES cells[65] include retina cells,[66,67] cardiomyocytes,[32,68] neurons,[69,70] hematopoietic cells,[71,72] hepatic cells,[73–75] trophoblasts,[76,77] pancreatic insulin-producing cells,[31] vascular endothelial cells,[30,78,79] pituitary hormone–producing cells,[30] and osteoblasts.[80,81]

Somatic or Adult Stem Cells

In general, the regenerative capacity of adult tissues depends on tissue-specific stem-cell populations that maintain stable numbers by self-renewal and possess the ability to differentiate into distinct cell lineages. Regeneration and renewal in adult mammals has been studied in several organs, including blood, mammary glands, gut, brain, skin, muscle, and hair. These tissues contain adult stem cells such as hematopoietic, endothelial, mammary, intestinal, neural, skin, muscle, and hair-follicle stem cells. Similarly, teeth and supporting structures contain multiple lineages of somatic stem cells, including:

1. mesenchymal stem cells isolated from the dental pulp of permanent teeth, termed Dental Pulp Stem Cells (DPSC)[82] and from the dental pulp of exfoliated deciduous teeth termed Stem cells from Human Exfoliated Deciduous teeth (SHED)[83]
2. mesenchymal stem cells isolated from the periodontal ligament[84]
3. mesenchymal stem cells isolated from the apical end of developing tooth roots, termed Stem Cells from the Apical Papilla (SCAP),[85–87] and
4. epithelial stem cells isolated from the labial cervical loop of rodent incisors.[88–91]

In primates, incisors cease growth once their roots are completely formed, whereas in rodents the incisors continue to grow throughout postnatal life because of the presence of epithelial and mesenchymal stem cells that have the capacity to self-renew and differentiate into all of the cell types of adult teeth, including ameloblasts, odontoblasts, and the stratum Intermedium (SI). Thus, rodent incisors provide a model for determination of signaling mechanisms that coordinate cell-fate decisions, stem cell self-renewal, and maintenance. The labial cervical loop (CL), but not the lingual CL, of rodent incisors contains stem cells that give rise to ameloblasts and the SI (**Fig. 1**).[92] Labeling experiments demonstrated that cells in the dental epithelium move in a proximal to distal direction.[93] In the labial CL, the stem-cell progeny contribute to a population of transit-amplifying (T-A) cells (see **Fig. 1**A, B). T-A cells undergo several rounds of cell division before they move distally and differentiate into ameloblasts. The incisor epithelia seem to function as a conveyor belt, moving cells from a proximal, undifferentiated source to regularly repopulate the tooth with specialized cell types.

Identification of organ-/tissue-specific adult stem-cell populations can be challenging, because stem cells often reside in heterogeneous niches intermingled with support cells. A useful characteristic of stem cells that has aided in their identification in vivo is the relatively slow cell-division kinetics of many stem cells relative to surrounding tissue.[94] Slow-cycling cell populations have largely been identified through label-retention experiments, traditionally using 5-bromo-2′-deoxyuridine (BrdU) incorporation, because cells that divide slowly do not dilute the BrdU label as quickly as their rapidly dividing neighbors. Using this technique, BrdU label-retaining cells (LRCs) were identified in the labial CL of cultured perinatal incisors and in adult incisors in situ. Another approach to label retention is the use of transgenic mice harboring a tetracycline-sensitive, histone H2B conjugated with a green fluorescent protein cassette (H2B-GFP) under the control of a tissue-specific transactivator (see **Fig. 1**C, D).[95] Expression of H2B-GFP is initially activated in all cells of the tissue of interest followed by a "chase" period when the transgene is repressed by exposure of the animal to doxycycline, such that dividing cells dilute the label. This technique

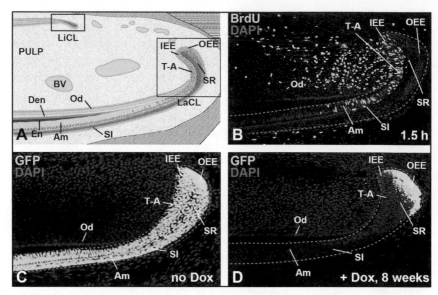

Fig. 1. Mouse epithelial cervical loop stem cells. (*A*) Sagittal view of mandibular mouse incisors shows 2 stem-cell compartments in the lingual (liCL) and labial (laCL) cervical loops. The transit-amplifying (T-A) cells and ameloblasts (Am) arise from inner enamel epithelium (IEE), whereas the outer enamel epithelium (OEE) houses the label-retaining cells (LRCs) in the laCL. The LRCs are putative dental epithelial stem cells. D, dentin; E, enamel; Od, odontoblasts; SI, stratum intermedium; SR, stellate reticulum. (*B*) BrdU labeling (1.5 hours) of rapidly proliferating cells in the T-A region of laCL epithelium and adjacent mesenchyme. (*C, D*) Images from incisors of *Krt5*-tTA; H2B-GFP mice. In the absence of doxycycline (no Dox; *C*), GFP is present in all CL epithelial cells expressing *Krt5* including OEE, IEE, SR, SI, and Am. In the presence of doxycycline (+Dox; *D*) for 8 weeks, H2B-GFP expression was turned off, leading to the retention of GFP in the slowly proliferating LRCs of the OEE.

was used to identify LRCs in the outer enamel epithelium of the adult labial CL.[91] The LRCs of the dental epithelium expressed *Gli1*, a target gene of sonic hedgehog (SHH) signaling, and lineage-tracing experiments demonstrated that the *Gli1*-expressing cells were indeed stem cells.[91]

Understanding the regulation of adult stem-cell populations is key to the future use of such cells for clinical therapies. How stem cells are maintained at the appropriate number, what signals regulate their differentiation, and how they are established within the context of the developing organism are important questions in stem-cell research. Many signaling molecules and pathways are implicated in the development and homeostasis of stem cells. These signaling components include SHH, WNT, NOTCH, bone morphogenetic protein (BMP), and fibroblast growth factor (FGF) superfamily proteins that are important regulators of stem cell self-renewal and differentiation.[88,90,92,96–98] During the development of epithelial-mesenchymal-derived organs such as teeth, these proteins mediate critical interactions between epithelial and mesenchymal cells that lead to the various stages of tooth development (**Fig. 2**). Gene-expression data on growth factors and bioactive molecules at each stage of tooth development can be found at www.bite-it.helsinki.fi. An extensive review of dental stem cells and growth factors is provided in articles elsewhere in this issue.

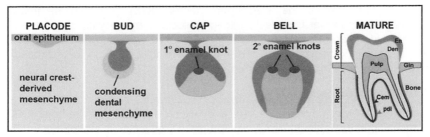

Fig. 2. Schematic of molar development. (1) Placode stage: thickening of oral epithelium and invagination into the neural crest–derived mesenchyme. (2) Bud stage: neural crest–derived mesenchymal cells condense around the epithelial bud. (3) Cap stage: the primary enamel knot, a signaling center, is formed in the epithelial cap. (4) Bell stage. The secondary enamel knots, the future sites of cusps, are present. At the tip of the future cusps, the dental papilla mesenchymal cells, adjacent to the inner enamel epithelium, differentiate into dentin-producing cells, odontoblasts. Once the odontoblasts lay down the dentin matrix, the inner enamel epithelial cells, adjacent to odontoblasts, differentiate into enamel-producing cells (ameloblasts) and secrete enamel matrix. This process continues until the tooth crown is completely formed. (5) Mature tooth: once the crown is completely formed with mineralized enamel and dentin, the tooth erupts while the roots and periodontal supporting structures are continuously formed until the closure of the apical end of the tooth roots.

CELL-REPROGRAMMING TECHNIQUES

ES cells possess the capacity to multiply indefinitely. Under an appropriate microenvironment, these cells can differentiate into any cell types and are very useful in research and clinical applications in tissue engineering and regenerative medicine. However, undifferentiated ES cells have the potential to form tumors.[99–101] The derivation of human ES cells with matched immunogenotypes from fertilized human embryos also raises ethical issues. By contrast, somatic stem cells or adult stem cells have limited applications. These cells are capable of generating cell types of the tissue in which the cells reside but not cells of a very different origin. For example, hematopoietic stem cells are blood-forming adult stem cells that give rise to various blood cells but not cells of different tissues.

The challenges of working with human ES cells and somatic stem cells in part led to the development of new techniques for obtaining stem cells. Two such techniques are transdifferentiation and induced pluripotent stem cells.

Transdifferentiation

This process converts a given cell type directly into another specialized cell type without bringing the cells back to a pluripotent state. The success of this approach was shown for the conversion between two closely related cell types. For example, a transcription factor, MyoD, was used to convert dermal fibroblasts, chondroblasts, gizzard smooth muscle cells, and pigmented retinal epithelial cells into elongated postmitotic mononucleated striated myoblasts.[102] Similarly, adult mesenchymal stem cells from teeth and bone marrow were shown to normally differentiate only into other mesenchymal cell types such as chondrocytes and adipocytes.[82,103] However, a combination of 3 neural transcription factors, ASCL1, BRN2, and MYT1L, converted mouse embryonic and postnatal fibroblasts into functional neurons in vitro.[104] Furthermore, the transcription factor OCT4 and cytokine treatment converts human dermal fibroblasts into granulocytic, monocytic, megakaryocytic, and erythroid lineage cells.[105] Another set of transcription factors, C/EBPβ and C/EBPα, were used to convert fibroblasts into macrophages.[106] Even so, the transdifferentiation approach remains an area of great debate.

Induced Pluripotent Stem Cells

This technique was developed using a quartet of transcription factors, OCT3/4 (Pou5f1), SOX2, KLF4, and c-MYC, to reprogram somatic cells into pluripotent stem cells.[107–109] The first induced pluripotent stem (iPS) cells were developed from adult mouse cells by Yamanaka and Takahashi in 2006[107,108] and from adult human cells by the same group in 2007.[110] This breakthrough discovery provided a new way to dedifferentiate cells while maintaining donor-specific immunocharacteristics necessary to prevent rejection by the immune system. The iPS cells possess almost identical properties to the ES cells in that they can multiply almost indefinitely without losing their potential to differentiate into any cells of the 3 germ layers: endoderm, mesoderm, and ectoderm.[110,111]

iPS cells can be produced from both normal and diseased tissues. For example, iPS cells were derived from human amniotic fluid cells collected for diagnosis from patients with β-thalassemia[112] and those from cystic fibrosis lung removed from patients.[113] Instead of transdifferentiation, this approach is also useful to reprogram adult stem cells to generate specialized cells of different origins. For example, endothelial CD34$^+$ progenitor cells were derived from the iPS cells of bone marrow,[114] and functional neurons were produced from the iPS cells of skin dermal fibroblasts.[115]

STRATEGIES FOR SELECTIVE REMOVAL OF UNDIFFERENTIATED STEM CELLS

Challenges in the clinical application of stem-cell–based therapies are not only to differentiate the cells into the desired specialized cell types but also to establish strategies to remove residual undifferentiated cells to prevent tumor formation. Both positive and negative selection systems have been proposed, including:

- Engineered human ES cells to express herpes simplex virus thymidine kinase so that the ES cells can be killed by ganciclovir at concentrations that are nonlethal to other cell types[116–118]
- Magnetic activated cell sorting using antibodies for differentiation markers for positive selection and/or a selective killing of residual undifferentiated cells by the cytotoxic monoclonal antibody mAb 84.[119–121]

SCAFFOLDS IN TISSUE ENGINEERING

The type of scaffolding material that stem cells will require to generate specific tissues is an area of great interest. The 2 basic methods for tissue engineering are a top-down approach and a bottom-up approach. The more traditional method is the top-down approach, whereby cells are seeded in a preformed 3D scaffold made from polymer, natural porous materials, or decellularized native extracellular matrix. In the bottom-up approach, various methods have been used to aggregate cells to form distinct subunits that could eventually be used as building blocks to engineer whole organs. Examples of these methods are cell printing, microwells, cell sheets, and self-assembled hydrogels. This section describes the various types of scaffold materials used in tissue engineering, the types of methods in which these materials are used (top-down vs bottom-up), and a few examples of how these materials are being applied to dental pulp regeneration. An extensive review of scaffolds in dental tissue generation is provided in an article elsewhere in this issue.

Scaffold Materials

Whether the approach is top-down or bottom-up, the role of a scaffold is to provide support for delivering cells and/or growth factors to the proposed site of tissue regeneration. Toward these goals, there are important features to consider in scaffold selection, including the physical and mechanical aspects of the material, its biocompatibility, and its degradation timeline. These physical aspects of a 3D scaffold include the porosity (pore volume fraction of the scaffold), pore size (pore diameter), pore structure (shape), and all aspects that can influence how well the cells adhere to the material.[122–124] Hydrogels are polymeric structures that are crosslinked and swell in water. For a hydrogel, important aspects include swelling behavior and diffusivity of the hydrogel.

Important mechanical properties of a scaffold material include the viscoelasticity and the tensile strength. For dental regeneration purposes, the tensile strength may be not as important as the viscoelastic properties of the scaffold materials. In general, scaffold materials should reflect the microenvironment of target tissues/organs to facilitate cell growth and ultimately integration to the host. A beneficial clinical feature for dental pulp regeneration would be if the scaffold is injectable, as are some of the natural scaffold materials and hydrogels. In these cases, the gelation time would need to be taken in to consideration when seeding cells in a scaffold for implantation into a host.

An essential clinical feature for scaffold selection is biocompatibility. Naturally derived scaffold materials have the advantage that they are generally well tolerated, do not lead to immunogenic response, and do not involve the use of harsh chemicals during processing. However, a major drawback is the lack of control over the pore size and heterogeneity of the scaffold.

The degradation process of the scaffold is important, and should closely follow the rate of tissue regeneration. When using synthetic polymers, the release of acidic degradation products must be taken into consideration, as well as the resulting drop in pH in the surrounding microenvironment and how that affects the immune response, surrounding tissue, and other factors. Ceramics and bioactive glasses have only recently been studied in terms of how their dissolution products affect cell behavior, and further research is needed to completely understand the mechanism by which the cells and these by-products react.[125]

Synthetic Scaffolds

Biodegradable scaffold materials

Polyglycolic acid (PGA) is a simple, linear, aliphatic polyester that was first used as a biodegradable suture. The PGA suture was brought to market under the trade name Dexon. PGA in scaffolds was first introduced in the 1980s, alone as a mesh to investigate renal injury,[126] and blended with Dacron (polyethylene terephthalate), to study tendon and ligament repair.[127–129] Large-scale production of fibrous PGA scaffolds with consistent porosity was achieved in the early 1990s, which was used to regenerate cartilaginous tissue.[130] The degradation rate was studied in vitro, whereby only 30% of the polymer remained after 8 weeks.

The first copolymer mixture to gain approval from the Food and Drug Administration was the mixture of PGA with a more hydrophobic polymer, polylactic acid (PLA).

This copolymer, poly(lactic-co-glycolic acid) (PLGA) was first available as a suture material under the trade name Vicryl in 1974. PLGA scaffolds were used in the early 1990s toward engineering bone[131] and liver,[132] and were famously used in the tissue engineering of cartilage in the shape of a human ear.[133] PLGA in a 50:50 mixture has a degradation time of about 8 weeks.[134] PLGA can also be blended with other polymers as well as natural materials, such as gelatin,[131] which was used to study trabecular bone regeneration.

PLA is another biodegradable aliphatic polyester, more hydrophobic than PGA. There are 2 racemic isoforms, poly-L-lactic acid (PLLA) and poly-D-lactic acid (PDLA). The racemic mixture can be termed poly-D,L-lactic acid (PDLLA) or simply PLA, without indication of which chiral form is present. PLA in scaffolds is usually found in a copolymer mixture (see above), although a few early studies looked at the use of PLA scaffolds for cartilage repair[135] and nerve regeneration.[136] PLLA fibrous scaffolds maintained integrity for a 42-day period, during which PDLLA fibrous scaffolds shrunk significantly after only 3 days.[137]

Poly(ε-caprolactone) (PCL) is a slowly degrading polymer that was first tested as a bulk material for dermal fibroblast growth.[138] PCL scaffolds have been used toward tissue engineering efforts in bone, either alone[139,140] or combined with hydroxyapatite (HA).[141] PCL scaffolds are attractive for the longer term, as it degrades over 2 years.[142,143]

Non-biodegradable scaffold materials

In addition to biodegradable scaffolds, nonbiodegradable scaffolds have also been investigated for tissue-engineering purposes. These materials in some cases can be osseointegrated and are well tolerated by the body.

Polymethyl methacrylate (PMMA) is biocompatible and has been studied for its potential in drug delivery[144] and dermal fillers,[145] but a few studies have been done on its potential as a 3D scaffold,[146] toward bone and cartilage repair,[145,147] as well as a template for nerve regereration.[148]

Polytetrafluoroethylene (PTFE), more commonly known by its commercial name Teflon, is a polymer made up of repeating carbon and fluorine subunits. It has been extensively studied for its use in vascular grafts.[149] Tissue-engineering efforts using this material outside of vascular work have been sparse, although successful culture of adipocytes[150] and cartilage from the temporomandibular joint have been reported.[151]

Polydimethylsiloxane (PDMS) is a silicon-based polymer, most commonly used in soft lithography processing of microfluidic devices. PDMS scaffolds have been used in tissue engineering of the heart,[152,153] bone,[154,155] liver,[156] and muscle.[157]

Other synthetic scaffold materials

Polyethylene glycol (PEG)-based scaffolds are the most widely used hydrogels. These scaffolds have been synthesized as copolymer solutions and come in variable weights. Poly(2-hydroxyethyl methacrylate) has been used since the late 1960s as a contact-lens material.[158] Studies using the material as a hydrogel for cell encapsulation/tissue engineering began in the 1980s and have been used toward the regeneration of several tissues, including spinal cord/nerve,[159] cardiac tissue,[160] bone,[161] and skin.[162] There have been a few published studies of this material and composites in dental applications, discussed in the section on dental pulp regeneration. Polyvinyl alcohol has long been used to investigate islet encapsulation,[163–166] and has been used as a drug-delivery material[167] and in tissue engineering of the cornea[168] and cartilage.[169]

Naturally Derived Materials

Naturally derived scaffolds

There are several naturally derived materials used as either a coating, alone as a hydrogel, or in combination with synthetic materials.

Alginate is a hydrogel comprising 1,4-linked β-D-mannuronic acid and α-L-guluronic acid, typically derived from brown seaweed and also bacteria.[170] The advantages of alginate are its biocompatibility, low toxicity, and slow gelling time (20–60 minutes), depending on the concentration and temperature.[171] Disadvantages of the material are the inability to control its degradation rate in vivo and its low viscoelasticity, although this can be improved by increased crosslinking or addition of other substances, such as HA.[172] Several studies using alginate and alginate/HA mixtures have been performed in bone and cartilage tissue engineering.[173,174]

Agarose is well known for its use in nucleic acid electrophoresis, but it is also a useful hydrogel for cell encapsulation. It has been used in neuronal[148,175] and cartilage[176,177] tissue engineering, as well as in composites for engineering of bone[173] and cornea[178] with HA and fibrin, respectively.

Chitosan is a polymer derived from the deacetylation of chitin, the major component of crustacean exoskeletons. It can be formulated into an injectable hydrogel, and has been used in the study of epithelial wound healing,[179] repair after myocardial infarction,[180] and for intestinal[181] and central nervous system[182] tissue engineering. Chitosan is also used as a copolymer with other natural materials[183–185] and synthetic materials.[186,187]

Collagen, fibrin, gelatin, hyaluronic acid, and pectin have been used as natural materials in conjunction with one of the other materials described previously, and are discussed here only regarding their contributions toward dental tissue engineering.

Bioceramics and Metals

Bioceramics and metals have long been used as implant materials for joint and tooth replacement. HA is a natural bioceramic constituting various hard tissues such as bone, dentin, and enamel.[188] The HA-based materials have been widely used for dental tissue and bone engineering[141,145,173,174] and are often used in conjunction with tricalcium phosphate (TCP).[189–191]

Titanium is the most widely used metal for implants because of its biocompatibility and a capacity to osteointegrate, a beneficial feature for dental implants. Titanium can be coated with various polymers.

3D Organ Printing

3D organ printing involves 3 sequential steps: (1) preprocessing or development of blueprints for organs, (2) processing or actual organ printing, and (3) postprocessing or organ conditioning and accelerated organ maturation. The 3D cell printers can print single cells or cell aggregates onto the previously printed successive layers of thermosensitive gels in a layer-by-layer fashion. These sequential layers are assembled to create the 3D organ.[192–194] Recently, a new technique termed micro-masonry was introduced for the formation of engineered tissues or organs in 3 dimensions. The shape-controlled PEG microgels are mixed in a prepolymer solution and spread onto the surface of a template made from PDMS. The microgels assemble and closely pack to form a brick-wall–like structure on the surface of the template. The microgels are then illuminated to crosslink the polymer and create a 3D replica of the PDMS template. Cells can be incorporated into the prepolymer solution with a high survival rate ($83.1\% \pm 2.3\%$).[195]

SCAFFOLDS IN DENTAL PULP TISSUE ENGINEERING

Humans have long used both natural and synthetic materials as replacements for lost teeth. The earliest known dental implant was made of iron and found in a Roman male, believed to be dated around 200 CE.[196] The first tooth made from a natural material was found in a Mayan woman, estimated around 600 CE, and was made of nacre, or mother of pearl, from sea shells.[197] Although dental implants continue to be used today, more recently tissue engineering has been used to recreate dental tissues. Not surprisingly, both natural and synthetic materials have been explored for this use, each with encouraging results. In dental tissue engineering, a wide variety of biomaterials have been used such as human bone derivatives, natural porous materials, bioceramics, and synthetic polymers.

Synthetic Scaffolds

The most extensively studied scaffold system for dental tooth regeneration is the use of biodegradable PGA scaffolds. The first reported studies maintained human adult dental pulp on a PGA scaffold for more than 60 days in culture.[198] Follow-up studies used PGA scaffolds with human dental pulp and found upregulation of type I collagen, fibronectin, and several BMPs and their receptors, suggesting the capacity of this scaffold to maintain cell vitality and support the differentiation of human dental pulp cells.[199]

More recently, mixtures of PGA with both synthetic copolymers and other macromolecules were used for dental tissue engineering. PLGA scaffolds have 2 different pore sizes: 150 to 180 μm and 180 to 300 μm. These scaffolds were evaluated in rabbits using autologous DPSCs and were shown to induce osteodentin formation after subcutaneous implantation for 2 and 6 weeks.[200]

PGA scaffolds were compared with β-tricalcium phosphate (B-TCP), fibrin, and collagen scaffolds for their capacity to grow dental structures when seeded with tooth germs from 6-month-old minipigs.[201] On fibrin and collagen gels, the porcine third molar tooth bud maintains its epithelial structure, resembling tooth buds, whereas on PGA and B-TCP, the implanted tooth buds produce more dentin-like material.

The mixtures of PGA fiber mesh scaffolds with porous or nonporous HA/B-TCP were used to seed porcine dental pulp–derived cells and were implanted subcutaneously for 6 weeks. Newly-formed hard tissues were observed in all implants but the dentin-like structure with expression of dentin sialoprotein (DSP), collagen type I, osteonectin, and bone sialoprotein (BSP) was only seen in the PGA-cell implants with porous HA/beta-tricalcium phosphate.[202]

PGA/PLLA and PLGA scaffolds were used in pioneering work in which scaffolds were formed in tooth molds, seeded with porcine third molar dissociated tooth buds, and allowed to grow in the omenta of athymic rats. After 20, 25, and 30 weeks, tooth-like structures containing pulp, dentin, and enamel were observed, with surrounding cells expressing BSP and amelogenin.[203] Similar results were obtained by seeding rat tooth bud cells on both PGA and PLGA scaffolds for 12 weeks in the omentum[204] or rat jaw.[205]

Studies comparing PLGA with HA, B-TCP, or calcium carbonate hydroxyapatite found that human DPSCs proliferated best on PLGA with B-TCP and were able to form mineralized structures. After 4 to 5 weeks, the rat tooth bud cells differentiated and expressed DSP.[180]

PCL scaffolds were used for the regeneration of various mineralized tissues such as bone, cartilage, and dentin.[206–209] The PCL scaffolds support adhesion, proliferation, and odontoblastic differentiation. The incorporation of HA into PCL scaffolds enhances odontoblastic differentiation of human DPSCs.[209]

PEG is also known as polyethylene oxide or polyoxyethylene. These scaffold materials can support cell growth and differentiation as well as decelerate the degradation of fibrin, thus creating a new hybrid material, PEGylated fibrin gel, for cell delivery.[210]

Naturally Derived Materials

Naturally derived scaffolds

Alginate has been used in dental engineering to deliver cells and/or growth factors. The alginate hydrogel with either transforming growth factor (TGF)-β1 or acid treatment was applied to slices of human teeth with vital dentin-pulp complex tissues and maintained in culture. Hydrogel with TGF-β1 or acid treatment, but not the untreated control hydrogel, induced dentin matrix secretion and formation of new odontoblast-like cells in the human tooth slices.[211]

Collagens, particularly type I collagen, are major constituents of dentin and have been used to provide a 3D culture environment for various types of cells, including stem cells from the dental pulp.[212] Compared with other natural scaffold products including gelatin and chitosan, the dental pulp cells cultured in the type I and III collagen gel exhibited a higher degree of odontoblastic differentiation as shown by alkaline phosphatase activity and expression of osteocalcin, dentin sialophosphoprotein (DSPP), and dentin matrix protein 1 (DMP1).[212–216] Collagen gel can be used alone or in combination with growth factors (eg, TGF-β1, BMP4, FGF2)[217] and other scaffold materials such as chitosan.[218]

Chitosan/HA blend (polyelectrolyte complex) was used for compatibility studies with mesenchymal stem cells. In a 2:1 blend (HA/chitosan), cells were viable for 72 hours and no cytotoxicity was apparent.[185] The same group used chitosan/pectin scaffolds for bone regeneration with similarly positive results.[184] Chitosan/collagen scaffolds adsorbed with BMP7 were seeded with human adult dental pulp cells and stained positive for dentin matrix proteins DSPP and DMP1, whereas scaffolds without BMP7 were negative.[218]

Hyaluronic acid sponges were used as 3D scaffolds for the regeneration of dental pulp. In comparison with the collagen sponge, the hyaluronic acid sponge can support cell growth in culture and in vivo from the amputated dental pulp of rat molars, with fewer immunologic reactions as shown by expression of inflammatory cytokines tumor necrosis factor (TNF)-α and interleukin-6, as well as leukocyte infiltration.[219] However, when used as an injectable hyaluronic acid gel for soft-tissue augmentation, adverse hypersensitivity reactions were reported, due to impurities and bacterial contamination.[220]

Fibrin consists of the blood proteins fibrinogen and thrombin, which are produced naturally in the body after injury to establish hemostasis and enhance wound healing. Because of these properties, fibrin glue, fibrin sealant, and fibrin in other forms were produced to aid bleeding control, speed wound healing, cover holes instead of sutures, and provide slow-release delivery of antibiotics or other drugs. Because of their biocompatibility, biodegradability, simple preparation, and manipulation, fibrin scaffolds have been used for multiple purposes (eg, filling in bone cavities, vascular graft, and repairing injuries to urinary tract, liver, and lung) and are also available as mixtures with other polymers such as fibrin-PEG blend.[210,221–225] Fibrin hydrogel allows the incorporation of growth factors and bioactive molecules via a heparin-binding delivery system, cell seeding through inkjet printing, and self-assembly through a magnetically influenced technique.[225] Blood clots have been used as natural scaffolds for bone healing in the tooth-extraction socket as well as for dental pulp regeneration/revascularization in immature necrotic teeth. Fibrin glue and platelet-rich fibrin can be prepared from whole blood before surgery. The mixture of these 2 components was used as a scaffold for reassembly of porcine tooth bud cells implanted in the extraction socket. After 36 weeks, these implants developed into a complete tooth or an unerupted tooth crown.[226] The mixtures of fibrin and other polymers such as PEGylated fibrin scaffold aid in handling the material. The PEGylated fibrin scaffold is injectable, tunable, degradable, and compatible with dental stem cells. It induces osteoblastic and odontoblastic differentiation as well as the formation of dentin-like collagenous matrix and vascularized pulp-like structure after transplantation in vivo.[226]

Nanostructured Films and Self-assembled Peptides

Recently, investigators have been examining scaffold microtopography and nanotopography as a determinant for successful dentin regeneration. Scaffold nanotopography and molecular self-assembly offer new directions for the fabrication of tissues with similar cell and matrix organization to the native tissues at the nanoscale.[227] This nanotechnology can be used not only for tissue engineering but also for the delivery of antimicrobial and/or anti-inflammatory drugs, which will be beneficial for endodontic regeneration. For example, the PGA scaffold was incorporated with an anti-inflammatory peptide, α-melanocortin (α-MSH). The PGA/α-MSH scaffold promotes the adhesion and proliferation of human pulp fibroblasts while inhibiting inflammatory responses.[228] In another study, the nanostructured, self-assembling peptides were used as a carrier for the anti-inflammatory drug K5, which inhibits the production of inflammatory cytokines TNF-α and prostaglandin E_2 from macrophages.[229] More detailed studies are needed to evaluate the effects of these peptides on various cell types in the dental pulp and the formation of dentin in a more clinical relevant setting.

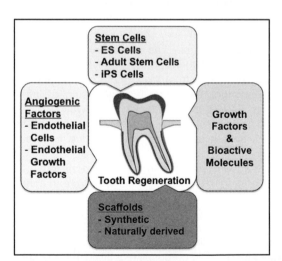

Fig. 3. Key components of organ/tissue engineering. Key components include (1) stem cells (ie, embryonic stem cells, ES cells; somatic/adult stem cells; induced pluripotent stem cells, iPS cells) or any cells with the capacity to form the desired tissue/organ; (2) angiogenic factors to enhance vascularization of the engineered tissue/organ; (3) growth factors and/or bioactive molecules such as those in the fibroblast growth factor, bone morphogenetic protein, sonic hedgehog, Wnt, and Notch signaling pathways; and (4) scaffold to deliver cells and drugs. Together with embedded growth factors and/or bioactive molecules, the scaffold provides a microenvironment that supports the development and differentiation of stem cells into specialized cells to form the target tissue/organ.

SUMMARY

The emergence of tissue engineering and regenerative medicine shed new light on the treatment of patients with degenerative disorders. These approaches combine tools from a variety of fields such as stem-cell biology, biomaterials, and developmental biology. Whereas regenerative medicine places more emphasis on cell-based therapy, particularly stem cells, to repair or replace damaged tissues/organs, tissue engineering focuses on using biomaterials with or without cells to make bioartificial tissues or organs. Various sources of stem cells have been identified and used to generate the desired specialized cell or tissue types. These stem cells are classified into 3 main types: ES cells, somatic/adult stem cells, and induced pluripotent stem cells. In addition, endothelial cells and their paracrine factors such as vascular endothelial growth factor were shown to play important roles in mediating angiogenesis to nurture engineered tissues or organs and facilitate host integration. Other growth factors and bioactive molecules such as those included in the FGF, BMP, Shh, Wnt, and Notch signaling pathways dictate various aspects of tooth morphogenesis and maturation, and thus can be used to guide the formation of engineered tooth tissues/organs in the manner recapitulating development. These key components are summarized in **Fig. 3**.

Finally, in order to apply stem-cell–based therapies to the treatment of diseases, the appropriate microenvironment must be identified to guide the development of stem cells through the following 6 steps:

1. To increase survival of stem cells in the recipient/transplant.
2. To integrate the transplanted cells into the surrounding tissue without harming the recipient; research strategies must be created to avoid the problem of immune rejection without long-term use of immunosuppressive drugs.
3. To increase the proliferation of stem cells to generate sufficient amounts of tissue.
4. To induce the differentiation of stem cells into the desired cell type(s).
5. To maintain the differentiated cells and retain their functions throughout the recipient's life.
6. To remove unwanted cells.

ACKNOWLEDGMENTS

The authors thank Dr Kerstin Seidel for help with figures, and members of the Klein and Desai laboratories for helpful discussions.

REFERENCES

1. Kim BS, Nikolovski J, Bonadio J, et al. Engineered smooth muscle tissues: regulating cell phenotype with the scaffold. Exp Cell Res 1999;251:318–28.
2. Stock UA, Vacanti JP. Tissue engineering: current state and prospects. Annu Rev Med 2001;52:443–51.
3. Hutmacher DW, Goh JC, Teoh SH. An introduction to biodegradable materials for tissue engineering applications. Ann Acad Med Singapore 2001;30:183–91.
4. Gloria A, De Santis R, Ambrosio L. Polymer-based composite scaffolds for tissue engineering. J Appl Biomater Biomech 2010;8:57–67.
5. Novotny L, Crha M, Rauser P, et al. Novel biodegradable polydioxanone stents in a rabbit airway model. J Thorac Cardiovasc Surg 2012;143:437–44.
6. Neeley WL, Redenti S, Klassen H, et al. A microfabricated scaffold for retinal progenitor cell grafting. Biomaterials 2008;29:418–26.

7. Tao S, Young C, Redenti S, et al. Survival, migration and differentiation of retinal progenitor cells transplanted on micro-machined poly(methyl methacrylate) scaffolds to the subretinal space. Lab Chip 2007;7:695–701.

8. Tao SL, Desai TA. Aligned arrays of biodegradable poly(epsilon-caprolactone) nanowires and nanofibers by template synthesis. Nano Lett 2007;7:1463–8.

9. Horst M, Madduri S, Gobet R, et al. Engineering functional bladder tissues. J Tissue Eng Regen Med 2012. [Epub ahead of print].

10. Mhashilkar A, Atala A. Editorial: effective bio-economic approaches for stem cell therapy and regenerative medicine. Curr Stem Cell Res Ther 2012;7:1.

11. Hutmacher DW. Scaffolds in tissue engineering bone and cartilage. Biomaterials 2000;21:2529–43.

12. Guarino V, Causa F, Netti PA, et al. The role of hydroxyapatite as solid signal on performance of PCL porous scaffolds for bone tissue regeneration. J Biomed Mater Res B Appl Biomater 2008;86:548–57.

13. Yokoo T, Fukui A, Kobayashi E. Application of regenerative medicine for kidney diseases. Organogenesis 2007;3:34–43.

14. Woolf AS, Palmer SJ, Snow ML, et al. Creation of a functioning chimeric mammalian kidney. Kidney Int 1990;38:991–7.

15. Herman AR. The history of skin grafts. J Drugs Dermatol 2002;1:298–301.

16. Green H, Kehinde O, Thomas J. Growth of cultured human epidermal cells into multiple epithelia suitable for grafting. Proc Natl Acad Sci U S A 1979;76:5665–8.

17. Grafting of burns with cultured epithelium prepared from autologous epidermal cells. Lancet 1981;1:75–8.

18. Burke JF, Yannas IV, Quinby WC Jr, et al. Successful use of a physiologically acceptable artificial skin in the treatment of extensive burn injury. Ann Surg 1981;194:413–28.

19. Yannas IV, Burke JF, Orgill DP, et al. Wound tissue can utilize a polymeric template to synthesize a functional extension of skin. Science 1982;215:174–6.

20. Bell E, Ehrlich HP, Buttle DJ, et al. Living tissue formed in vitro and accepted as skin-equivalent tissue of full thickness. Science 1981;211:1052–4.

21. Bell E, Ehrlich HP, Sher S, et al. Development and use of a living skin equivalent. Plast Reconstr Surg 1981;67:386–92.

22. Brittberg M, Lindahl A, Nilsson A, et al. Treatment of deep cartilage defects in the knee with autologous chondrocyte transplantation. N Engl J Med 1994; 331:889–95.

23. Berthiaume F, Maguire TJ, Yarmush ML. Tissue engineering and regenerative medicine: history, progress, and challenges. Annu Rev Chem Biomol Eng 2011;2:403–30.

24. Norotte C, Marga FS, Niklason LE, et al. Scaffold-free vascular tissue engineering using bioprinting. Biomaterials 2009;30:5910–7.

25. Uygun BE, Soto-Gutierrez A, Yagi H, et al. Organ reengineering through development of a transplantable recellularized liver graft using decellularized liver matrix. Nat Med 2010;16:814–20.

26. Shito M, Tilles AW, Tompkins RG, et al. Efficacy of an extracorporeal flat-plate bioartificial liver in treating fulminant hepatic failure. J Surg Res 2003;111:53–62.

27. McGuigan AP, Sefton MV. The influence of biomaterials on endothelial cell thrombogenicity. Biomaterials 2007;28:2547–71.

28. Asahara T, Murohara T, Sullivan A, et al. Isolation of putative progenitor endothelial cells for angiogenesis. Science 1997;275:964–7.

29. Masuda H, Asahara T. Post-natal endothelial progenitor cells for neovascularization in tissue regeneration. Cardiovasc Res 2003;58:390–8.

30. Zeng Y, Liu YS. Vascular endothelial cells and pituitary hormone producing cells derived from embryonic stem cells therapy for hypopituitarism. Med Hypotheses 2011;77:680–1.
31. Jaramillo M, Banerjee I. Endothelial cell co-culture mediates maturation of human embryonic stem cell to pancreatic insulin producing cells in a directed differentiation approach. J Vis Exp 2012;61:e3759.
32. Kado M, Lee JK, Hidaka K, et al. Paracrine factors of vascular endothelial cells facilitate cardiomyocyte differentiation of mouse embryonic stem cells. Biochem Biophys Res Commun 2008;377:413–8.
33. Sun J, Zhou W, Ma D, et al. Endothelial cells promote neural stem cell proliferation and differentiation associated with VEGF activated Notch and Pten signaling. Dev Dyn 2010;239:2345–53.
34. Sekine H, Shimizu T, Hobo K, et al. Endothelial cell coculture within tissue-engineered cardiomyocyte sheets enhances neovascularization and improves cardiac function of ischemic hearts. Circulation 2008;118:S145–52.
35. Nyman S, Lindhe J, Karring T, et al. New attachment following surgical treatment of human periodontal disease. J Clin Periodontol 1982;9:290–6.
36. Al Ghamdi AS, Shibly O, Ciancio SG. Osseous grafting part I: autografts and allografts for periodontal regeneration—a literature review. J Int Acad Periodontol 2010;12:34–8.
37. AlGhamdi AS, Shibly O, Ciancio SG. Osseous grafting part II: xenografts and alloplasts for periodontal regeneration a literature review. J Int Acad Periodontol 2010;12:39–44.
38. Izumi Y, Aoki A, Yamada Y, et al. Current and future periodontal tissue engineering. Periodontol 2000 2011;56:166–87.
39. Villar CC, Cochran DL. Regeneration of periodontal tissues: guided tissue regeneration. Dent Clin North Am 2010;54:73–92.
40. Darby I. Periodontal materials. Aust Dent J 2011;56(Suppl 1):107–18.
41. Javed F, Al-Askar M, Al-Rasheed A, et al. Significance of the platelet-derived growth factor in periodontal tissue regeneration. Arch Oral Biol 2011;56:1476–84.
42. Murakami S. Periodontal tissue regeneration by signaling molecule(s): what role does basic fibroblast growth factor (FGF-2) have in periodontal therapy? Periodontol 2000 2011;56:188–208.
43. Kitamura M, Akamatsu M, Machigashira M, et al. FGF-2 stimulates periodontal regeneration: results of a multi-center randomized clinical trial. J Dent Res 2011;90:35–40.
44. Hughes FJ, Ghuman M, Talal A. Periodontal regeneration: a challenge for the tissue engineer? Proc Inst Mech Eng H 2010;224:1345–58.
45. Amin HD, Olsen I, Knowles JC, et al. Differential effect of amelogenin peptides on osteogenic differentiation in vitro: identification of possible new drugs for bone repair and regeneration. Tissue Eng Part A 2012;18(11–12):1193–202.
46. Nokhbehsaim M, Deschner B, Winter J, et al. Interactions of regenerative, inflammatory and biomechanical signals on bone morphogenetic protein-2 in periodontal ligament cells. J Periodontal Res 2011;46:374–81.
47. Kakehashi S, Stanley HR, Fitzgerald RJ. The effects of surgical exposures of dental pulps in germ-free and conventional laboratory rats. Oral Surg Oral Med Oral Pathol 1965;20:340–9.
48. Cox CF, Bergenholtz G, Heys DR, et al. Pulp capping of dental pulp mechanically exposed to oral microflora: a 1-2 year observation of wound healing in the monkey. J Oral Pathol 1985;14:156–68.

49. Kling M, Cvek M, Mejare I. Rate and predictability of pulp revascularization in therapeutically reimplanted permanent incisors. Endod Dent Traumatol 1986;2:83–9.
50. Ohman A. Healing and sensitivity to pain in young replanted human teeth. An experimental, clinical and histological study. Odontol Tidskr 1965;73:166–227.
51. Andreasen JO, Borum MK, Jacobsen HL, et al. Replantation of 400 avulsed permanent incisors. 2. Factors related to pulpal healing. Endod Dent Traumatol 1995;11:59–68.
52. Provenza DV. The blood vascular supply of the dental pulp with emphasis on capillary circulation. Circ Res 1958;6:213–8.
53. Matthews JI, Dorman HL, Bishop JG. Fine structures of the dental pulp. J Dent Res 1959;38:940–6.
54. Cell biology/introduction/cell size. WIKIBOOKS. Available at: http://en.wikibooks.org/wiki/Cell_Biology/Introduction/Cell_size. Accessed May 31, 2012.
55. Banchs F, Trope M. Revascularization of immature permanent teeth with apical periodontitis: new treatment protocol? J Endod 2004;30:196–200.
56. Jung IY, Lee SJ, Hargreaves KM. Biologically based treatment of immature permanent teeth with pulpal necrosis: a case series. J Endod 2008;34:876–87.
57. Cotti E, Mereu M, Lusso D. Regenerative treatment of an immature, traumatized tooth with apical periodontitis: report of a case. J Endod 2008;34:611–6.
58. Thibodeau B, Trope M. Pulp revascularization of a necrotic infected immature permanent tooth: case report and review of the literature. Pediatr Dent 2007;29:47–50.
59. Bose R, Nummikoski P, Hargreaves K. A retrospective evaluation of radiographic outcomes in immature teeth with necrotic root canal systems treated with regenerative endodontic procedures. J Endod 2009;35:1343–9.
60. Iwaya SI, Ikawa M, Kubota M. Revascularization of an immature permanent tooth with apical periodontitis and sinus tract. Dent Traumatol 2001;17:185–7.
61. Reynolds K, Johnson JD, Cohenca N. Pulp revascularization of necrotic bilateral bicuspids using a modified novel technique to eliminate potential coronal discolouration: a case report. Int Endod J 2009;42:84–92.
62. Evans MJ, Kaufman MH. Establishment in culture of pluripotential cells from mouse embryos. Nature 1981;292:154–6.
63. Martin GR. Isolation of a pluripotent cell line from early mouse embryos cultured in medium conditioned by teratocarcinoma stem cells. Proc Natl Acad Sci U S A 1981;78:7634–8.
64. Thomson JA, Itskovitz-Eldor J, Shapiro SS, et al. Embryonic stem cell lines derived from human blastocysts. Science 1998;282:1145–7.
65. Odorico JS, Kaufman DS, Thomson JA. Multilineage differentiation from human embryonic stem cell lines. Stem Cells 2001;19:193–204.
66. Klimanskaya I, Hipp J, Rezai KA, et al. Derivation and comparative assessment of retinal pigment epithelium from human embryonic stem cells using transcriptomics. Cloning Stem Cells 2004;6:217–45.
67. Lund RD, Wang S, Klimanskaya I, et al. Human embryonic stem cell-derived cells rescue visual function in dystrophic RCS rats. Cloning Stem Cells 2006;8:189–99.
68. Laflamme MA, Chen KY, Naumova AV, et al. Cardiomyocytes derived from human embryonic stem cells in pro-survival factors enhance function of infarcted rat hearts. Nat Biotechnol 2007;25:1015–24.
69. Kriks S, Shim JW, Piao J, et al. Dopamine neurons derived from human ES cells efficiently engraft in animal models of Parkinson's disease. Nature 2011;480:547–51.

70. Chambers SM, Fasano CA, Papapetrou EP, et al. Highly efficient neural conversion of human ES and iPS cells by dual inhibition of SMAD signaling. Nat Biotechnol 2009;27:275–80.
71. Kaufman DS, Hanson ET, Lewis RL, et al. Hematopoietic colony-forming cells derived from human embryonic stem cells. Proc Natl Acad Sci U S A 2001; 98:10716–21.
72. Ledran MH, Krassowska A, Armstrong L, et al. Efficient hematopoietic differentiation of human embryonic stem cells on stromal cells derived from hematopoietic niches. Cell Stem Cell 2008;3:85–98.
73. Cai J, Zhao Y, Liu Y, et al. Directed differentiation of human embryonic stem cells into functional hepatic cells. Hepatology 2007;45:1229–39.
74. Lavon N, Yanuka O, Benvenisty N. Differentiation and isolation of hepatic-like cells from human embryonic stem cells. Differentiation 2004;72:230–8.
75. Takayama K, Inamura M, Kawabata K, et al. Efficient generation of functional hepatocytes from human embryonic stem cells and induced pluripotent stem cells by HNF4alpha transduction. Mol Ther 2012;20:127–37.
76. Gerami-Naini B, Dovzhenko OV, Durning M, et al. Trophoblast differentiation in embryoid bodies derived from human embryonic stem cells. Endocrinology 2004;145:1517–24.
77. Chen G, Ye Z, Yu X, et al. Trophoblast differentiation defect in human embryonic stem cells lacking PIG-A and GPI-anchored cell-surface proteins. Cell Stem Cell 2008;2:345–55.
78. Wang ZZ, Au P, Chen T, et al. Endothelial cells derived from human embryonic stem cells form durable blood vessels in vivo. Nat Biotechnol 2007;25: 317–8.
79. Levenberg S, Golub JS, Amit M, et al. Endothelial cells derived from human embryonic stem cells. Proc Natl Acad Sci U S A 2002;99:4391–6.
80. Arpornmaeklong P, Wang Z, Pressler MJ, et al. Expansion and characterization of human embryonic stem cell-derived osteoblast-like cells. Cell Reprogram 2010;12:377–89.
81. Lee KW, Yook JY, Son MY, et al. Rapamycin promotes the osteoblastic differentiation of human embryonic stem cells by blocking the mTOR pathway and stimulating the BMP/Smad pathway. Stem Cells Dev 2010;19:557–68.
82. Gronthos S, Mankani M, Brahim J, et al. Postnatal human dental pulp stem cells (DPSCs) in vitro and in vivo. Proc Natl Acad Sci U S A 2000;97:13625–30.
83. Miura M, Gronthos S, Zhao M, et al. SHED: stem cells from human exfoliated deciduous teeth. Proc Natl Acad Sci U S A 2003;100:5807–12.
84. Seo BM, Miura M, Gronthos S, et al. Investigation of multipotent postnatal stem cells from human periodontal ligament. Lancet 2004;364:149–55.
85. Sonoyama W, Liu Y, Fang D, et al. Mesenchymal stem cell-mediated functional tooth regeneration in swine. PLoS One 2006;1:e79.
86. Sonoyama W, Liu Y, Yamaza T, et al. Characterization of the apical papilla and its residing stem cells from human immature permanent teeth: a pilot study. J Endod 2008;34:166–71.
87. Huang GT, Sonoyama W, Liu Y, et al. The hidden treasure in apical papilla: the potential role in pulp/dentin regeneration and bioroot engineering. J Endod 2008;34:645–51.
88. Wang XP, Suomalainen M, Felszeghy S, et al. An integrated gene regulatory network controls stem cell proliferation in teeth. PLoS Biol 2007;5:e159.
89. Thesleff I, Wang XP, Suomalainen M. Regulation of epithelial stem cells in tooth regeneration. C R Biol 2007;330:561–4.

90. Klein OD, Lyons DB, Balooch G, et al. An FGF signaling loop sustains the generation of differentiated progeny from stem cells in mouse incisors. Development 2008;135:377–85.
91. Seidel K, Ahn CP, Lyons D, et al. Hedgehog signaling regulates the generation of ameloblast progenitors in the continuously growing mouse incisor. Development 2010;137:3753–61.
92. Harada H, Kettunen P, Jung HS, et al. Localization of putative stem cells in dental epithelium and their association with Notch and FGF signaling. J Cell Biol 1999;147:105–20.
93. Smith CE, Warshawsky H. Cellular renewal in the enamel organ and the odontoblast layer of the rat incisor as followed by radioautography using 3H-thymidine. Anat Rec 1975;183:523–61.
94. Fuchs E. The tortoise and the hair: slow-cycling cells in the stem cell race. Cell 2009;137:811–9.
95. Tumbar T, Guasch G, Greco V, et al. Defining the epithelial stem cell niche in skin. Science 2004;303:359–63.
96. van der Flier LG, Clevers H. Stem cells, self-renewal, and differentiation in the intestinal epithelium. Annu Rev Physiol 2009;71:241–60.
97. Blanpain C, Lowry WE, Pasolli HA, et al. Canonical notch signaling functions as a commitment switch in the epidermal lineage. Genes Dev 2006;20:3022–35.
98. Blanpain C, Fuchs E. Epidermal stem cells of the skin. Annu Rev Cell Dev Biol 2006;22:339–73.
99. Arnhold S, Klein H, Semkova I, et al. Neurally selected embryonic stem cells induce tumor formation after long-term survival following engraftment into the subretinal space. Invest Ophthalmol Vis Sci 2004;45:4251–5.
100. Asano T, Sasaki K, Kitano Y, et al. In vivo tumor formation from primate embryonic stem cells. Methods Mol Biol 2006;329:459–67.
101. Nussbaum J, Minami E, Laflamme MA, et al. Transplantation of undifferentiated murine embryonic stem cells in the heart: teratoma formation and immune response. FASEB J 2007;21:1345–57.
102. Choi J, Costa ML, Mermelstein CS, et al. MyoD converts primary dermal fibroblasts, chondroblasts, smooth muscle, and retinal pigmented epithelial cells into striated mononucleated myoblasts and multinucleated myotubes. Proc Natl Acad Sci U S A 1990;87:7988–92.
103. Janebodin K, Horst OV, Ieronimakis N, et al. Isolation and characterization of neural crest-derived stem cells from dental pulp of neonatal mice. PLoS One 2011;6:e27526.
104. Vierbuchen T, Ostermeier A, Pang ZP, et al. Direct conversion of fibroblasts to functional neurons by defined factors. Nature 2010;463:1035–41.
105. Szabo E, Rampalli S, Risueno RM, et al. Direct conversion of human fibroblasts to multilineage blood progenitors. Nature 2010;468:521–6.
106. Feng R, Desbordes SC, Xie H, et al. PU.1 and C/EBPalpha/beta convert fibroblasts into macrophage-like cells. Proc Natl Acad Sci U S A 2008;105:6057–62.
107. Yamanaka S, Takahashi K. Induction of pluripotent stem cells from mouse fibroblast cultures. Tanpakushitsu Kakusan Koso 2006;51:2346–51 [in Japanese].
108. Takahashi K, Yamanaka S. Induction of pluripotent stem cells from mouse embryonic and adult fibroblast cultures by defined factors. Cell 2006;126:663–76.
109. Takahashi K, Okita K, Nakagawa M, et al. Induction of pluripotent stem cells from fibroblast cultures. Nat Protoc 2007;2:3081–9.

110. Takahashi K, Tanabe K, Ohnuki M, et al. Induction of pluripotent stem cells from adult human fibroblasts by defined factors. Cell 2007;131:861–72.
111. Yamanaka S. Strategies and new developments in the generation of patient-specific pluripotent stem cells. Cell Stem Cell 2007;1:39–49.
112. Fan Y, Luo Y, Chen X, et al. Generation of human beta-thalassemia induced pluripotent stem cells from amniotic fluid cells using a single excisable lentiviral stem cell cassette. J Reprod Dev 2012. [Epub ahead of print].
113. Mou H, Zhao R, Sherwood R, et al. Generation of multipotent lung and airway progenitors from mouse ESCs and patient-specific cystic fibrosis iPSCs. Cell Stem Cell 2012;10:385–97.
114. Xu Y, Liu L, Zhang L, et al. Efficient commitment to functional CD34+ progenitor cells from human bone marrow mesenchymal stem-cell-derived induced pluripotent stem cells. PLoS One 2012;7:e34321.
115. Oki K, Tatarishvili J, Woods J, et al. Human Induced pluripotent stem cells form functional neurons and improve recovery after grafting in stroke-damaged brain. Stem Cells 2012;30(6):1120–33.
116. Schuldiner M, Itskovitz-Eldor J, Benvenisty N. Selective ablation of human embryonic stem cells expressing a "suicide" gene. Stem Cells 2003;21:257–65.
117. Naujok O, Kaldrack J, Taivankhuu T, et al. Selective removal of undifferentiated embryonic stem cells from differentiation cultures through HSV1 thymidine kinase and ganciclovir treatment. Stem Cell Rev 2010;6:450–61.
118. Hara A, Aoki H, Taguchi A, et al. Neuron-like differentiation and selective ablation of undifferentiated embryonic stem cells containing suicide gene with Oct-4 promoter. Stem Cells Dev 2008;17:619–27.
119. Schriebl K, Satianegara G, Hwang A, et al. Selective removal of undifferentiated human embryonic stem cells using magnetic activated cell sorting followed by a cytotoxic antibody. Tissue Eng Part A 2012;18:899–909.
120. Choo AB, Tan HL, Ang SN, et al. Selection against undifferentiated human embryonic stem cells by a cytotoxic antibody recognizing podocalyxin-like protein-1. Stem Cells 2008;26:1454–63.
121. Lim DY, Ng YH, Lee J, et al. Cytotoxic antibody fragments for eliminating undifferentiated human embryonic stem cells. J Biotechnol 2011;153:77–85.
122. Goldstein AS, Zhu G, Morris GE, et al. Effect of osteoblastic culture conditions on the structure of poly(DL-lactic-co-glycolic acid) foam scaffolds. Tissue Eng 1999;5:421–34.
123. O'Brien FJ, Harley BA, Yannas IV, et al. The effect of pore size on cell adhesion in collagen-GAG scaffolds. Biomaterials 2005;26:433–41.
124. Zeltinger J, Sherwood JK, Graham DA, et al. Effect of pore size and void fraction on cellular adhesion, proliferation, and matrix deposition. Tissue Eng 2001;7:557–72.
125. Hoppe A, Guldal NS, Boccaccini AR. A review of the biological response to ionic dissolution products from bioactive glasses and glass-ceramics. Biomaterials 2011;32:2757–74.
126. Mounzer AM, McAninch JW, Schmidt RA. Polyglycolic acid mesh in repair of renal injury. Urology 1986;28:127–30.
127. Cabaud HE, Feagin JA, Rodkey WG. Acute anterior cruciate ligament injury and repair reinforced with a biodegradable intraarticular ligament. Experimental studies. Am J Sports Med 1982;10:259–65.
128. Rodkey WG, Cabaud HE, Feagin JA, et al. A partially biodegradable material device for repair and reconstruction of injured tendons. Experimental studies. Am J Sports Med 1985;13:242–7.

129. Townley CO, Fumich RM, Shall LM. The free synovial graft as a shield for collagen ingrowth in cruciate ligament repair. Clin Orthop Relat Res 1985;(197):266–71.
130. Freed LE, Vunjak-Novakovic G, Biron RJ, et al. Biodegradable polymer scaffolds for tissue engineering. Biotechnology (N Y) 1994;12:689–93.
131. Thomson RC, Yaszemski MJ, Powers JM, et al. Fabrication of biodegradable polymer scaffolds to engineer trabecular bone. J Biomater Sci Polym Ed 1995;7:23–38.
132. Wintermantel E, Cima L, Schloo B, et al. Angiopolarity: a new design parameter for cell transplantation devices and its application to degradable systems. ASAIO Trans 1991;37:M334–6.
133. Cao Y, Vacanti JP, Paige KT, et al. Transplantation of chondrocytes utilizing a polymer-cell construct to produce tissue-engineered cartilage in the shape of a human ear. Plast Reconstr Surg 1997;100:297–302 [discussion: 303–4].
134. Singhal AR, Agrawal CM, Athanasiou KA. Salient degradation features of a 50:50 PLA/PGA scaffold for tissue engineering. Tissue Eng 1996;2:197–207.
135. Chu CR, Coutts RD, Yoshioka M, et al. Articular cartilage repair using allogeneic perichondrocyte-seeded biodegradable porous polylactic acid (PLA): a tissue-engineering study. J Biomed Mater Res 1995;29:1147–54.
136. Evans GR, Brandt K, Widmer MS, et al. In vivo evaluation of poly(L-lactic acid) porous conduits for peripheral nerve regeneration. Biomaterials 1999;20: 1109–15.
137. Li WJ, Cooper JA Jr, Mauck RL, et al. Fabrication and characterization of six electrospun poly(alpha-hydroxy ester)-based fibrous scaffolds for tissue engineering applications. Acta Biomater 2006;2:377–85.
138. Doyle V, Pearson R, Lee D, et al. An investigation of the growth of human dermal fibroblasts on poly-L-lactic acid in vitro. J Mater Sci Mater Med 1996;7:381–5.
139. Corden TJ, Jones IA, Rudd CD, et al. Physical and biocompatibility properties of poly-epsilon-caprolactone produced using in situ polymerisation: a novel manufacturing technique for long-fibre composite materials. Biomaterials 2000;21:713–24.
140. Calvert JW, Marra KG, Cook L, et al. Characterization of osteoblast-like behavior of cultured bone marrow stromal cells on various polymer surfaces. J Biomed Mater Res 2000;52:279–84.
141. Marra KG, Szem JW, Kumta PN, et al. In vitro analysis of biodegradable polymer blend/hydroxyapatite composites for bone tissue engineering. J Biomed Mater Res 1999;47:324–35.
142. Pitt CG, Chasalow FI, Hibionada YM, et al. Aliphatic polyesters. 1. The degradation of poly(epsilon-caprolactone) in vivo. J Appl Polym Sci 1981;26:3779–87.
143. Pitt CG, Gratzl MM, Kimmel GL, et al. Aliphatic polyesters. 2. The degradation of poly(DL-lactide), poly(epsilon-caprolactone), and their copolymers in vivo. Biomaterials 1981;2:215–20.
144. Bettencourt A, Almeida AJ. Poly(methyl methacrylate) particulate carriers in drug delivery. J Microencapsul 2012;29(4):353–67.
145. Rogers-Foy JM, Powers DL, Brosnan DA, et al. Hydroxyapatite composites designed for antibiotic drug delivery and bone reconstruction: a caprine model. J Invest Surg 1999;12:263–75.
146. Liu Y, Ji Y, Ghosh K, et al. Effects of fiber orientation and diameter on the behavior of human dermal fibroblasts on electrospun PMMA scaffolds. J Biomed Mater Res A 2009;90:1092–106.
147. Arevalo-Silva CA, Eavey RD, Cao Y, et al. Internal support of tissue-engineered cartilage. Arch Otolaryngol Head Neck Surg 2000;126:1448–52.

148. Lynam D, Bednark B, Peterson C, et al. Precision microchannel scaffolds for central and peripheral nervous system repair. J Mater Sci Mater Med 2011;22: 2119–30.
149. Peck M, Gebhart D, Dusserre N, et al. The evolution of vascular tissue engineering and current state of the art. Cells Tissues Organs 2012;195:144–58.
150. Kral JG, Crandall DL. Development of a human adipocyte synthetic polymer scaffold. Plast Reconstr Surg 1999;104:1732–8.
151. Springer IN, Fleiner B, Jepsen S, et al. Culture of cells gained from temporomandibular joint cartilage on non-absorbable scaffolds. Biomaterials 2001;22: 2569–77.
152. Patel AA, Desai TA, Kumar S. Microtopographical assembly of cardiomyocytes. Integr Biol (Camb) 2011;3:1011–9.
153. Ayala P, Desai TA. Integrin alpha3 blockade enhances microtopographical down-regulation of alpha-smooth muscle actin: role of microtopography in ECM regulation. Integr Biol (Camb) 2011;3:733–41.
154. Kim EJ, Boehm CA, Mata A, et al. Post microtextures accelerate cell proliferation and osteogenesis. Acta Biomater 2010;6:160–9.
155. Mata A, Kim EJ, Boehm CA, et al. A three-dimensional scaffold with precise micro-architecture and surface micro-textures. Biomaterials 2009;30:4610–7.
156. Leclerc E, Sakai Y, Fujii T. Microfluidic PDMS (polydimethylsiloxane) bioreactor for large-scale culture of hepatocytes. Biotechnol Prog 2004;20:750–5.
157. Fujita H, Shimizu K, Nagamori E. Novel method for fabrication of skeletal muscle construct from the C2C12 myoblast cell line using serum-free medium AIM-V. Biotechnol Bioeng 2009;103:1034–41.
158. Refojo MF. Contact lens materials. Int Ophthalmol Clin 1973;13:263–77.
159. Hejcl A, Lesny P, Prodny M, et al. Biocompatible hydrogels in spinal cord injury repair. Physiol Res 2008;57(Suppl 3):S121–32.
160. Madden LR, Mortisen DJ, Sussman EM, et al. Proangiogenic scaffolds as functional templates for cardiac tissue engineering. Proc Natl Acad Sci U S A 2010; 107:15211–6.
161. Netti PA, Shelton JC, Revell PA, et al. Hydrogels as an interface between bone and an implant. Biomaterials 1993;14:1098–104.
162. Young CD, Wu JR, Tsou TL. High-strength, ultra-thin and fiber-reinforced pHEMA artificial skin. Biomaterials 1998;19:1745–52.
163. Aung T, Inoue K, Kogire M, et al. Comparison of various gels for immobilization of islets in bioartificial pancreas using a mesh-reinforced polyvinyl alcohol hydrogel tube. Transplant Proc 1995;27:619–21.
164. Aung T, Inoue K, Kogire M, et al. Improved insulin release from a bioartificial pancreas using mesh-reinforced polyvinyl alcohol hydrogel tube: immobilization of islets in agarose gel. Transplant Proc 1994;26:790–1.
165. Qi Z, Shen Y, Yanai G, et al. The in vivo performance of polyvinyl alcohol macroencapsulated islets. Biomaterials 2010;31:4026–31.
166. Qi M, Gu Y, Sakata N, et al. PVA hydrogel sheet macroencapsulation for the bioartificial pancreas. Biomaterials 2004;25:5885–92.
167. Taheri A, Atyabi F, Dinarvnd R. Temperature-responsive and biodegradable PVA: PVP k30:poloxamer 407 hydrogel for controlled delivery of human growth hormone (hGH). J Pediatr Endocrinol Metab 2011;24:175–9.
168. Bakhshandeh H, Soleimani M, Hosseini SS, et al. Poly (epsilon-caprolactone) nanofibrous ring surrounding a polyvinyl alcohol hydrogel for the development of a biocompatible two-part artificial cornea. Int J Nanomedicine 2011;6: 1509–15.

169. Bodugoz-Senturk H, Macias CE, Kung JH, et al. Poly(vinyl alcohol)-acrylamide hydrogels as load-bearing cartilage substitute. Biomaterials 2009;30:589–96.
170. Smidsrod O, Skjak-Braek G. Alginate as immobilization matrix for cells. Trends Biotechnol 1990;8:71–8.
171. Drury JL, Dennis RG, Mooney DJ. The tensile properties of alginate hydrogels. Biomaterials 2004;25:3187–99.
172. Yuan Z, Nie H, Wang S, et al. Biomaterial selection for tooth regeneration. Tissue Eng Part B Rev 2011;17:373–88.
173. Khanarian NT, Haney NM, Burga RA, et al. A functional agarose-hydroxyapatite scaffold for osteochondral interface regeneration. Biomaterials 2012;33(21): 5247–58.
174. Khanarian NT, Jiang J, Wan LQ, et al. A hydrogel-mineral composite scaffold for osteochondral interface tissue engineering. Tissue Eng Part A 2012;18:533–45.
175. Balgude AP, Yu X, Szymanski A, et al. Agarose gel stiffness determines rate of DRG neurite extension in 3D cultures. Biomaterials 2001;22:1077–84.
176. Rotter N, Aigner J, Naumann A, et al. Behavior of tissue-engineered human cartilage after transplantation into nude mice. J Mater Sci Mater Med 1999;10: 689–93.
177. Hung CT, Lima EG, Mauck RL, et al. Anatomically shaped osteochondral constructs for articular cartilage repair. J Biomech 2003;36:1853–64.
178. Alaminos M, Del Carmen Sanchez-Quevedo M, Munoz-Avila JI, et al. Construction of a complete rabbit cornea substitute using a fibrin-agarose scaffold. Invest Ophthalmol Vis Sci 2006;47:3311–7.
179. Obara K, Ishihara M, Ishizuka T, et al. Photocrosslinkable chitosan hydrogel containing fibroblast growth factor-2 stimulates wound healing in healing-impaired db/db mice. Biomaterials 2003;24:3437–44.
180. Liu ZQ, Wang HB, Wang Y, et al. The influence of chitosan hydrogel on stem cell engraftment, survival and homing in the ischemic myocardial microenvironment. Biomaterials 2012;33:3093–106.
181. Zakhem E, Raghavan S, Gilmont RR, et al. Chitosan-based scaffolds for the support of smooth muscle constructs in intestinal tissue engineering. Biomaterials 2012;33:4810–7.
182. Pakulska MM, Ballios BG, Shoichet MS. Injectable hydrogels for central nervous system therapy. Biomed Mater 2012;7:024101.
183. Hong Y, Gong Y, Gao C, et al. Collagen-coated polylactide microcarriers/chitosan hydrogel composite: injectable scaffold for cartilage regeneration. J Biomed Mater Res A 2008;85:628–37.
184. Coimbra P, Ferreira P, de Sousa HC, et al. Preparation and chemical and biological characterization of a pectin/chitosan polyelectrolyte complex scaffold for possible bone tissue engineering applications. Int J Biol Macromol 2011;48: 112–8.
185. Coimbra P, Alves P, Valente TA, et al. Sodium hyaluronate/chitosan polyelectrolyte complex scaffolds for dental pulp regeneration: synthesis and characterization. Int J Biol Macromol 2011;49:573–9.
186. Sahoo SK, Panda AK, Labhasetwar V. Characterization of porous PLGA/PLA microparticles as a scaffold for three dimensional growth of breast cancer cells. Biomacromolecules 2005;6:1132–9.
187. Li C, Wang L, Yang Z, et al. A viscoelastic chitosan-modified three-dimensional porous poly(L-lactide-co-epsilon-caprolactone) scaffold for cartilage tissue engineering. J Biomater Sci Polym Ed 2012;23:405–24.
188. Eastoe JE. Organic matrix of tooth enamel. Nature 1960;187:411–2.

189. Zheng L, Yang F, Shen H, et al. The effect of composition of calcium phosphate composite scaffolds on the formation of tooth tissue from human dental pulp stem cells. Biomaterials 2011;32:7053–9.
190. Ebrahimian-Hosseinabadi M, Ashrafizadeh F, Etemadifar M, et al. Evaluating and modeling the mechanical properties of the prepared PLGA/nano-BCP composite scaffolds for bone tissue engineering. J Mater Sci Tech 2011;27: 1105–12.
191. Arinzeh TL, Tran T, McAlary J, et al. A comparative study of biphasic calcium phosphate ceramics for human mesenchymal stem-cell-induced bone formation. Biomaterials 2005;26:3631–8.
192. Mironov V, Boland T, Trusk T, et al. Organ printing: computer-aided jet-based 3D tissue engineering. Trends Biotechnol 2003;21:157–61.
193. Boland T, Mironov V, Gutowska A, et al. Cell and organ printing 2: fusion of cell aggregates in three-dimensional gels. Anat Rec A Discov Mol Cell Evol Biol 2003;272:497–502.
194. Jakab K, Norotte C, Marga F, et al. Tissue engineering by self-assembly and bio-printing of living cells. Biofabrication 2010;2:022001.
195. Fernandez JG, Khademhosseini A. Micro-masonry: construction of 3D structures by microscale self-assembly. Adv Mater 2010;22:2538–41.
196. Crubezy E, Murail P, Girard L, et al. False teeth of the Roman world. Nature 1998; 391:29.
197. Bobbio A. The first endosseous alloplastic implant in the history of man. Bull Hist Dent 1972;20:1–6.
198. Mooney DJ, Powell C, Piana J, et al. Engineering dental pulp-like tissue in vitro. Biotechnol Prog 1996;12:865–8.
199. Buurma B, Gu K, Rutherford RB. Transplantation of human pulpal and gingival fibroblasts attached to synthetic scaffolds. Eur J Oral Sci 1999; 107:282–9.
200. El-Backly RM, Massoud AG, El-Badry AM, et al. Regeneration of dentine/pulp-like tissue using a dental pulp stem cell/poly(lactic-co-glycolic) acid scaffold construct in New Zealand white rabbits. Aust Endod J 2008;34:52–67.
201. Ohara T, Itaya T, Usami K, et al. Evaluation of scaffold materials for tooth tissue engineering. J Biomed Mater Res A 2010;94:800–5.
202. Tonomura A, Mizuno D, Hisada A, et al. Differential effect of scaffold shape on dentin regeneration. Ann Biomed Eng 2010;38:1664–71.
203. Young CS, Terada S, Vacanti JP, et al. Tissue engineering of complex tooth structures on biodegradable polymer scaffolds. J Dent Res 2002;81: 695–700.
204. Duailibi MT, Duailibi SE, Young CS, et al. Bioengineered teeth from cultured rat tooth bud cells. J Dent Res 2004;83:523–8.
205. Duailibi SE, Duailibi MT, Zhang W, et al. Bioengineered dental tissues grown in the rat jaw. J Dent Res 2008;87:745–50.
206. Savarino L, Baldini N, Greco M, et al. The performance of poly-epsilon-caprolactone scaffolds in a rabbit femur model with and without autologous stromal cells and BMP4. Biomaterials 2007;28:3101–9.
207. Williams JM, Adewunmi A, Schek RM, et al. Bone tissue engineering using poly-caprolactone scaffolds fabricated via selective laser sintering. Biomaterials 2005;26:4817–27.
208. Li WJ, Tuli R, Okafor C, et al. A three-dimensional nanofibrous scaffold for cartilage tissue engineering using human mesenchymal stem cells. Biomaterials 2005;26:599–609.

209. Yang X, Yang F, Walboomers XF, et al. The performance of dental pulp stem cells on nanofibrous PCL/gelatin/nHA scaffolds. J Biomed Mater Res A 2010;93: 247–57.
210. Galler KM, Cavender AC, Koeklue U, et al. Bioengineering of dental stem cells in a PEGylated fibrin gel. Regen Med 2011;6:191–200.
211. Dobie K, Smith G, Sloan AJ, et al. Effects of alginate hydrogels and TGF-beta 1 on human dental pulp repair in vitro. Connect Tissue Res 2002;43:387–90.
212. Kim NR, Lee DH, Chung PH, et al. Distinct differentiation properties of human dental pulp cells on collagen, gelatin, and chitosan scaffolds. Oral Surg Oral Med Oral Pathol Oral Radiol Endod 2009;108:e94–100.
213. Mizuno M, Miyamoto T, Wada K, et al. Type I collagen regulated dentin matrix protein-1 (Dmp-1) and osteocalcin (OCN) gene expression of rat dental pulp cells. J Cell Biochem 2003;88:1112–9.
214. Srisuwan T, Tilkorn DJ, Al-Benna S, et al. Revascularization and tissue regeneration of an empty root canal space is enhanced by a direct blood supply and stem cells. Dent Traumatol 2012. [Epub ahead of print].
215. Yamauchi N, Yamauchi S, Nagaoka H, et al. Tissue engineering strategies for immature teeth with apical periodontitis. J Endod 2011;37:390–7.
216. Yamauchi N, Nagaoka H, Yamauchi S, et al. Immunohistological characterization of newly formed tissues after regenerative procedure in immature dog teeth. J Endod 2011;37:1636–41.
217. Srisuwan T, Tilkorn DJ, Al-Benna S, et al. Survival of rat functional dental pulp cells in vascularized tissue engineering chambers. Tissue Cell 2012;44:111–21.
218. Yang X, Han G, Pang X, et al. Chitosan/collagen scaffold containing bone morphogenetic protein-7 DNA supports dental pulp stem cell differentiation in vitro and in vivo. J Biomed Mater Res A 2012. [Epub ahead of print].
219. Inuyama Y, Kitamura C, Nishihara T, et al. Effects of hyaluronic acid sponge as a scaffold on odontoblastic cell line and amputated dental pulp. J Biomed Mater Res B Appl Biomater 2010;92:120–8.
220. Friedman PM, Mafong EA, Kauvar AN, et al. Safety data of injectable nonanimal stabilized hyaluronic acid gel for soft tissue augmentation. Dermatol Surg 2002; 28:491–4.
221. Atrah HI. Fibrin glue. BMJ 1994;308:933–4.
222. Evans LA, Ferguson KH, Foley JP, et al. Fibrin sealant for the management of genitourinary injuries, fistulas and surgical complications. J Urol 2003;169:1360–2.
223. Feinstein AJ, Varela JE, Cohn SM, et al. Fibrin glue eliminates the need for packing after complex liver injuries. Yale J Biol Med 2001;74:315–21.
224. Bastarache JA. The complex role of fibrin in acute lung injury. Am J Physiol Lung Cell Mol Physiol 2009;296:L275–6.
225. Ahmed TA, Dare EV, Hincke M. Fibrin: a versatile scaffold for tissue engineering applications. Tissue Eng Part B Rev 2008;14:199–215.
226. Yang KC, Wang CH, Chang HH, et al. Fibrin glue mixed with platelet-rich fibrin as a scaffold seeded with dental bud cells for tooth regeneration. J Tissue Eng Regen Med 2011. [Epub ahead of print].
227. Reches M, Gazit E. Controlled patterning of aligned self-assembled peptide nanotubes. Nat Nanotechnol 2006;1:195–200.
228. Fioretti F, Mendoza-Palomares C, Helms M, et al. Nanostructured assemblies for dental application. ACS Nano 2010;4:3277–87.
229. Yang WS, Park YC, Kim JH, et al. Nanostructured, self-assembling peptide K5 blocks TNF-alpha and PGE(2) production by suppression of the AP-1/p38 pathway. Mediators Inflamm 2012;2012:489810.

Pulpal and Periradicular Response to Caries

Current Management and Regenerative Options

Sami M.A. Chogle, BDS, DMD, MSD[a,b,c,*], Harold E. Goodis, DDS[b,d,e],
Bassam Michael Kinaia, DDS, MS[f,g,h]

KEYWORDS

- Pulp capping • Vital pulp therapy • Tertiary dentin • Pulp exposure
- Periapical pathology • Periradicular lesion • Periodontal regeneration

KEY POINTS

- The pulp-dentin complex is a strategic and dynamic barrier to various insults that plague the dentition. Researchers have yet to understand the complete potential of this constantly shifting junction and its components, the predentin, dentinal tubules, odontoblast layer; their processes; and the vascular and neural elements.
- The most common cause of injury to the pulp-dentin complex is the carious breakdown of the enamel and dentin, leading to pathologic changes in the pulp and periradicular area.
- In recent years, there has been a change in the restorative management of caries. Classically, complete removal of caries was a basic principle strictly taught for many years in dental schools. The current emphasis, however, is on strategies to preserve dentin and protect the pulp, sometimes with incomplete removal of caries.

INTRODUCTION

The dentin and pulp function physiologically as a single unit, the pulp-dentin complex. This complex is a dynamic tissue that responds to mechanical, bacterial, or chemical

Conflict of Interest: The authors declare that there is no conflict of interest related to this article.

[a] Postgraduate Program in Endodontics, Endodontics Department, The Boston University Institute for Dental Research and Education, PO Box 505097, Dubai Healthcare City, Dubai, United Arab Emirates; [b] Department of Endodontics, The Goldman School of Dental Medicine, Boston, MA, USA; [c] Department of Endodontics, Case School of Dental Medicine, Cleveland, OH, USA; [d] The Boston University Institute for Dental Research and Education, PO Box 505097, Dubai Healthcare City, Dubai, United Arab Emirates; [e] Department of Endodontics, The University of California School of Dentistry, San Francisco, CA, USA; [f] Postgraduate Periodontology Program, Periodontology Department, The Boston University Institute for Dental Research and Education, PO Box 505097, Dubai Healthcare City, Dubai, United Arab Emirates; [g] Department of Periodontology and Oral Biology, The Goldman School of Dental Medicine, Boston, MA, USA; [h] University of Detroit Mercy – School of Dentistry, Detroit, MI, USA
* Corresponding author. 3149 Sebor Road, Shaker Heights, OH 44120.
E-mail address: sxc89@case.edu

irritation in several ways to decrease that irritation.[1] The vitality and dentin repair potential of the pulp are dependent on the survival of the odontoblasts beneath the site of injury.[2] Apart from dentinogenesis, odontoblasts also play important roles as defense cells[3] and as thermal and mechanical sensory receptors.[4,5] Thus, the net effect of caries or a restorative procedure on the pulp is the result of a complex interaction of many factors. These factors include the thickness and permeability of the intervening dentin, the health of the underlying pulp, mechanical injury to odontoblast processes during cavity preparation, the possible toxicity of the restorative material, and microbial leakage.[6]

Although caries are the principal reason for placement of initial restorations, it is important to discriminate between pulp management of a carious insult and the events that can affect the pulp in the absence of caries. The latter include injurious events that occur after deep cavity preparation[7] or bacterial leakage from restorations.[8] This article summarizes current understanding of the management of carious insults to the pulp and the subsequent effects on the periradicular tissues as they relate to current views on tissue regeneration.

PULP RESPONSE TO CARIES

Contrary to most connective tissues, the dental pulp does not tolerate injury easily and is more vulnerable for 3 reasons: (1) it is a large volume of tissue with a small volume of blood supply; (2) it is a terminal circulation with few, if any, collateral vessels; and (3) it is confined in calcified tissue walls.[9,10] As a result, early caries lesions produce cytoplasmic changes in the odontoblasts that are evident at the ultrastructural level.[11] Before an active lesion reaches the dentinoenamel junction, a significant reduction in the cytoplasm-to-nucleus ratio of odontoblasts and a concomitant reduction in predentin thickness have been observed.[12] The dynamics of caries progression cannot be explained solely on a chemical basis and are influenced by interaction between the metabolic activities of the bacterial biofilms and the response from odontoblasts. Generation of microbial metabolic products and matrix degradation products and the release of growth factors from the dentin extracellular matrix influence disease progression. At the same time, the tubular characteristics of dentin and the extent of tubular sclerosis derived from the reactionary response of the pulp-dentin complex affect the permeability of dentin.[13,14] Due to this variability in caries progression, there is no single response to the disease. Rather, the pulp-dentin complex exhibits a broad spectrum of responses that represents a summation of injury, defense, and repair events.[15] The relative contributions and interactions of these interrelated responses are critical in determining the fate of the pulp-dentin complex and its ability to survive the caries assault. Although discussion of these interactions and their is beyond the scope of this article, a few examples provide a brief overview.

A positive hydrostatic pressure from the pulpal circulation results in outward fluid flow when tubules are exposed. Outward fluid flow is a transudate of plasma and may contribute to pulpal protection because it contains proteins (immunoglobulins, albumin, and fibrinogen) and minerals (calcium and phosphates).[14] Outward fluid flow also limits the rate of diffusion of noxious agents in a pulpal direction.[16] To initiate injury, bacterial acids, soluble plaque metabolic products, and cell wall components have to diffuse pulpward against an outward flow of dentinal fluid.[17] Although outward fluid flow reduces the rates of permeation of microbial and chemical solutes,[18] endotoxins derived from the lipopolysaccharides may be observed in vital pulps of human carious teeth.[19] Alternatively, the buffering action of dentin (0.6 mm or thicker) can effectively buffer bacterial acids found in carious dentin, such as lactic and acetic acids, and avoid direct injury to the pulp.[20] Taken together, these findings may explain why injury responses to the odontoblasts and subodontoblastic cells are apparent in active carious lesions that involve more than a quarter of the thickness of enamel.[21]

In response to the carious insult, the pulp-dentin complex initiates both innate[22] and adaptive immune response.[23] Innate immunity plays an important role in shallow caries after the initial enamel caries reaches the dentinoenamel junction. During this initial stage, pulpal responses are likely low grade and chronic.[24] The transition from innate to adaptive immunity probably occurs in irreversibly inflamed pulps that are separated by less than 2 mm of deep carious dentin.[25] This transition may also be influenced by repair reactions involving dentinal sclerosis and tertiary dentinogenesis, which modify the permeability of the dentin matrix.

When the pulp is subjected to a gradually progressive insult, a major part of the pulp's response is the deposition of minerals within the dentinal tubules, occluding the tubules against further ingress of noxious stimuli. Caries lesions may progress slowly or rapidly or become arrested. Consequently, sclerosis of the dentinal tubules is either absent or minimal in rapidly progressing active lesions. In the absence of complete occlusion or with minimal tubular occlusion, rapid diffusion of the metabolic and degradation products could overwhelm the pulp's defensive responses and result in pulpal inflammation, absence of tertiary dentinogenesis, and severe pulpal injury.[26] Conversely, a transparent zone of sclerotic dentin observed at the base of the caries-affected dentin can reduce dentin permeability and impede the diffusion of bacterial products or solubilized matrix components along the tubules, thereby delaying lesion progression. Because the thickness of this zone is higher in slow progressing and arrested lesions,[27] this form of defense and healing of pulp tissue are more favorable in response to slowly progressing or arrested lesions.[28]

Additionally, the pulp-dentin complex may react to stimuli with tertiary dentin formation. Unlike primary and secondary dentinogenesis, tertiary dentinogenesis is a focused reaction in the vicinity of the dentin that is directly affected by the caries process. Recent reports have redefined tertiary dentinogenesis in relation to the nature of the injury. The term, *reactionary dentinogenesis*, has been adopted to describe the secretion of a tertiary dentin matrix by primary odontoblasts that have survived injury to the tooth (**Fig. 1**). This is a wound healing reaction to produce circumpulpal dentin in response to slowly progressing dentinal caries.[29] Conversely, reparative dentinogenesis refers to the secretion of tertiary dentin after the death of the primary odontoblasts underlying the injury, after the differentiation of odontoblast-like cells (**Fig. 2**).[15,30] Reparative dentin formation occurs in response to deep dentinal caries and represents a more complex sequence of biologic events compared to reactionary dentinogenesis, including progenitor cell recruitment and differentiation.[31] When the pulp is exposed in advanced lesions, reparative dentinogenesis results in dentin bridge formation, which restores the functional integrity of the pulp-dentin complex. In actively progressing advanced lesions involving pulpal exposure, however, the inflammatory reactions may become acute and uncontrolled as bacteria approach and penetrate the pulp. Although inflammation is regarded as a defense response, severe reactions can result from continued ingress of bacteria, producing irreversible destruction of the pulp that eventually results in pulpal necrosis and development of periradicular lesions.[32]

VITAL PULP THERAPY

Vital pulp therapy is aimed at sealing the pulp after injury and stimulating the formation of tertiary dentin.[33] This can be achieved through direct and indirect pulp capping, pulpotomy, and other therapies that protect the pulp from the chemical, bacterial, mechanical, and thermal insults due to attrition, erosion, caries, restoration

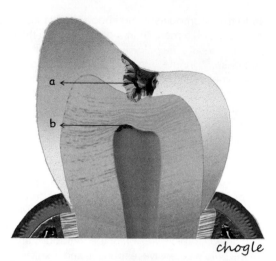

Fig. 1. Illustration of a tooth with caries involving the superficial layer of dentin. Bioactive molecules are released by cariously involved dentin (a), which increase secretory activity of odontoblasts and result in deposition of reactionary dentin (b).

procedures, and restoration placement.[34] The dental pulp, when exposed, may respond favorably to application of a variety of materials used in pulp capping procedures.[35] Many studies have confirmed the formation of hard tissue over the site of the exposure.[36–40] This may demonstrate that the dental pulp has an intrinsic capacity to heal. The clinical outcomes differ, however, in their inferences as to the predictability of hard tissue formation. The factors affecting the outcome of pulpal capping procedures may be categorized broadly as those related to the pulp exposure and the material used to seal the exposure.

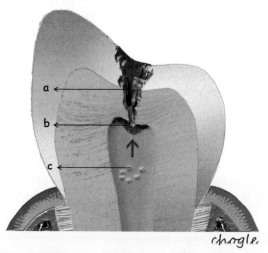

Fig. 2. Illustration of a tooth with caries involving the pulp-dentin complex leading to death of underlying odontoblasts. Bioactive molecules are released by cariously involved dentin (a) into the subjacent pulp and cause proliferation/differentiation of precursor cells (c). These odontoblast-like cells migrate to site of pulpal injury and deposit reparative dentin matrix (b).

Indirect Pulp Treatment

When the bacterial penetration reaches less than a 0.75 mm away from the pulp, the degree of pulpal disease becomes extreme. In other words, the pulp remains reasonably intact if there is at least 0.75 mm or more of intact, bacteria-free dentin between the caries lesion and the pulp. This may be due to the increase in number of tubules per unit area, the tubule diameter increase closer to the pulp,[41] and the ability of the bacterial by-products (enzymes, toxins, and so forth) to penetrate the remaining tubular distance causing pulpitis. When the majority of the caries are removed, except for the deepest layer overlying some intact dentin, then the bulk of the lactic acid–producing complex is eliminated (**Fig. 3**). Additionally, it has been hypothesized that if the source of nutrition for the cariogenic bacteria is eliminated, the organisms would die, resulting in an arrested carious lesion.

In an indirect pulp treatment procedure, stepwise excavation of caries lesions in the permanent dentition involves 2 main steps. The initial removal of gross caries and subsequent placement of a material, in an attempt to deprive bacteria of a substrate,

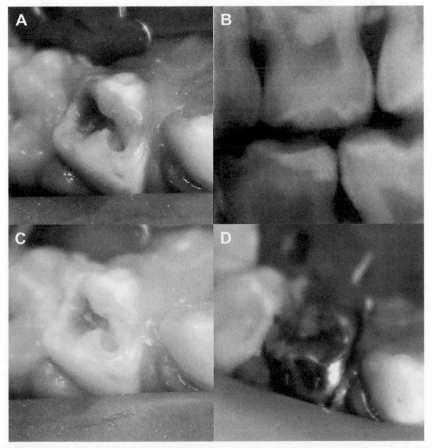

Fig. 3. Indirect pulp capping procedure. (*A*) Preoperative clinical view of primary first molar. (*B*) Preoperative radiograph. (*C*) Clinical view after gross caries débridement. (*D*) Permanent restoration with glass ionomer and stainless steel crown. (*Courtesy of* Dr Manal Al Halabi, BDS, MS.)

prevent a direct carious pulpal exposure, and remineralize the remaining caries lesion, with a subsequent return to normal tissue pH.[42] In vitro studies of severely carious teeth, however, found that clinical observations of dentin color changes and mineral increases in the remaining carious dentin do not always represent a change in the bacterial content.[43] Although the microbiologic bioburden may be reduced, it is still present. In a clinical setting, retaining a layer of carious dentin (indirect procedures) presents the dilemma most clinicians face in deciding how to treat these lesions. Continued research and clinical trials are needed to develop the appropriate case selection guidelines, treatment approaches, and materials needed to maximize clinical success.

Pulp Exposure

The classic studies of Kakehashi and colleagues[44] demonstrate bacterial infection as a critical etiologic factor for pulpal necrosis. The extent of damage from microbial contamination may vary based on the size and chronicity of the exposure, pulp status, and material used to seal the exposure.

Several studies suggest that the size of the pulpal exposure may influence case selection because large pulpal exposures may have greater risk of microleakage and be difficult to restore.[45,46] ppartial pulpotomies after traumatic crown fractures, however, have demonstrated a 96% success rate with close to 3-year follow-up, including pulpal exposures ranging from 0.5 mm to 4.0 mm.[47] Thus, the size of the exposure may not play a major role, at least within this range.

The duration of pulpal contamination, although important, remains a controversial factor in terms of successful pulp capping. Many clinicians believe that longer periods of contamination by oral microorganisms and debris reduce the chance of success. This is supported by results from animal studies that indicate that the success of $Ca(OH)_2$ pulp capping is reduced from 93% to 56% when microbial contamination is extended from 1 hour to 7 days.[48-50] Alternatively, clinical studies in younger patients with up to 3 months of pulp exposure demonstrate a 93% radiographic success rate for partial pulpotomy at a mean follow-up of 4.5 years.[47,51] As a result, the superficial pulp in younger patients seems more resistant to bacterial invasion than the mature pulp in older patients. Furthermore, the size of the pulp chamber and root canal systems of younger patients mitigates toward a larger volume of pulpal tissue, hence greater success in younger patients.

The inflammatory response of the pulp to bacteria and their by-products and the trauma of caries removal may increase the amount of bleeding of exposed dental pulp tissue. This can adversely affect the effective seal against bacterial invasion and lead to development of a chronic inflammatory infiltrate and inhibition of tertiary dentin formation. Therefore, the use of a hemostatic agent may be useful in vital pulp procedures to clot the capillaries within the subjacent pulp tissue.[46] Several studies have examined the use of hemostatic agents placed over the exposure to halt hemorrhage with conflicting results, such as sodium hypochlorite, ferric sulfate, and chlorhexidine digluconate.[52-55] Further work should better define the use of these agents, especially when used in combination with other materials, such as mineral trioxide aggregate (MTA), that is now suggested for these procedures.

Materials of Pulp Capping

For a successful outcome in vital pulp therapy, the healing response must demonstrate rapid hard tissue formation at the pulp-material interface with minimal inflammatory response. This desirable healing process should occur when any substance is applied directly to the pulpal exposure site that is capable of stimulating dentinogenesis.[56] One study using a cell culture model system reported that calcium hydroxide

(Ca[OH]₂)inhibited macrophage function and reduced inflammatory reactions when used in direct pulp capping and pulpotomy procedures.[57] In another study, an adhesive system applied to exposed human pulp tissue caused large areas of neutrophil infiltration and death of odontoblasts, thereby inhibiting pulp repair.[58] Together, these studies suggest that the sealing ability of the agent, the method of placement (eg, minimizing the impaction of pulp capping agents in dental pulp), and the chemical nature of the pulp capping material are all critical factors in desirable pulpal healing.

Calcium hydroxide

The introduction of Ca(OH)₂, from a historical perspective, played an important role in the development of vital pulp therapy. Recently, it has been shown that calcium ions released from Ca(OH)₂ stimulate fibronectin synthesis by dental pulp cells, which in turn may induce the differentiation of pulp progenitor cells into mineralized tissue-producing phenotypes.[59] Cross-sections of pulps treated for more than 6 weeks demonstrated a superior amorphous layer of tissue debris and Ca(OH)₂, a middle layer of a coarse meshwork of fibers identified as fibrodentin, and an inner layer showing tubular osteodentin.[60] Apart from the ability to form a dentin bridge in the subjacent pulp tissue, Ca(OH)₂ has demonstrated additional benefits, such as antimicrobial characteristics. In a primate study with a 1-year to 2-year follow-up, Ca(OH)₂-induced dentin bridge formation occurred in 78 of 91 (85%) exposed and contaminated dental pulps, whereas 10% of the pulps in the study sample became necrotic. Despite the successful use of Ca(OH)₂ as a pulp capping agent for 60 years,[61] predictable outcomes remain a problem. For example, a retrospective study that examined Ca(OH)₂ pulp capping of carious exposures in 123 teeth, revealed that 45% failed in the 5-year group and 80% failed in the 10-year group.[62] Additionally a summary of several primate studies involving direct pulp capping with Ca(OH)₂ reported several inflamed and infected pulps after a follow-up period of 1 years to 2 years.[63] The investigators questioned the long-term efficacy of commercially available Ca(OH)₂ bases, particularly in light of the potential for microleakage.[63] This has led to newer studies comparing it with other materials. One such material, MTA, has generated great interest for direct pulp capping and vital pulp therapy.

Mineral trioxide aggregate

MTA is the material of choice for correcting procedural errors as well as for root-end filling material in apicoectomy procedures. In both instances, the material has been shown e tissue compatible, encouraging the formation of new cementum-like hard tissue with restoration of the periodontal ligament, and is considered to have significant osteogenic potential.[64–66] MTA is currently the alternative material for Ca(OH)₂ in direct pulp capping procedures (**Fig. 4**). MTA was compared with Ca(OH)₂ in young permanent teeth undergoing apexogenesis (coronal pulpotomy, retention of root system vital pulp tissue, and immature root formation).[67] Two of 14 teeth in the Ca(OH)₂ group failed because of pain and swelling, whereas all in the MTA group seemed successfully treated. When MTA and Ca(OH)₂ were compared in direct pulp capping procedures in dog teeth,[68] MTA presented a higher success rate than Ca(OH)₂, with a lower occurrence of infection and pulpal necrosis. A more recent randomized clinical trial compared the pulpal responses with iatrogenic pulpotomy performed in healthy human teeth using MTA or Dycal.[69] Pulpal wounds treated with MTA were mostly free from inflammation after 1 week and covered with a compact hard tissue barrier within 3 months whereas teeth treated with Dycal revealed distinctly less consistent formation of a hard tissue barrier and presence of pulpal inflammation at up to 3 months. Collectively, the results of all these studies indicate

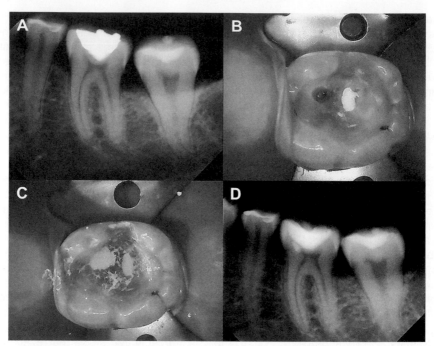

Fig. 4. Direct pulp capping procedure. (*A*) Preoperative radiograph of #19 with secondary decay underneath restoration. (*B*) Exposure of mesial pulp horn after complete caries débridement under rubber dam isolation. (*C*) Placement of MTA over exposure. (*D*) Follow-up (3-month) radiograph with normal clinical testing. (*Courtesy of* Dr Sameeha Al Marzouqi, DDS.)

that MTA is as successful as or more successful than Ca(OH)$_2$ in vital pulp therapy procedures.[70,71]

Glass ionomer and adhesives

Contrary to some favorable responses reported with the use of resin-modified glass ionomers in primates,[72] poor responses have been reported in human teeth. Intentional mechanical exposures in human teeth that were capped with resin-modified glass ionomers were found to exhibit moderate to intense inflammatory pulpal responses, including large necrotic zones, lack of dentin bridge formation, and impaired healing.[73] As with dentin adhesives, recently available data suggest that these are unacceptable and contraindicated as direct pulp capping agents.[74–76] The critical argument against resin-based pulp capping procedures is not about the hard tissue barrier but the persistence of intense inflammation and foreign body reactions that frequently accompany the application of such procedures.

Bioactive materials

The past several years have seen a change in thinking from attempting to induce pulp repair through irritation to the use of substances that mimic normal developmental processes in response to cellular signaling mechanisms. Briefly, dentin contains many peptides and signaling molecules within a mineralized matrix. These molecules are released in response to pulpal injury.[77] They include many of the same molecules that are expressed during embryonic tooth development and are again expressed in dental tissues in response to pathologic conditions.[78] Because the pulp-dentin complex demonstrates great regenerative potential, a suitable bioactive substance could recruit a population of multipotent mesenchymal progenitor cells to produce new hard tissue. Investigations of these bioactive substances, although in their infancy, include the roles of stem cells and genetic recruitment. These strategies involve selective activation of genes and other proteins necessary in dentinogenesis and can generate new, biologically based approaches to pulpal healing.[31]

PERIRADICULAR DISEASE

Anatomically, the periodontium anastamoses with the dental pulp through the apical foramen and other apical foramina. Such anastamoses create pathways for exchange of microorganisms in disease conditions. The classic studies of Kakehashi and colleagues[44] showed the pathologic role of bacteria in pulpal exposures leading to periradicular involvement of the endodontic infection. In the presence of bacteria, exposed rat pulp tissue was completely necrotic with formation of periradicular abscesses by the fourteenth day. The response of the periradicular tissues to microbial insult is similar to that of other connective tissues in the body. The immune-inflammatory reaction occurs in response to microbial toxins, noxious metabolic by-products, and disintegrated pulp tissue in the root canal system.[79,80] Unfortunately, the microbial biofilm formed in the apical end of a necrotic root canal system is shielded from host defenses and antibiotic therapy due to absence of blood circulation. Consequently, healing of wounded periradicular tissues becomes difficult, and bacterial toxins and noxious metabolic by-products continuously pass into the periapical area and irritate the periapical tissues, leading to continued periradicular tissue destruction (**Fig. 5**).

Apical Periodontitis and Periodontal Disease

The cause and pathogenesis of apical periodontitis and periodontal disease are similar. Both diseases display bacterial infection and involve pathologic changes of alveolar bone, periodontal ligament, and cementum. Marginal periodontitis affects

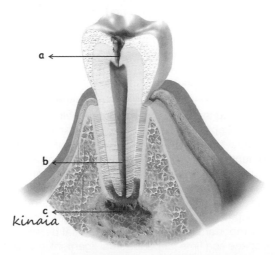

kinaia

Fig. 5. Illustration of a tooth with advanced caries (a) involving the pulp-dentin complex leading to pulp necrosis (b) and periapical tissue destruction (c).

the coronal periodontal tissues, whereas apical periodontitis affects apical periodontal tissues. Bone loss is one of characteristic feature with crestal bone loss in periodontal disease and apical resorption in apical periodontitis. Apical periodontitis, however, does not have a direct communication with the oral cavity and the main source of pathogenesis originates through the root canal system. Periodontal disease, alternatively, has a direct communication with the microflora of the oral cavity, making it more difficult to isolate.[81] The intimate relationship between the root canal system and the periodontium results in multiple pathways connecting the pulpal and the periodontal tissues where microbial by-products may affect neighboring tissues. A primary endodontic lesion may be complicated with secondary periodontal involvement or a concomitant periodontal disease on the same tooth.[82,83] Even though pathology involving pulpal and/or periodontal tissues may be separate disease entities, each primary disease may mimic characteristics as well as etiologically influence the progression of the other, often making diagnosis and treatment planning in such cases a challenge for clinicians. An interdisciplinary approach is often used to establish the appropriate treatment plan.

Management and Treatment Options

Despite the location (apically, crestally, or a combination) of the diseased tissues, treatment options aim to repair and regenerate the lost structures. Various treatment methods have been proposed, ranging from the use of bone grafts,[84] guided tissue regeneration (GTR),[85,86] molecular biologic agents (enamel matrix derivatives),[87] and growth and differentiation factors[88,89] to the promising use of stem cells[90,91] (see the article elsewhere in this issue by Sedgley and colleagues). Bone grafts generally resulted in repair that is healing of a wound by tissues that do not fully restore the architecture or the function of the lost part (ie, healing by long junctional epithelium).[92] GTR, enamel matrix derivatives, and growth and differentiation factors heal by regeneration that constitutes the reproduction of a lost or injured part. GTR is a procedure that attempts to regenerate lost periradicular structures through differential tissue responses by using a barrier (**Fig. 6**).[93] Therefore, restoration of the periodontal apparatus occurs by regeneration of connective tissue, cementum, and bone rather than epithelium. Healing by regeneration is favorable compared with repair, because the goal of periodontal therapy is to restore the periodontal tissues to their original biologic structure. Although many materials have been used to regenerate the lost structures, the concept of GTR remains the major principle in the treatment methodology used today to manage periodontal-endodontic tissue/bony defects.

Guided Tissue Regeneration

GTR constitutes the reproduction of a lost or injured tissue. Melcher[94] suggested that 4 different cell types dictate the type of periodontal healing that occurs. These cells originate from the gingival epithelial tissue, lamina propria of connective tissue, alveolar bone, and periodontal ligament. Cells derived from periodontal ligament and alveolar bone have the potential to heal by true regeneration compared with cells from the lamina propria of gingiva or gingival epithelial tissue. Understanding barrier-mediated selective cell repopulation gave rise to the concept of epithelial exclusion to restore lost periodontal tissue and obtain new attachments. In periodontal disease, the crestal region Is primarily affected because it is exposed to the microflora of the oral cavity The use of a barrier is important to isolate the periodontal defect from the soft tissues and allow adequate space and time for periodontal ligament and alveolar bone cells to reconstitute the lost periodontal attachment apparatus. GTR therapy in intrabony and furcation defects has been used with favorable results.[85,86]

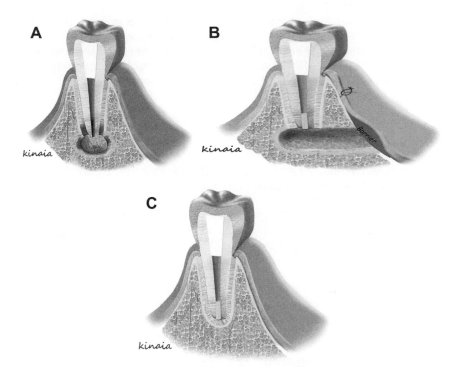

Fig. 6. (*A*) Illustration of post-treatment periapical disease on a tooth with previous endodontic therapy and permanent restoration. (*B*) Illustration of surgical management of post-treatment periapical disease with periapical curettage, apical resection, root-end preparation and filling, and GTR with barrier to allow periodontal tissues regeneration. (*C*) Illustration of healing after surgical treatment using GTR.

In endodontic periradicular lesions, however, the confined nature of the periradicular defect is isolated from the oral cavity. The surrounding tissue also contains progenitor stem cells that can divide and proliferate into periodontal ligament cells, cemento-blasts,[90] and osteoblasts,[91] regenerating the lost or damaged tissues. Consequently, several studies debate the use of GTR in apical periodontitis. In small-sized lesions, the periradicular tissue may regenerate naturally whereas large lesions may heal with fibrous tissue and scar.[81,95] A recent systematic review by Tsesis and colleagues[95] eval-uated the efficacy of GTR in endodontic surgery. The review included 5 studies defining small periapical lesions as those measuring less than 10 mm and large lesions equal to or more than 10 mm. Generally, small lesions healed better than large lesions but the results were not statistically significant ($P = .06$). Both small and large lesions treated with GTR, however, demonstrated greater healing compared with no GTR use. The results were statistically significant for both small ($P = .005$) and large ($P = .001$) lesions with GTR use. With regard to the extent of the lesion, GTR achieved better results in through-and-through lesions ($P = .02$) compared with lesions breaking through the buccal or lingual wall only ($P = .27$). Taken collectively, when there is a communication of the peri-apical lesion (through-and-through lesion), GTR procedure is of greater potential benefit.

SUMMARY

Treatment techniques and other therapy considerations associated with management of pulp and periradicular injury are constantly under review. Ongoing research is under way to better understand intricacies related to caries, pulp, and periradicular responses. Significant advances in understanding of the molecular basis of the pulpal and periradicular injury and healing response should lead to significant new, biologically based pulp therapies. In this issue, readers can gain insight into clinical practices and techniques, current understanding, and future directions for regenerative medicine for the field of endododontics.

REFERENCES

1. Goldberg M, Farges JC, Lacerda-Pinheiro S, et al. Inflammatory and immunological aspects of dental pulp repair. Pharmacol Res 2008;58:137–47.
2. About I, Murray PE, Franquin JC, et al. The effect of cavity restoration variables on odontoblast cell number and dental repair. J Dent 2001;29:109–17.
3. Farges JC, Keller JF, Carrouel F, et al. Odontoblasts in the dental pulp immune response. J Exp Zool B Mol Dev Evol 2009;312B:425–36.
4. Magloire H, Couble ML, Thillichon·Prince B, et al. Odontoblast: a mechanosensory cell. J Exp Zool B Mol Dev Evol 2009;312B:416–24.
5. Son AR, Yang YM, Hong JH, et al. Odontoblast TRP channels and thermo/mechanical transmission. J Dent Res 2009;88:1014–9.
6. Mjör IA, Odont D. Pulp-dentin biology in restorative dentistry. Part 2: initial reactions to preparation of teeth for restorative procedures. Quintessence Int 2001;32:537–51.
7. Wisithphrom K, Murray Pf, About I, et al. Interactions between cavity preparation and restoration events and their effects on pulp vitality. Int J Periodontics Restorative Dent 2006;26:596–605.
8. Bergenholtz G. Evidence for bacterial causation of adverse pulpal responses in resin-based dental restorations. Crit Rev Oral Biol Med 2000;11:467–80.
9. Stanley HR. Pulpal response to dental techniques and materials. Dent Clin North Am 1971;15:115–26.
10. Kim S. Microcirculation of the dental pulp in health and disease. J Endod 1985;11:465–71.
11. Magloire H, Joffre A, Couble ML, et al. Ultrastructural alterations of human odontoblasts and collagen fibers in the pulpal border zone beneath early caries lesions. Cell Mol Biol 1981;27:437–43.
12. Bjørndal L, Darvann T, Thylstrup A. A quantitative light microscopic study of the odontoblast and subodontoblastic reactions to active and arrested enamel caries without cavitation. Caries Res 1998;32:59–69.
13. Mjör IA. Dentin permeability: the basis for understanding pulp reactionsand adhesive technology. Braz Dent J 2009;20:3–16.
14. Pashley DH, Pashley H, Carvalho RM, et al. The effects of dentin permeability on restorative dentistry. Dent Clin North Am 2002;46:211–45.
15. Smith AJ. Pulpal responses to caries and dental repair. Caries Res 2002;36:223–32.
16. Puapichartdumrong P, Ikeda H, Suda H. Outward fluid flow reduces inward diffusion of bacterial lipopolysaccharide across intact and demineralised dentine. Arch Oral Biol 2005;50:707 13.
17. Hahn CL, Liewehr FR. Relationships between caries bacteria, host responses and clinical signs and symptoms of pulpitis. J Endod 2007;33:213–9.
18. Pashley DH, Matthews WG. The effects of outward forced convective flow on inward diffusion in human dentine *in vitro*. Arch Oral Biol 1993;38:577–82.

19. Khabbaz MG, Anastasiadis PL, Sykaras SN. Determinat ion of endotoxins in the vital pulp of human carious teeth: association with pulpal pain. Oral Surg Oral Med Oral Pathol 2001;91:587–93.
20. Camps J, Pashley DH. Buffering action of human dentin *in vitro*. J Adhes Dent 2000;2:39–50.
21. Brännström M, Lind PO. Pulpal response to early dental caries. J Dent Res 1965; 44:1045–50.
22. Hahn CL, Liewehr FR. Innate immune responses of the dental pulp to caries. J Endod 2007;33:643–51.
23. Hahn CL, Liewehr FR. Update on the adaptive immune responses of the dental pulp. J Endod 2007;33:773–81.
24. Trowbridge HO. Pathogenesis of pulpitis resulting from dental caries. J Endod 1981;7:52–60.
25. Reeves R, Stanley HR. The relationship of bacterial penetration and pulpal pathosis in carious teeth. Oral Surg Oral Med Oral Pathol 1966;22:59–65.
26. Bjørndal L. The caries process and its effect on the pulp: the science is changing and so is our understanding. J Endod 2008;34(Suppl 7):52–5.
27. Zheng L, Hilton JF, Habelitz S, et al. Dentin caries activity status related to hardness and elasticity. Eur J Oral Sci 2003;111:243–52.
28. Bjørndal L, Mjör IA. Pulp-dentin biology in restorative dentistry, Part 4: dental caries-characteristics of lesions and pulpal reactions. Quintessence Int 2001; 32:717–36.
29. Duque C, Hebling J, Smith AJ, et al. Reactionary dentinogenesis after app lying restorative materials and bioactive dentin matrix molecules as liners in deep cavities prepared in nonhuman primate teeth. J Oral Rehabil 2006;33:452–61.
30. Tooloo O, Laurent P, Zygouritsas S, et al. Activation of human dental pulp progenitor/stem cells in response to odontoblast injury. Arch Oral Biol 2005; 50:103–8.
31. Sloan AJ, Smith AJ. Stem cells and the dental pulp: potential roles in dentine regeneration and repair. Oral Dis 2007;13:151–7.
32. Bergenholtz G. Pathogenic mechanisms in pulpal disease. J Endod 1990;16: 98–101.
33. Tziafas D, Smith AJ, Lesot H. Designing new treatment strategies in vital pulp therapy. J Dent 2000;28:77–92.
34. Burke FM, Samarawickrama DY. Progressive changes in the pulpo-dentinal complex and their clinical consequences. Gerodontology 1995;12:57–66.
35. Tjäderhane L. The mechanism of pulpal wound healing. Aust Endod J 2002;28: 68–74.
36. Cvek M, Cleaton-Jones PE, Austin JC, et al. Pulp reactions to exposure after experimental crown fractures or grinding in adult monkeys. J Endod 1982;8:391–7.
37. Zander HA, Glass RL. The healing of phenolized pulp exposure. Oral Surg Oral Med Oral Pathol 1949;2:803–10.
38. Mastenon JB. Inherent healing potential of the dental pulp. Br Dent J 1966;120: 430–6.
39. Torneck CD, Moe H, Howley TP. The effect of calcium hydroxide on porcine pulp fibroblasts *in vitro*. J Endod 1983;9:131–5.
40. Cox CF, Bergenholtz G, Fitzgerald M, et al. Capping of the dental pulp mechanically exposed to the oral microflora-A 5-week observation of wound healing in the monkey. J Oral Pathol 1982;11:327–39.
41. Cvek M. A clinical report on partial pulpotomy and capping with calcium hydroxide in permanent incisors with complicated crown fracture. J Endod 1978;4:232–7.

42. Mejilre I, Cvek M. Partial pulpotomy in young permanent teeth with deep carious lesions. Endod Dent Traumatol 1993;9:238–42.
43. Isermann GT, Kaminski EJ. Pulpal response to minimal exposure in presence of bacteria and Dycal. J Endod 1979;5:322–7.
44. Kakehashi S, Stanley HR, Fitzgerald RJ. The effects of surgical exposures of dental pulps in germ-free and conventional laboratory rats. Oral Surg Oral Med Oral Pathol 1965;20:340–9.
45. Segura JJ, Llamas R, Rubio-Manzanares AJ, et al. Calcium hydroxide inhibits substrate adherence capacity of macrophages. J Endod 1997;23:444–7.
46. Hebling J, Giro EM, Costa CA. Biocompatibility of an adhesive system applied to exposed human dental pulp. J Endod 1999;25:676–82.
47. Hafez AA, Cox CF, Tarim B, et al. An in vivo evaluation of hemorrhage control using sodium hypochlorite and direct capping with a one- or two- component adhesive system in exposed nonhuman primate pulps. Quintessence Int 2002;33:261–72.
48. Accorinte Mde L, Loguercio AD, Reis A, et al. Response of human pulp capped with a bonding agent after bleeding control with hemostatic agents. Oper Dent 2005;30:147–55.
49. Accorinte Mde L, Loguercio AD, Reis A, et al. Effects of hemostatic agents on the histomorphologic response of human dental pulp capped with calcium hydroxide. Quintessence Int 2007;38:843–52.
50. Silva AF, Tarquinio SB, Demarco FF, et al. The influence of haemostatic agents on healing of healthy human dental pulp tissue capped with calcium hydroxide. Int Endod J 2006;39:309–16.
51. Pitt Ford TR. Pulpal response to Procal for capping exposures in dog's teeth. J Br Endod Soc 1979;12:67–72.
52. Pitt Ford TR. Pulpal response to a calcium hydroxide material for capping exposures. Oral Surg Oral Med Oral Pathol 1985;59:194–7.
53. Brännstrom M, Nyborg H, Strömberg T. Experiments with pulp capping. Oral Surg Oral Med Oral Pathol 1979;48:347–52.
54. Heys DR, Cox CF, Heys RJ, et al. Histological considerations of direct pulp capping agents. J Dent Res 1981;60:1371–9.
55. Cox CF, Bergenholtz G, Heys DR, et al. Pulp capping of dental pulp mechanically exposed to oral microflora: a 1-2 year observation of wound healing in the monkey. J Oral Pathol 1985;14:156–68.
56. Stanley HR. Criteria for standardizing and increasing credibility of direct pulp capping studies [special issue]. Am J Dent 1998;11:S17–34.
57. Franz FE, Holz J, Baume LJ. Ultrastructure (SEM) of dentine bridging in the human dental pulp. J Biol Buccale 1984;12:239–46.
58. Nair PN, Duncan HF, Pitt Ford TR, et al. Histological, ultrastructural and quantitative investigations on the response of healthy human pulps to experimental capping with mineral trioxide aggregate: a randomized controlled trial. Int Endod J 2008;41:128–50.
59. Cox CF, Sübay RK, Ostro E, et al. Tunnel defects in dentin bridges: their formation following direct pulp capping. Oper Dent 1996;21:4–11.
60. Ziafras D, Belibasakis G, Veis A, et al. Dentin regeneration in vital pulp therapy: design principles. Adv Dent Res 2001;15:96–100.
61. Barthel CR, Rosenkranz B, Leuenberg A, et al. Pulp capping of carious exposures: treatment outcome after 5 and 10 years: a retrospective study. J Endod 2000;26:525–8.
62. Murray PE, Garcia-Godoy F. The incidence of pulp healing defects with direct capping materials. Am J Dent 2006;19:171–7.

63. do Nascimento AB, Fontana UF, Teixeria HM, et al. Biocompatibility of a resin-modified glass-ionomer cement applied as pulp capping in human teeth. Am J Dent 2000;13:28–34.

64. Accorinte ML, Loguercio AD, Reis A, et al. Response of human pulps capped with different self-etch adhesive systems. Clin Oral Investig 2008;12:119–27.

65. Cui C, Zhou X, Chen X, et al. The adverse effect of self-etching adhesive systems on dental pulp after direct pulp capping. Quintessence Int 2009;40: e26–34.

66. Başak F, Vural IM, Kaya E, et al. Vasorelaxant effect of a self-etch adhesive system through calcium antagonistic action. J Endod 2008;34:1202–6.

67. Salako N, Joseph B, Ritwik P, et al. Comparison of bioactive glass, mineral trioxide aggregate, ferric sulfate, and formocresol as pulpotomy agents in rat molar. Dent Traumatol 2003;19:314–20.

68. El-Meligy OA, Avery DR. Comparison of mineral trioxide aggregate and calcium hydroxide as pulpotomy agents in young permanent teeth (apexogenesis). Pediatr Dent 2006;28:399–404.

69. Witherspoon DE. Vital pulp therapy with new materials: new directions and treatment perspectives-Permanent teeth. J Endod 2008;34(Suppl 7):S25–8.

70. Bogen G, Kim JS, Bakland LK. Direct pulp capping with mineral trioxide aggregate: an observational study. J Am Dent Assoc 2008;139:305–15.

71. Silva TA, Rosa AL, Lara VS. Dentin matrix proteins and soluble factors: intrinsic regulatory signals for healing and resorption of dental and periodontal tissues. Oral Dis 2004;10:63–74.

72. About I, Mitsiadis TA. Molecular aspects of tooth pathogenesis and repair: *in vivo* and *in vitro* models. Adv Dent Res 2001;15:59–62.

73. Marshall GW Jr, Marshall SJ, Kinney JH, et al. The dentin substrate: structure and properties related to bonding. J Dent 1997;25:441–58.

74. Cox CF, Halez AA, Akimoto N, et al. Biocompatibility of primer, adhesive and resin composite systems on non-exposed and exposed pulps on non-human primate teeth [special issue]. Am J Dent 1998;11:S55–63.

75. Bönecker M, Toi C, Cleaton-Jones P. *Mutans Streptococci* and *lactobacilli* in carious dentin before and after a traumatic restorative treatment. J Dent 2003; 31:413–28.

76. Washington JT, Schneiderman E, Spears R, et al. Biocompatibility and osteogenic potential of new generation endodontic materials established by using primary osteoblasts. J Endod 2011;37:1166–70.

77. Zairi A, Lambrianidis T, Pantelidou O, et al. Periradicular tissue responses to biologically active molecules or MTA when applied in furcal perforation of dogs' teeth. Int J Dent 2012;2012:257832.

78. Al-Hiyasat AS, Al-Sa'Eed OR, Darmani H. Quality of cellular attachment to various root-end filling materials. J Appl Oral Sci 2012;20:82–8.

79. Möller AJ, Fabricius L, Dahlén G, et al. Influence on periapical tissues of indigenous oral bacteria and necrotic pulp tissue in monkeys. Scand J Dent Res 1981; 89:475–84.

80. Fabricius L, Dahlén G, Ohman AE, et al. Predominant indigenous oral bacteria isolated from infected root canals after varied times of closure. Scand J Dent Res 1982;90:134–44.

81. Lin L, Chen M, Ricucci D, et al. Guided tissue regeneration in periapical surgery. J Endod 2010;36:618–25.

82. Simon JH, Glick DH, Frank AL. The relationship of endodontic-periodontic lesions. J Periodontol 1972;43:202–8.

83. Rotstein I, Simon JH. Diagnosis, prognosis and decision-making in the treatment of combined periodontal-endodontic lesions. Periodontol 2000 2004;34: 165–203.
84. Schallhorn RG. Present status of osseous grafting procedures. J Periodontol 1977;48(9):570–6.
85. Murphy KG, Gunsolley JC. Guided tissue regeneration for the treatment of periodontal intrabony and furcation defects. A systematic review. Ann Periodontol 2003;8(1):266–302.
86. Kinaia BM, Steiger J, Neely AL, et al. Treatment of class II molar furcation involvement: meta-analyses of reentry results. J Periodontol 2011;82(3):413–28.
87. Esposito M, Grusovin M, Papanikolaou N, et al. Enamel matrix derivative (Emdogain) for periodontal tissue regeneration in intrabony defects. A Cochrane systematic review. Eur J Oral Implantol 2009;2:247–66.
88. Howell TH, Fiorellini JP, Paquette DW, et al. A phase I/II clinical trial to evaluate a combination of recombinant human platelet-derived growth factor-BB and recombinant human insulin-like growth factor-I in patients with periodontal disease. J Periodontol 1997;68(12):1186–93.
89. Sigurdsson TJ, Lee MB, Kubota K, et al. Periodontal repair in dogs: recombinant human bone morphogenetic protein-2 significantly enhances periodontal regeneration. J Periodontol 1995;66(2):131–8.
90. Gronthos S, Zannettino AC, Hay SJ, et al. Molecular and cellular characterization of highly purified stromal stem cells derived from human bone marrow. J Cell Sci 2003;116:1827–35.
91. Seo BM, Miura M, Gronthos S, et al. Investigation of multipotent postnatal stem cells from human periodontal ligament. Lancet 2004;364(9429):149–55.
92. The American Academy of Periodontology. Glossary of periodontal terms. 4th edition. Chicago: The American Academy of Periodontology; 2001. p. 47.
93. The American Association of Endodontics. Glossary of endodontic terms. 7th edition. Chicago: The American Academy of Periodontology; 2003. p. 26.
94. Melcher AH. On the repair potential of periodontal tissues. J Periodontol 1976; 47(5):256–60.
95. Tsesis I, Rosen E, Tamse A, et al. Effect of guided tissue regeneration on the outcome of surgical endodontic treatment: a systematic review and meta-analysis. J Endod 2011;37(8):1039–45.

Regenerative Therapy
A Periodontal-Endodontic Perspective

Bassam Michael Kinaia, DDS, MS[a,b,c,*], Sami M.A. Chogle, BDS, DMD, MSD[d,e,f], Atheel M. Kinaia, DDS[g], Harold E. Goodis, DDS[e,h,i]

KEYWORDS

- Regeneration • Periodontal-endodontic • Dental pulp • Bone substitutes
- Growth factors • Stem cells

KEY POINTS

- Periodontal and endodontic diseases are inflammatory responses to microorganisms leading to periodontal and pulpal tissue damage and loss. Regenerative therapies aim to restore the lost structures to vitality and function.
- Various materials and treatments methods, such as bone grafts, guided tissue regeneration, enamel materials derivatives, growth and differentiation factors, and stem cells research, have been used.
- Although the current materials and methods demonstrated favorable clinical results, true and complete biological regeneration of the damaged or injured structures is not yet attainable.

INTRODUCTION

Periodontal disease is a destructive inflammatory process affecting the periodontal attachment apparatus of the teeth, leading to irreversible loss of bone and periodontal ligament (PDL).[1] Similarly in endodontics, a progressive injury (ie, caries) to the dental

Conflict of Interest: The authors declare that there is no conflict of interest related to this paper.
[a] Postgraduate Periodontology Program, Periodontology Department, The Boston University Institute for Dental Research and Education, PO Box 505097, Dubai Healthcare City, Dubai, United Arab Emirates; [b] Department of Periodontology and Oral Biology, The Goldman School of Dental Medicine, Boston, MA, USA; [c] University of Detroit Mercy - School of Dentistry, Detroit, MI, USA; [d] Postgraduate Program in Endodontics, Endodontics Department, The Boston University Institute for Dental Research and Education, PO Box 505097, Dubai Healthcare City, Dubai, United Arab Emirates; [e] Department of Endodontics, The Goldman School of Dental Medicine, Boston, MA, USA; [f] Department of Endodontics, Case School of Dental Medicine, Cleveland, OH, USA; [g] Advanced Education in General Dentistry Program, The European University, PO Box 505097, Dubai Healthcare City, Dubai, United Arab Emirates; [h] The Boston University Institute for Dental Research and Education, PO Box 505097, Dubai Healthcare City, Dubai, United Arab Emirates; [i] Department of Endodontics, The University of California School of Dentistry, San Francisco, CA, USA
* Corresponding author. 2452 Westmont Cr. Sterling Heights, MI 48310.
E-mail address: kinaia@perio.org

Dent Clin N Am 56 (2012) 537–547
doi:10.1016/j.cden.2012.05.002
0011-8532/12/$ – see front matter © 2012 Elsevier Inc. All rights reserved.

pulp stimulates an inflammatory response leading to pulpal necrosis and periapical tissue involvement manifested in periradicular tissue breakdown. Various treatment methods have been proposed for the treatment of periodontal disease. In the 1950s and 1960s, treatments ranged from conservative therapy, such as curettage and open flap debridement, to surgical treatment procedures, such as gingivectomy, root amputation, hemi-section, and tunneling. Regardless of the treatment method used, healing occurred by repair (ie, long junctional epithelium) rather than regeneration of the lost tissues of the periodontal attachment apparatus. The introduction of bone grafts[2–4] in the 1970s and 1980s and the concept of guided tissue regeneration (GTR)[5–7] offered new treatment options to regenerate lost periodontal tissues.[8–10] In the 1990s and 2000s, enamel matrix derivatives (EMDs),[11] platelet-derived growth factor (PDGF),[12,13] insulinlike growth factor (IGF-I),[14] and bone morphogenetic proteins (BMPs)[15] have given a new dimension to periodontal regeneration with promising clinical results. The aim of periodontal treatment is complete regeneration of the lost or damaged tissues. Despite the success of the above-mentioned materials and methods, this aim has been partially but not completely established. At present, stem cells (SCs) represent a new era in regenerative therapy with the aim of complete regeneration. This article chronologically reviews the regenerative therapies used in periodontal and endodontic fields with emphasis on periodontal regeneration.

HEALING
Endodontic Repair Versus Regeneration

In pulpal injury, if the original odontoblasts survive and react by secreting tertiary dentin matrices, complete regeneration and return of the damaged vital pulp tissue to its normal form and function is possible via reactionary dentinogenesis.[16] Conversely, reparative dentin formation occurs in response to deep dentinal caries and represents a much more complex sequence of biologic events beginning with apoptosis of the odontoblasts in the area of injury, including progenitor cell recruitment and differentiation.[17] When the pulp is exposed in advanced lesions, reparative dentinogenesis may result in dentin bridge formation, which restores only the functional integrity of the pulpodentin complex. In the case of a periradicular lesion due to pulpal necrosis, usually the lesion would heal to form and function after conventional endodontic therapy. However, in some instances, the lesion may persist or not completely heal despite adequate therapy. Generally, a persistent periapical radiolucent lesion would indicate ongoing disease. On occasion, unresolved periapical radiolucency may represent healing by remnants of the lesion, which may be mistaken as a sign of failed endodontic treatment.[18,19] These types of lesions usually occur when the lesion penetrates both the buccal and lingual cortical plates (ie, communicating lesion). In such cases, the form and functional healing of the periradicular tissues are replaced by a fibrous tissue repair of the area, which persists as a radiolucency alluding to persistent disease of the apical region.

Periodontal Repair Versus Regeneration

Periodontally, repair is healing of a wound by tissue that does not fully restore the architecture or the function of the lost part as in healing by long junctional epithelium.[1] Regeneration constitutes the reproduction of a lost or injured part. Periodontally, GTR is a procedure that attempts to regenerate the lost periodontal structures through differential tissue responses by using a barrier (ie, membrane).[1] Thus, restoration of the periodontal apparatus occurs by the regeneration of connective tissue, cementum, and alveolar bone rather than epithelium. Healing by regeneration is favorable compared with repair because the goal of periodontal therapy is to restore the periodontal tissues to their original biological structure. Many materials and methods have been used to accomplish regeneration, including bone grafts, GTR, EMDs, growth factors, and SCs.

REGENERATIVE THERAPY
Bone Grafts

Bone grafts are used as fillers in periodontal defects and aid in healing by repair. Bone grafts are used because of their osteogenic (autograft), osteoinductive (allograft), or osteoconductive (xenograft/alloplast) properties.[20] Osteogenic materials stimulate the formation of new bones because they contain bone-forming cells and progenitor cells. Osteoinductive materials stimulate progenitor SCs in the surrounding tissue immediately adjacent to the defect to regenerate the lost structures.[21,22] In contrast, osteoconductive materials serve as scaffolds for bone growth within the existing bony walls and passively promote healing.[3] Although bone grafts demonstrated adequate clinical results, the healing mainly occurred by repair (long junctional epithelium), rather than regeneration of the PDL (**Fig. 1**).[6,23]

Bone grafts are also used in the treatment of apical periodontitis and more specifically, in periradicular surgery. Freeze-dried bone allografts (FDBA) were used in osseous defects after the removal of periapical lesions. The results showed that FDBA had an osteogenic potential and, for the most part, bone regeneration occurred.[24] Although the previously mentioned studies were beneficial in healing of periodontal and periradicular defects, complete true regeneration did not occur.

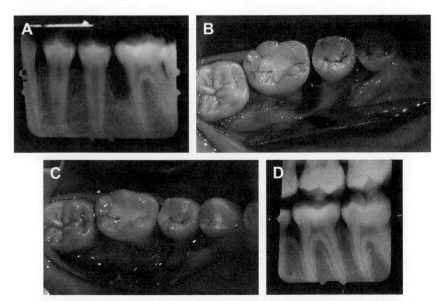

Fig. 1. Bone allograft material for treatment of intrabony periodontal defect. (*A*) Preoperative radiograph of intrabony periodontal defect #19. (*B*) Clinical picture showing surgical exposure of the defect extending mesiolingually. (*C*) Bone allograft material filling the defect. (*D*) Follow-up radiograph (18 months) showing the presence of adequate bone fill. (*Courtesy of* Bassam M. Kinaia, DDS, MS, Boston University Institute for Dental Research and Education, Dubai Healthcare City, Dubai, UAE.)

Guided Tissue Regeneration

Melcher[5] suggested that there are 4 different cell types dictating the type of periodontal healing that occurs. These cells originate from the gingival epithelial tissue, lamina propria of connective tissue, alveolar bone, and PDL. Cells derived from PDL and bone posses the potential to heal by true regeneration when compared with cells from lamina propria of gingiva or gingival epithelial tissue that heal by repair (**Fig. 2**).[5] Understanding barrier mediated selective cell repopulation gave rise to the concept of epithelial exclusion to restore lost periodontal tissue and obtain new attachment. Bowers and colleagues[6] published a histologic report on the formation of new periodontal attachment apparatus in humans. The study included teeth with intrabony defects that needed to be extracted because of advanced periodontal disease. The investigators performed flap curettage, crown removal, and submersion of the vital root beneath the mucosa with biopsies obtained at 6 months after treatment. The submersion of the teeth allowed epithelial exclusion similar to GTR. New attachment occurred in the submerged group indicating regeneration. Healing by long junctional epithelium was observed on the nonsubmerged teeth, indicating repair. Further, regeneration of new attachment apparatus, cementum, and bone was more likely in submerged, intrabony grafted defects with demineralized FDBA. New attachment in

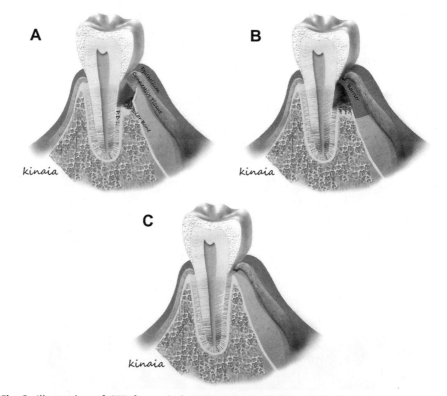

Fig. 2. Illustration of GTR for periodontal intrabony defect. (*A*) Epithelium and connective tissue migration into periodontal intrabony defect with PDL tissue and alveolar bone loss. (*B*) Membrane to exclude the soft tissue coronally to allow selective PDL and alveolar bone regeneration. (*C*) Ideal outcome of GTR showing complete reconstruction of the periodontal attachment apparatus. (*Courtesy of* Bassam M. Kinaia, DDS, MS, Boston University Institute for Dental Research and Education, Dubai Healthcare City, Dubai, UAE.)

grafted sites measured 1.76 mm compared with 0.76 mm in nongrafted sites. The investigators concluded that healing with a new attachment was more predictable for submerged teeth and more likely when a bone graft was added.[23] The literature demonstrated that GTR was biologically possible with promising clinical results in intrabony and furcation defects.[9,10]

Although the concept of GTR was primarily established in periodontal regeneration, it also has been applied in surgical endodontic treatment (**Fig. 3**). A recent systematic review by Tsesis and colleagues[25] evaluated the efficacy of GTR in endodontic surgery. They found that large communicating lesions healed better with GTR compared with those without GTR ($P = .02$). However, GTR in small confined lesions was of no added benefit ($P = .27$). The use of a resorbable membrane was more favorable than nonresorbable membranes ($P = .02$), a finding that was similar to that obtained in the regeneration of periodontal furcation defects.[10] Therefore, when a periapical lesion is confined, GTR may not be necessary. If there is a large communication of the periapical lesion, GTR would be of potential benefit.[26] Despite the success of GTR in periodontal and endodontic treatments, complete regeneration of the periodontal attachment apparatus is not always predictable.[25] Thus, advances in molecular biology, such as EMDs and growth factors, offer a new area of research with the hope of complete regeneration.

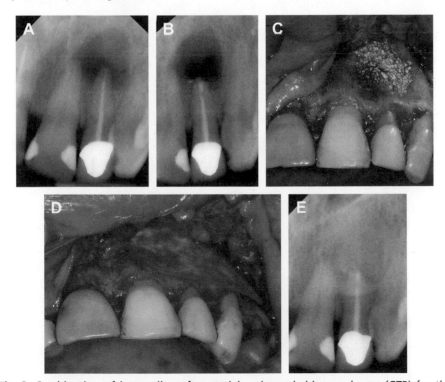

Fig. 3. Combination of bone allograft material and resorbable membrane (GTR) for the treatment of apical periodontitis. (*A*) Periapical radiolucency on #10 after treatment (RCT completed 15 years ago). (*B*) Immediate postsurgical radiograph showing retrograde fill. (*C*) Bone allograft material added. (*D*) Resorbable membrane placed. (*E*) Follow-up radiograph (6 months) showing adequate bone fill. (*Courtesy of* Bassam M. Kinaia, DDS, MS, and Sami Chogle, BDS, DMD, MSD, Boston University Institute for Dental Research and Education, Dubai Healthcare City, Dubai, UAE.)

Enamel Matrix Derivatives

Advances in molecular biology set the stage for a new era in periodontal regeneration for complete regeneration (**Fig. 4**). Studies reported that treatment of intrabony defects with EMDs led to decreased probing depth, increased clinical attachment level (CAL), increased bone-fill, and periodontal regeneration.[27] EMD contains amelogenins among other enamel matrix proteins that mimic the cementogenesis process during root formation.[28] These proteins, in primate studies, have demonstrated stimulation of the surrounding undifferentiated mesenchymal cells into cementoblasts to form acellular cementum, a process similar to the formation of the inner layer of Hertwig epithelial root sheath during tooth development.[29] Once the cementum is formed, collagen fibers attach from the adjacent PDL leading to the restoration of the periodontal attachment apparatus.[28] Although not consistent, EMD creates a favorable environment at the cellular level for periodontal regeneration by improving the attachment as well as differentiation of PDL fibroblasts compared with gingival fibroblasts.[30] Similarly, the amelogenins are involved in the differentiation of odontoblasts during development indicating that they may play a role in odontogenesis. Nakamura and colleagues[31] examined the effect of EMD on pulpal wound healing in an animal study using premolars. They found that EMD formed dentinlike hard tissue with the presence

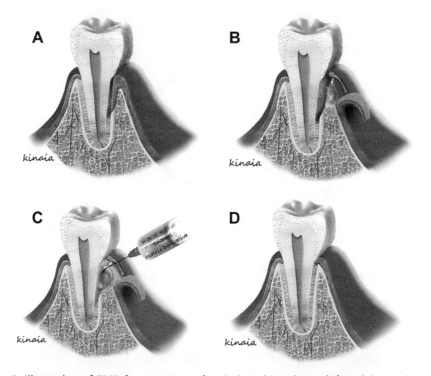

Fig. 4. Illustration of EMD for treatment of periodontal intrabony defect. (*A*) Apical migration of epithelium and connective tissue into periodontal intrabony defect with PDL tissue and alveolar bone loss. (*B*) Diseased root surface and periodontal defect are surgically exposed. (*C*) Enamel matrix derivatives added to repair the defect. (*D*) Ideal outcome showing complete reconstruction of the periodontal attachment apparatus. (*Courtesy of* Bassam M. Kinaia, DDS, MS, Boston University Institute for Dental Research and Education, Dubai Healthcare City, Dubai, UAE.)

of formative cells outlining the pulpal wound. EMD had a 2-fold better reparative potential of the pulpal wound compared with the control (calcium-hydroxide) group. At the microbiological level, EMD selectively inhibited the growth of gram-negative pathogens although exhibiting no effect on gram-positive pathogens.[32] EMD mainly creates a positive environment, but it does not contain a specific growth factor that can be useful to enhance regeneration.[33] More recent advances in regenerative therapies include the use of growth and differentiation factors for periodontal and endodontic regeneration.

Growth and Differentiation Factors

Growth and differentiation factors play an important role in regulating wound-healing events, such as chemotaxis, cell adhesion, proliferation, and differentiation.[34] These factors include platelet-derived growth factor (PDGF), vascular endothelial growth factor (VEGF), transforming growth factors (TGF) α and β, acidic and basic fibroblast growth factors, epidermal growth factor, IGF-I, IGF-II, cementum-derived growth factor, parathyroid hormone-related protein, and BMPs.[35] See the article by Kim and colleagues in this issue for further details on growth and differentiation factors.

At present, the most used factors are PDGF, IGF, and BMPs. PDGFs are dimeric glycoproteins comprising 2 A (-AA), 2 B (-BB) chains, or a combination of the 2 (-AB) chains. PDGF-BB has been used in intrabony periodontal defects with significant improvement in clinical outcomes demonstrated as CAL gain, bone growth, and percentage bone fill.[13,36] IGF is a protein with 2 ligands (IGF-1 and IGF-2). Howell and colleagues[14] reported CAL gain, periodontal probing depth (PPD) reduction, and bone gain with use of a combination of IGF-1 and PDGF-BB. Further, a pulp-capping study in rat molars by Lovschall and colleagues[37] reported a positive effect of IGF-1 in dentin repair. IGF-1 improved the reparative dentinogenesis in injured dental pulps. Contrary to the Lovschall study, Regan and colleagues[38] evaluated the use of the PDGF and IGF combination in periapical surgery and reported no regeneration of the periapical tissues. PDGF and IGF have shown promising results in periodontal regeneration but their results are controversial in endodontic regeneration.[13,14,36–38]

BMPs are differentiating factors belonging to the TGF-β superfamily. They play a major role in differentiation, cell migration, proliferation, and apoptosis. At present, there are more than 20 BMPs with BMP-2 (osteogenic protein-2 [OP-2]), BMP-3 (osteogenin), and BMP-7 (osteogenic protein-1 [OP-1]) being the most useful in regenerative therapy.[39] In 2007, the Food and Drug Administration approved the use of INFUSE Bone Graft containing BMP in dental regeneration.[40] BMP-2 and -3 have shown potential in correcting intrabony and furcation bone loss. However, BMP-2 has been associated with ankylosis histologically.[15] Therefore, these molecules are generally reserved for use around implants or for guided bone regeneration.[41] However, BMP-7 has been used successfully in periodontal regeneration with no ankylosis.[42] Similarly, animal studies reported the differentiation of pulp cells into odontoblasts leading to the formation of osteodentin when using BMP-2[43] and BMP-7.[44] The current regenerative methods have shown adequate clinical results, but complete regeneration as of yet is not predictably achievable. New research emphasizes the use of SCs with the aim and hope of complete regeneration of the original periodontal and endodontic tissues.

Stem Cells

Although growth and differentiating factors have shown positive clinical results, they possess a short biologic half-life that may limit their use in complete regeneration of lost or damaged tissues. Therefore, constant release of these factors may be essential for complete periodontal regeneration. SCs are readily present in human tissues offering new horizons for complete regeneration. Dental SCs are primarily found in the dental pulp and PDL. Three dental SC populations have been identified based on their origin: dental pulp SCs (DPSCs), SCs from human exfoliated deciduous teeth (SHED), and PDLSCs .[45,46] DPSC's and SHEDs are further discussed in the article by Sedgley and colleagues in this issue.

Several preclinical studies have been reported on PDLSCs. In 1 study, PDLSCs were isolated from extracted human third molar PDLs and transplanted into immuno-compromised mice and rats.[47] PDLSCs differentiated into cementoblastlike cells, adipocytes, and collagen-forming cells and generated cementum/PDLlike tissues. PDLSCs are similar to DPSCs and SHED in their expression of surface markers of STRO-1 and CD146/MUC18. Further, they are superior to bone mesenchymal stromal SCs (BMSSCs) in their high proliferation rate and differentiation capacity.[46] Lin and colleagues[48] examined human periodontium of molar teeth. The investigators used SC markers STRO-1, CD146, and CD44, and were able to identify PDLSCs in the regenerated tissue, indicating their involvement in periodontal regeneration. Another marker that has been seen in BMSSCs recruitment is stromal cell–derived factor-1 (SDF-1). A recent study by Du and colleagues,[49] reported significant proliferation and stimulated the migration of PDLSCs at concentrations of 100 and 400 ng/mL of SDF-1. This process suggests that SDF-1 may play a role in periodontal tissue regeneration in addition to the previous cell markers mentioned. PDLSCs require a scaffold such as hydroxyapatite/tricalcium phosphate to generate periodontal tissues.

PDL progenitor cells (PDLPs) are alternative cell sources to PDLSCs. PDLPs have been shown to play a role in periodontal regeneration because both are driven from the PDL. SCs differentiate into progenitor cells, which are more developmentally committed, yet are undifferentiated in comparison to those cells that have differentiated into specialized tissue cells. Fen and colleagues[50] examined the use of PDLPs in the treatment of human intrabony periodontal defects and compared it to PDLSCs. PDLPs were transplanted in defects measuring more than 6 mm depth in 3 patients. PDLPs were similar to PDLSCs in their high proliferation rate and multipotent differentiation, resulting in therapeutic periodontal regeneration.[50] This study represents one of the early clinical studies examining the use of stem/progenitor cells in periodontal regeneration in humans.

FUTURE DIRECTIONS

Although the current research in regenerative therapy is very promising, complete biological regeneration of periodontal and endodontic tissues is not yet predictably obtained. Bone grafts generally result in repair rather than regeneration. GTR is a sound principle, but it does not always regenerate the lost tissues predictably and completely. EMDs and growth and differentiation factors have a short biological half-life limiting their use for complete regeneration. SCs possess great potential for complete regeneration but still needs to be demonstrated as effective in human clinical trials. Future directions involve the fabrication of vehicles and scaffolds that are able to have a sustained release of growth factors and SCs with the aim of complete and true biological regeneration to restore the original tissues. See the article by Goodis and colleagues in this issue for an update on scaffolds for pulp regeneration.

REFERENCES

1. The American Academy of Periodontology. Glossary of periodontal terms. 4th edition. Chicago; 2001. p. 42–7.

2. Schallhorn RG, Hiatt WH, Boyce W. Iliac transplants in periodontal therapy. J Periodontol 1970;41(10):566–80.
3. Schallhorn RG. Present status of osseous grafting procedures. J Periodontol 1977;48(9):570–6.
4. Mellonig JT, Bowers GM, Bright RW, et al. Clinical evaluation of freeze-dried bone allografts in periodontal osseous defects. J Periodontol 1976;47(3):125–31.
5. Melcher AH. On the repair potential of periodontal tissues. J Periodontol 1976; 47(5):256–60.
6. Bowers GM, Chadroff B, Carnevale R, et al. Histologic evaluation of new attachment apparatus formation in humans. Part I. J Periodontol 1989;60(12):664–74.
7. Becker W, Becker BE, Berg L, et al. New attachment after treatment with root isolation procedures: report for treated Class III and Class II furcations and vertical osseous defects. Int J Periodontics Restorative Dent 1988;8(3):8–23.
8. Reynolds MA, Aichelmann-Reidy ME, Branch-Mays GL, et al. The efficacy of bone replacement grafts in the treatment of periodontal osseous defects. A systematic review. Ann Periodontol 2003;8(1):227–65.
9. Murphy KG, Gunsolley JC. Guided tissue regeneration for the treatment of periodontal intrabony and furcation defects. A systematic review. Ann Periodontol 2003;8(1):266–302.
10. Kinaia BM, Steiger J, Neely AL, et al. Treatment of Class II molar furcation involvement: meta-analyses of reentry results. J Periodontol 2011;82(3):413–28.
11. Esposito M, Grusovin MG, Papanikolaou N, et al. Enamel matrix derivative (Emdogain) for periodontal tissue regeneration in intrabony defects. A Cochrane systematic review. Eur J Oral Implantol 2009;2(4):247–66.
12. Nevins M, Camelo M, Nevins ML, et al. Periodontal regeneration in humans using recombinant human platelet-derived growth factor-BB (rhPDGF-BB) and allogenic bone. J Periodontol 2003;74(9):1282–92.
13. Jayakumar A, Rajababu P, Rohini S, et al. Multi-centre, randomized clinical trial on the efficacy and safety of recombinant human platelet-derived growth factor with β-tricalcium phosphate in human intra-osseous periodontal defects. J Clin Periodontol 2011;38(2):163–72.
14. Howell TH, Fiorellini JP, Paquette DW, et al. A phase I/II clinical trial to evaluate a combination of recombinant human platelet-derived growth factor-BB and recombinant human insulin-like growth factor-I in patients with periodontal disease. J Periodontol 1997;68(12):1186–93.
15. Sigurdsson TJ, Lee MB, Kubota K, et al. Periodontal repair in dogs: recombinant human bone morphogenetic protein-2 significantly enhances periodontal regeneration. J Periodontol 1995;66(2):131–8.
16. Duque C, Hebling J, Smith AJ, et al. Reactionary dentinogenesis after applying restorative materials and bioactive dentin matrix molecules as liners in deep cavities prepared in nonhuman primate teeth. J Oral Rehabil 2006;33(6):452–61.
17. Sloan AJ, Smith AJ. Stem cells and the dental pulp: potential roles in dentine regeneration and repair. Oral Dis 2007;13(2):151–7.
18. Nair PN, Sjogren U, Figdor D, et al. Persistent periapical radiolucencies of root-filled human teeth, failed endodontic treatments, and periapical scars. Oral Surg Oral Med Oral Pathol Oral Radiol Endod 1999;87(5):617–27.
19. Love RM, Firth N. Histopathological profile of surgically removed persistent periapical radiolucent lesions of endodontic origin. Int Endod J 2009;42(3): 198–202.
20. Lindhe J, Karring T, Lang NP. Clinical periodontology and implant dentistry. Oxford (United Kingdom): Blackwell Munksgaard; 2003. p. 667.

21. Ellegaard B, Karring T, Listgarten M, et al. New attachment after treatment of interradicular lesions. J Periodontol 1973;44(4):209–17.
22. Ellegaard B. Bone grafts in periodontal attachment procedures. J Clin Periodontol 1976;3(5):1–54.
23. Bowers GM, Chadroff B, Carnevale R, et al. Histologic evaluation of new attachment apparatus formation in humans. Part II. J Periodontol 1989;60(12):675–82.
24. Saad AY, Abdellatief EM. Healing assessment of osseous defects of periapical lesions associated with failed endodontically treated teeth with use of freeze-dried bone allograft. Oral Surg Oral Med Oral Pathol 1991;71(5):612–7.
25. Tsesis I, Rosen E, Tamse A, et al. Effect of guided tissue regeneration on the outcome of surgical endodontic treatment: a systematic review and meta-analysis. J Endod 2011;37(8):1039–45.
26. Bashutski JD, Wang HL. Periodontal and endodontic regeneration. J Endod 2009;35(3):321–8.
27. Kalpidis CD, Ruben MP. Treatment of intrabony periodontal defects with enamel matrix derivative: a literature review. J Periodontol 2002;73(11):1360–76.
28. Hammarstrom L. Enamel matrix, cementum development and regeneration. J Clin Periodontol 1997;24(9 Pt 2):658–68.
29. Lindskog S. Formation of intermediate cementum. II: a scanning electron microscopic study of the epithelial root sheath of Hertwig in monkey. J Craniofac Genet Dev Biol 1982;2(2):161–9.
30. Lyngstadaas SP, Lundberg E, Ekdahl H, et al. Autocrine growth factors in human periodontal ligament cells cultured on enamel matrix derivative. J Clin Periodontol 2001;28(2):181–8.
31. Nakamura Y, Hammarstrom L, Lundberg E, et al. Enamel matrix derivative promotes reparative processes in the dental pulp. Adv Dent Res 2001;15:105–7.
32. Spahr A, Lyngstadaas SP, Boeckh C, et al. Effect of the enamel matrix derivative Emdogain on the growth of periodontal pathogens in vitro. J Clin Periodontol 2002;29(1):62–72.
33. Haase HR, Bartold PM. Enamel matrix derivative induces matrix synthesis by cultured human periodontal fibroblast cells. J Periodontol 2001;72(3):341–8.
34. Narayanan AS, Bartold PM. Biology of the periodontal connective tissues. Carol Stream (IL): Quintessence; 1998. p. 245–6.
35. AAP Position Paper. The potential role of growth and differentiation factors in periodontal regeneration. J Periodontol 1996;67(5):545–53.
36. Nevins M, Giannobile WV, McGuire MK, et al. Platelet-derived growth factor stimulates bone fill and rate of attachment level gain: results of a large multicenter randomized controlled trial. J Periodontol 2005;76(12):2205–15.
37. Lovschall H, Fejerskov O, Flyvbjerg A. Pulp-capping with recombinant human insulin-like growth factor I (rhIGF-I) in rat molars. Adv Dent Res 2001;15:108–12.
38. Regan JD, Gutmann JL, Iacopino AM, et al. Response of periradicular tissues to growth factors introduced into the surgical site in the root-end filling material. Int Endod J 1999;32(3):171–82.
39. Reddi AH. Bone morphogenetic proteins: from basic science to clinical applications. J Bone Joint Surg Am 2001;83(Suppl Pt 1):S1–6.
40. Wikesjo UM, Huang YH, Polimeni G, et al. Bone morphogenetic proteins: a realistic alternative to bone grafting for alveolar reconstruction. Oral Maxillofac Surg Clin North Am 2007;19(4):535–51, vi–vii.
41. Cochran DL, Schenk R, Buser D, et al. Recombinant human bone morphogenetic protein-2 stimulation of bone formation around endosseous dental implants. J Periodontol 1999;70(2):139–50.

42. van den Bergh JP, ten Bruggenkate CM, Groeneveld HH, et al. Recombinant human bone morphogenetic protein-7 in maxillary sinus floor elevation surgery in 3 patients compared to autogenous bone grafts. A clinical pilot study. J Clin Periodontol 2000;27(9):627–36.
43. Nakashima M. Induction of dentin formation on canine amputated pulp by recombinant human bone morphogenetic proteins (BMP)-2 and -4. J Dent Res 1994;73(9):1515–22.
44. Six N, Decup F, Lasfargues JJ, et al. Osteogenic proteins (bone sialoprotein and bone morphogenetic protein-7) and dental pulp mineralization. J Mater Sci Mater Med 2002;13(2):225–32.
45. Gronthos S, Mankani M, Brahim J, et al. Postnatal human dental pulp stem cells (DPSCs) in vitro and in vivo. Proc Natl Acad Sci U S A 2000;97(25):13625–30.
46. Seo BM, Miura M, Gronthos S, et al. Investigation of multipotent postnatal stem cells from human periodontal ligament. Lancet 2004;364(9429):149–55.
47. Seo BM, Miura M, Sonoyama W, et al. Recovery of stem cells from cryopreserved periodontal ligament. J Dent Res 2005;84(10):907–12.
48. Lin NH, Menicanin D, Mrozik K, et al. Putative stem cells in regenerating human periodontium. J Periodontal Res 2008;43(5):514–23.
49. Du L, Yang P, Ge S. Stromal cell-derived factor-1 significantly induces proliferation, migration, and collagen type I expression in a human periodontal ligament stem cell subpopulation. J Periodontol 2012;83(3):379–88.
50. Feng F, Akiyama K, Liu Y, et al. Utility of PDL progenitors for in vivo tissue regeneration: a report of 3 cases. Oral Dis 2010;16(1):20–8.

Dental Stem Cells and Their Sources

Christine M. Sedgley, MDS, MDSc, FRACDS, MRACDS(ENDO), PhD[a],*,
Tatiana M. Botero, DDS, MS[b]

KEYWORDS

- Dental pulp stem cells (DPSCs)
- Stem cells from human exfoliated deciduous teeth (SHED cells)
- Stem cells from root apical papilla (SCAP cells)
- Periodontal ligament stem cells (PDLSCs) • Dental follicle precursor cells (DFPCs)

KEY POINTS

- The search for more accessible mesenchymal stem cells than those found in bone marrow has propelled interest in dental tissues, which are rich sources of stem cells. Human dental stem/progenitor cells (collectively termed dental stem cells [DSCs]) that have been isolated and characterized include dental pulp stem cells, stem cells from exfoliated deciduous teeth, stem cells from apical papilla, periodontal ligament stem cells, and dental follicle progenitor cells.
- The common characteristics of these cell populations are the capacity for self-renewal and the ability to differentiate into multiple lineages (multipotency). In vitro and animal studies have shown that DSCs can differentiate into osseous, odontogenic, adipose, endothelial, and neural-like tissues.
- In recent studies, third molar dental pulp somatic cells have been reprogrammed to become induced pluripotent stem cells, and dental pulp pluripotentlike stem cells have been isolated from the pulps of third molar teeth.

INTRODUCTION

The aim of regenerative medicine and tissue engineering is to replace or regenerate human cells, tissue or organs, to restore or establish normal function.[1] The 3 key elements for tissue engineering are stem cells, scaffolds, and growth factors. Cell-based therapies are integral components of regenerative medicine that exploit the

The authors have nothing to disclose.
[a] Department of Endodontology, School of Dentistry, Oregon Health and Science University, 611 Southwest Campus Drive, Portland, OR 97239, USA; [b] Cariology, Restorative Sciences and Endodontics, School of Dentistry, University of Michigan, 1011 North University, Room 1376D, Ann Arbor, MI 48108-1078, USA
* Corresponding author.
E-mail address: sedgley@ohsu.edu

Dent Clin N Am 56 (2012) 549–561
http://dx.doi.org/10.1016/j.cden.2012.05.004
0011-8532/12/$ – see front matter © 2012 Elsevier Inc. All rights reserved.

dental.theclinics.com

inherent ability of stem cells to differentiate into specific cell types. The extension of basic stem cell science into translational therapies is already well established with artificial skin therapies,[2] whereas research is ongoing for cell-based therapies to target other diseases, including diabetes,[2] atherosclerosis,[3] and neurodegenerative diseases.[4] The search for more accessible mesenchymal stem cells (MSCs) than those found in bone marrow has propelled interest in dental tissues, which are rich sources of stem cells. This article provides an overview of stems cells and then focuses on dental stem cells (DSCs) and how recent developments have the potential to greatly impact the way DSCs might be used in future regenerative medicine applications that include regenerative endodontic therapies.

STEM CELLS
General Characteristics

Stem cells are undifferentiated embryonic or adult cells that continuously divide. A fundamental property of stem cells is self-renewal or the ability to go through numerous cycles of cell division while maintaining the undifferentiated state (**Box 1**). In addition, stem cells produce intermediate cell types (called progenitor or precursor cells) that have the capacity to differentiate into different cell types and generate complex tissues and organs.[5] Differentiation occurs when a stem cell acquires the features of a specialized cell (eg, odontoblast).

Stem cells can be either embryonic or adult (postnatal). Thomson and colleagues[6] first reported human embryonic stem cell lines in 1998. Embryonic stem cells are isolated from the blastocyst during embryonic development and give rise to the 3 primary germ layers: ectoderm, endoderm, and mesoderm. These cells are totipotent or pluripotent with an unlimited capacity to differentiate and can develop into each of the more than 200 cell types of the adult body (**Box 2**).

Adult stem cells exist throughout the body in different tissues, including bone marrow, brain, blood vessels, liver, skin, retina, pancreas, peripheral blood, muscle, adipose tissue, and dental tissues. They are localized to specific niches where the regulation of stem cell proliferation, survival, migration, fate, and aging occur.[5,7] Whether cells undergo either prolonged self-renewal or differentiation depends on intrinsic signals modulated by extrinsic factors in the stem cell niche.[8] An adult stem cell can divide and create another cell like itself, and also a cell more differentiated than itself, but the capacity for differentiation into other cell types is limited. This capability is described as being multipotent and is a distinguishing feature of adult stem cells compared with the pluripotency of embryonic stem cells. Although early research suggested that adult stem cells were limited in the types of tissues they produced, it is increasingly apparent that adult stem cells have greater plasticity than previously thought and can generate a tissue different to the site from which they were originally isolated.[9,10] An example with potential clinical applications is the ability of dental pulp cells to generate heart tissue in rats.[11]

Box 1	
Fundamental properties of stem cells	
Undifferentiated cells	Have not developed into a specialized cell type
Long-term self-renewal	The ability to go through numerous cycles of cell division while maintaining the undifferentiated state
Production of progenitor cells	Capacity to differentiate into specialized cell types (eg, odontoblast, osteoblast, adipocyte, fibroblast)

Box 2		
Stem cell potency		
Embryonic stem cells from inner cell mass of 3- to 5-day embryo (blastocyst)	Totipotent	Can give rise to all the cell types of the body, including those cells making the extraembryonic tissues (eg, placenta) Unlimited capacity to divide
Embryonic stem cells Induced pluripotent stem cells	Pluripotent	Can form derivatives of all the embryonic germ layers (ectoderm, mesoderm, and endoderm) from a single cell Can give rise to all of the various cell types of the body
Adult stem cells (postnatal)	Multipotent	Can give rise to more than one cell type of the body
Induced pluripotent stem cells	Pluripotent	Derived from somatic cells

MSCs

In 1963, hematopoietic stem cells giving rise to blood cells were identified in bone marrow.[12] Since then, it has been established that bone marrow is also the primary source for multipotent MSCs.[13] Bone marrow MSCs (BMMSCs) can differentiate into osteogenic, chondrogenic, adipogenic, myogenic, and neurogenic lineages. MSCs are found in many other tissues in the body, including umbilical cord blood, adipose tissue, adult muscle, and dental tissues[13]; are capable of differentiating into at least 3 cell lineages: osteogenic, chondrogenic, and adipogenic[14]; and can also differentiate into other lineages, such as odontogenic, when grown in a defined micro-environment in vitro.[13,14]

Definitive information on the location and distribution of MSCs is still being eluci-dated. However, it has been shown that MSCs can be found around blood vessel walls and perineurium as demonstrated by the immuno-colocalization of STRO-1/CD146 stem cell markers.[15] These observations have led to the proposal that MSCs arise from a perivascular stem cell niche[15,16] that provides an environment allowing the cells to retain their stemness.[14,17] Crisan and colleagues[15] demonstrated that human peri-vascular cells from diverse and multiple human tissues give rise to multi-lineage progenitor cells that exhibit the features of MSCs. Perivascular progenitor/stem cells can also proliferate in response to odontoblast injury by cavity preparation under ex vivo tooth culture conditions.[18]

Isolation, Identification, and Differentiation of MSCs

A fundamental approach to isolate MSCs in tissue samples involves the enzymatic digestion of tissue followed by the growth of isolated cells (expansion) in medium rich in growth factors.[19,20] The isolation of more immature stem cells involves a multi-step explant approach whereby pieces of tissue are first cultured until progenitor cells grow after which enzymatic digestion and expansion in media proceed.[7,21]

The identification of MSCs uses a series of in vitro tests. Colony-forming assays are used to confirm clonogenicity (the ability to generate identical stem cells with the appropriate cell morphology), which is a consistent characteristic of MSCs. Pheno-typic assays evaluate cell morphology or shape (eg, fibroblastic when flat and elon-gated) and cell behavior (eg, secretory). The possession of one or several cell surface markers found on cells in representative tissues is evaluated by flow cytome-try, which sorts cells with specific surface protein, such as STRO-1, found on stem cells that can differentiate into multiple mesenchymal lineages, including dental pulp cells (**Fig. 1**C, F, I).[14,22] DSCs can also express specific proteins associated with endothelium (CD106, CD146), perivascular tissues (α-smooth muscle actin, CD146, 3G5), bone, dentin and cementum (bone morphogenic protein [BMP], alkaline phosphatase, osteonectin, osteopontin, and bone sialoprotein), and fibroblasts (type I and III collagen).[23,24]

In vitro functional assays test putative MSCs for multipotency by confirming that differentiated cells demonstrate the appropriate phenotypic characteristics. Accordingly, the in vitro confirmation of the multipotency of dental pulp stem cells (DPSCs) can be demonstrated by the evidence of odontoblastlike differentiation (verified by the deposition of mineralized matrix and positive staining for dentin sialophosphoprotein), adipogenic differentiation (by the accumulation of lipid vacuoles), chondrogenic differentiation (by the production of collagen type II), and neurogenic differentiation (by neuronal-cell morphologies and markers).[25–31]

In vivo functional assays are used to confirm that stem cells implanted into a new environment (eg, immunodeficient mice) successfully integrate with adjacent cells, survive, and function as differentiated cells.[32] Several studies have demonstrated the formation of new pulp and dentinlike tissues following the insertion of DSCs

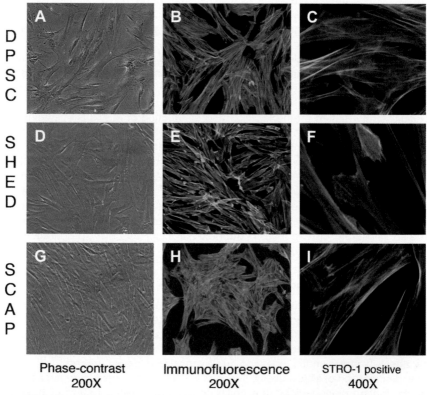

Fig. 1. Microphotographs showing morphology of stem cells in culture: DPSCs (*A*), SHED cells (*D*), and SCAP cells (*G*) (phase contrast, original magnification ×200). Microphotographs for cytoskeleton labeled for actin-F (*green fluorescent dye*), nuclei with DAPI (*blue fluorescent dye*), and STRO-1 positive cells (*red fluorescent dye*) for DPSCs (*B, C*), SHED cells (*E, F*), and SCAP cells (*H, I*) ([*B, E, H*] immunofluorescence, original magnification ×200; [*C, F, I*] STRO-1 positive, original magnification ×400). DPSC, dental pulp stem cells; SCAP, stem cells from apical papilla; SHED, stem cells from human exfoliated deciduous teeth.

seeded onto scaffolds in emptied human root canals or dentin disks embedded into immunocompromised mice; the resulting dentinogenesis is accomplished by odonto-blastlike cells derived from MSCs.[16,23,27,28,31–34]

Storage of Stem Cells

Adult stem cells can be obtained from individuals at any stage in life and, therefore, can provide a source of cells for autologous transplants.[35] Such procedures invariably require stem cell storage, which is achieved by cryopreservation in liquid nitrogen (−196°C). Stem cells can survive these low temperatures as long as they are dispersed in cryprotectants.[36,37] Human periodontal ligament stem cells (PDLSCs) have been successfully recovered after cryopreservation for 6 months; although the number of colonies was less than for fresh PDLSCs, the proliferation rate was similar.[37] Similarly, stem cells isolated from human third molar teeth and cryopreserved for at least 1 month retained STRO-1 marker expression and the potential to proliferate into neurogenic, adipogenic, osteogenic/odontogenic, myogenic, and chondrogenic pathways in inductive media.[36] Cryopreservation of intact teeth provides another potential storage method that can allow later extraction of stem cells demonstrating similar behavior as stem cells extracted from fresh teeth.[38,39]

DSCs

A tooth develops as a result of carefully orchestrated interactions between the oral epithelial ectodermal cells that form the enamel organ (for enamel formation) and cranial neural crest–derived mesenchymal cells that form the dental papilla and dental follicle. These MSCs give rise to the other components of the tooth: dentin, pulp, cementum, and periodontal ligament. Beginning in 2000,[23] several human dental stem/progenitor cells have been isolated and characterized (**Box 3**). These cells include human DPSCs from permanent teeth (see **Fig. 1A–C**),[23] stem cells from exfoliated deciduous teeth (SHED cells) (see **Fig. 1D–F**),[25] stem cells from apical papilla (SCAP cells) (see **Fig. 1G–I**),[27] PDLSCs,[40] and dental follicle precursor, or progenitor, cells (DFPCs).[41] Although MSCs from different DSCs form distinct populations,[24] among their common characteristics are the capacity for self-renewal and the ability to differentiate into at least 3 distinct lineages.[14,24] The regeneration/revascularization of pulpal tissues uses DSCs in partnership with growth factors, scaffolds, and vascular supply.[32,42,43]

DPSCs

DPSCs were first isolated from human permanent third molars in 2000.[23] The cells were characterized as clonogenic and highly proliferative. Colony formation frequency was high and produced densely calcified, albeit sporadic, nodules.[23] Dentin and pulplike tissues were generated following the transplantation of DPSCs in

Box 3	
Dental stem cells	
DFPCs	Dental follicle precursor cells
DPPSCs	Dental pulp pluripotentlike stem cells
DPSCs	Dental pulp stem cells
DSCs	Dental stem cells
PDLSCs	Periodontal ligament stem cells
PDLPs	Periodontal ligament progenitor cells
SCAP cells	Stem cells from apical papilla
SHED cells	Stem cells from human exfoliated deciduous teeth

hydroxyapatite/tricalcium phosphate (HA/TCP) scaffolds into immunodeficient mice.[23,24] A follow-up study confirmed that DPSCs fulfilled the criteria needed to be stem cells: an ability to differentiate into adipocytes and neural cells and odontoblasts (ie, multipotency) and self-renewal capabilities.[31] Additional studies have confirmed that DPSCs can also differentiate into osteoblast-, chondrocyte-, and myoblastlike cells and demonstrate axon guidance.[10,44–46]

It is now recognized that DSCs can play an important role in the balance of inflammation and repair/dentinogenesis during invasive caries lesions or pulp exposures.[47,48] Following odontoblast damage after caries or trauma, markers of inflammation and regeneration within the pulp tissue are differentially expressed,[47,49,50] with crosstalk between the inflammatory and regenerative processes considered to determine the outcome.[51] This notion is supported by in vitro observations of DPSCs migrating from the perivasculature toward the dentin surface following injury to the dentin matrix and differentiating into functional odontoblasts in response to EphB/ephrin signaling.[52,53] DPSCs have also been shown to express the bacterial recognition toll-like receptors, TLR4 and TLR2, and vascular endothelial growth factor in response to lipopolysaccharide, a product of gram-negative bacteria.[20,48,54] When compared with normal pulps, DPSCs in inflamed pulp tissues have reduced dentinogenesis activity,[55] and an in vitro investigation has shown reduced dentinogenic potential of DPSCs exposed to a high bacterial load that can be recovered after the inhibition of the bacterial recognition toll-like receptor TLR2.[48] Taken together, these studies support the existence of interactions between DSCs and immune cells in pulps affected by dental caries,[47] a better understanding of which has significant implications for the future management of teeth affected by dental caries.

In an effort to determine the fate of DPSCs exposed to root canal irrigants used in regenerative endodontic therapy procedures, dentin disks were preconditioned with different irrigants (5.25% sodium hypochlorite [NaOCl] or 17% ethylenediaminetetraacetic acid [EDTA]), seeded with DPSCs, and implanted subcutaneously into immunodeficient mice.[56] After 6 weeks, the differentiation of DPSCs into odontoblastlike cells was facilitated by the use of EDTA. In contrast, the use of NaOCl resulted in resorption lacunae at the cell-dentin interface.

SHED Cells

SHED cells are highly proliferative stem cells isolated from exfoliated deciduous teeth capable of differentiating into a variety of cell types, including osteoblasts, neural cells, adipocytes, and odontoblasts, and inducing dentin and bone formation.[25] Like DPSCs, SHED cells can generate dentin-pulplike tissues with distinct odontoblastlike cells lining the mineralized dentin-matrix generated in HA/TCP scaffolds implanted in immunodeficient mice.[24] However, SHED cells have a higher proliferation rate than DPSCs and BMMSCs, suggesting that they represent a more immature population of multipotent stem cells.[25,33,57] SHED cells have shown different gene expression profiles from DPSCs and BMMSCs; genes related to cell proliferation and extracellular matrix formation, such as transforming growth factor (TGF)-β, fibroblast growth factor (FGF)2, TGF-β2, collagen (Col) I, and Col III, are more highly expressed in SHED cells compared with DPSCs.[57]

In tissue engineering studies, odontoblastic and endothelial differentiation occurred when SHED cells were seeded in tooth slices/scaffold and implanted subcutaneously into immunodeficient mice.[33,34] The resultant tissues closely resembled those of human dental pulp, and tubular dentin mediated by dentin-derived BMP-2 protein was secreted.[33,58] These findings, together with those of other studies, suggest that SHED cells from exfoliated deciduous teeth may be an excellent resource for stem cell therapies, including autologous stem cell transplantation and tissue engineering.[7,25]

Regenerative endodontic therapy procedures should avoid compromising the attachment of stem cells to dentin. An in vitro study showed that the root canal irrigants 6% NaOCl and 2% chlorhexidine (CHX) were cytotoxic to SHED cells. In addition, the attachment of SHED cells to root canal dentin pretreated with NaOCl or CHX was reduced compared with negative controls (saline pretreatment).[59]

SCAP Cells

SCAP cells are found in the apical papilla located at the apices of developing teeth at the junction of the apical papilla and dental pulp.[27,60,61] The apical papilla is essential for root development. SCAP cells were first isolated in human root apical papilla collected from extracted human third molars.[27] The cells are clonogenic and can undergo odontoblastic/osteogenic, adipogenic, or neurogenic differentiation. Compared with DPSCs, SCAP cells show higher proliferation rates and greater expression of CD24, which is lost as SCAP cells differentiate and increase alkaline phosphate expression.[27,60,62]

SCAP cells seeded onto synthetic scaffolds consisting of poly-D,L-lactide/glycolide inserted into tooth fragments, and transplanted into immunodeficient mice, induced a pulplike tissue with well-established vascularity, and a continuous layer of dentinlike tissue was deposited onto the canal dentinal wall.[32] In a minipig, a bio-root was created by using autologous human SCAP cells seeded in an HA/TCP root-shaped carrier coated with Gelfoam (Pharmacia Canada Inc., Ontario, Canada) carrying PDLSCs that were implanted in the alveolar socket of a recent extracted anterior tooth.[27] After 4 months, the resulting bio-root was capable of supporting a porcelain crown and participating in normal tooth function.[27]

Root canal irrigants used in regenerative endodontic therapy procedures should ideally support cell survival, or at least not compromise survival. An in vitro study showed that 17% EDTA used alone supported SCAP cell survival better (89% survival) than when used with either 6% NaOCl (74% survival) or 2% CHX (0% survival).[63]

PDLSCs

McCulloch[64] reported the presence of progenitor/stem cells in the periodontal ligament of mice in 1985. Subsequently, the isolation and identification of multipotent MSCs in human periodontal ligaments were first reported in 2004.[40] Seo and colleagues[40] demonstrated the presence of clonogenic stem cells in enzymatically digested PDL and further showed that human PDLSCs transplanted into immunodeficient rodents generated a cementum/PDL-like structure that contributed to periodontal tissue repair. Later work showed that PDLSCs differentiation was promoted by Hertwig's epithelial root sheath cells in vitro.[65]

PDLSCs have the capability to differentiate into cementoblastlike cells, adipocytes, and fibroblasts that secrete collagen type I.[66] As with BMMSCs, PDLSCs can undergo osteogenic, adipogenic, and chondrogenic differentiation.[67] PDLSCs have also been shown to differentiate into neuronal precursors.[68] A recent retrospective pilot study showed evidence of the therapeutic potential of autologous periodontal ligament progenitor cells obtained from third molar teeth implanted on bone grafting material into intrabony defects in 2 patients.[69] After 32 to 70 months, a marked improvement was found in all sites. The progenitor cells behaved like PDLSCs, although they did not express the same markers.[69]

DFPCs

The dental follicle forms at the cap stage by ectomesenchymal progenitor cells. It is a loose vascular connective tissue that contains the developing tooth germ, and progenitors for periodontal ligament cells, cementoblasts, and osteoblasts. DFPCs were first isolated from the dental follicle of human third molars.[41]

Because DFPCs come from developing tissue, it is considered that they might exhibit a greater plasticity than other DSCs.[70] Indeed, different cloned DFPC lines have demonstrated great heterogeneity.[71] In addition, after transplantation in immunodeficient rodents, DFPCs differentiated into cementoblastlike[72,73] and osteogeniclike[74] cells, and surface markers compatible with those of fibroblasts were identified in human dental follicle tissues, suggesting the presence of immature PDL fibroblasts.[75] DFPCs were able to differentiate into odontoblasts in vitro, and four weeks after combining rat DFPCs with treated dentin matrix the root-like tissues stained positive for markers of dental pulp.[26,76] Both DFPCs and SHED cells can differentiate into neural cells; however, these are differentially expressed when the cells are grown under the same culture conditions.[77]

Induced Pluripotent Stem Cells and Dental Pulp Pluripotentlike Stem Cells

In breakthrough studies in 2006 and 2007, investigators described methods to reprogram somatic cells from mice,[78] and subsequently humans,[79,80] by the insertion of 4 genes (OCT3/4, SOX2, KLF4, and MYC) that reprogrammed the somatic cells and returned them to an embryolike state. The resultant induced pluripotent stem (iPS) cells have embryonic stem cell characteristics: they are capable of generating cells from each of the 3 embryonic germ layers and can propagate in culture indefinitely. The pluripotency of human stem cells can be tested in vitro by the aggregation and generation of embryoid bodies from cultured cells[81] and in vivo by teratoma formation after cells are injected subcutaneously into immunodeficient mice.[82] The use of MYC is now avoided because it might induce malignant tumor formation and, therefore, would be contraindicated for clinical application.[83]

Recent reports have described successful attempts to develop pluripotent stem cells from pulps recovered from deciduous teeth[7] and from third molar pulps.[84,85] Indeed, deriving iPS cells from deciduous teeth DPSCs was reported to be easier and more efficient compared with human fibroblasts.[7] Oda and colleagues[84] reported successfully reprogramming mesenchymal stromal cells derived from the pulps of young human third molars (obtained from patients aged 10, 13, and 16 years) by retroviral transduction of the transcription factors OCT3/4, SOX2, and KLF4. The resultant cells had high iPS clonal efficiency suggesting a potential role for dental pulp stromal cells in regenerative medicine. A recent report describes the isolation of dental pulp pluripotentlike stem cells (DPPSCs) from the pulps of human third molar pulp tissue obtained from 20 patients of different genders and ages ranging from 14 to 60 years.[85] When the cells were injected into nude mice, teratomalike structures developed that contained tissues derived from all 3 embryonic germ layers. Significantly, the investigators noted that even in older patients, there was always a population of DPPSCs present.[85]

Although iPS cells are not truly equal to embryonic stem cells,[86] and may even have a memory of the somatic tissue from which they were derived,[87] they have generated great interest for their many potential personalized regenerative therapeutic applications.[88] For example, disease-causing mutations could be repaired by reprogramming. Another potential application is to use iPS cells derived from patients with diseases for drug development and in vitro disease modeling.[89,90]

SUMMARY

The ready availability of DSCs makes them a viable source of adult MSCs for regenerative medicine applications. Human dental stem/progenitor cells that have been isolated and characterized include DPSCs, SHED cells, SCAP cells, PDLSCs, and DFPCs. Although much work is required for the translation of data from in vitro and animal studies to viable clinical applications, there are exciting possibilities for the use of DPSCs in tissue engineering and regenerative medicine applications within the root canal, the oral cavity, and in other parts of the body. Finally, the relative ease with which DSCs can be obtained, coupled with interest in stem cell banking,[91,92] will likely drive research that further elucidates their characteristics and potential applications.

REFERENCES

1. Dunnill P, Mason C. A brief definition of regenerative medicine. Regen Med 2008; 3:1–5.
2. Russ HA, Efrat S. Development of human insulin-producing cells for cell therapy of diabetes. Pediatr Endocrinol Rev 2011;9:590–7.
3. Goldschmidt-Clermont PJ, Dong C, Seo DM, et al. Atherosclerosis, inflammation, genetics, and stem cells: 2012 update. Curr Atheroscler Rep 2012;14(3):201–10.
4. Lunn JS, Sakowski SA, Hur J, et al. Stem cell technology for neurodegenerative diseases. Ann Neurol 2011;70:353–61.
5. Fuchs E, Segre JA. Stem cells: a new lease on life. Cell 2000;100:143–55.
6. Thomson JA, Itskovitz-Eldor J, Shapiro SS, et al. Embryonic stem cell lines derived from human blastocysts. Science 1998;282:1145–7.
7. Kerkis I, Caplan AI. Stem cells in dental pulp of deciduous teeth. Tissue Eng Part B Rev 2012;18:129–38.
8. Morrison SJ, Shah NM, Anderson DJ. Regulatory mechanisms in stem cell biology. Cell 1997;88:287–98.
9. Arthur A, Rychkov G, Shi S, et al. Adult human dental pulp stem cells differentiate toward functionally active neurons under appropriate environmental cues. Stem Cells 2008;26:1787–95.
10. Arthur A, Shi S, Zannettino AC, et al. Implanted adult human dental pulp stem cells induce endogenous axon guidance. Stem Cells 2009;27:2229–37.
11. Gandia C, Arminan A, Garcia-Verdugo JM, et al. Human dental pulp stem cells improve left ventricular function, induce angiogenesis, and reduce infarct size in rats with acute myocardial infarction. Stem Cells 2008;26:638–45.
12. Becker AJ, Mc CE, Till JE. Cytological demonstration of the clonal nature of spleen colonies derived from transplanted mouse marrow cells. Nature 1963;197:452–4.
13. Caplan AI. Mesenchymal stem cells. J Orthop Res 1991;9:641–50.
14. Huang GT, Gronthos S, Shi S. Mesenchymal stem cells derived from dental tissues vs. those from other sources: their biology and role in regenerative medicine. J Dent Res 2009;88:792–806.
15. Crisan M, Yap S, Casteilla L, et al. A perivascular origin for mesenchymal stem cells in multiple human organs. Cell Stem Cell 2008;3:301–13.
16. Shi S, Gronthos S. Perivascular niche of postnatal mesenchymal stem cells in human bone marrow and dental pulp. J Bone Miner Res 2003;18:696–704.
17. Schofield R. The relationship between the spleen colony-forming cell and the haemopoietic stem cell. Blood Cells 1978;4:7–25.
18. Tecles O, Laurent P, Zygouritsas S, et al. Activation of human dental pulp progenitor/stem cells in response to odontoblast injury. Arch Oral Biol 2005; 50:103–8.
19. Vemuri MC, Chase LG, Rao MS. Mesenchymal stem cell assays and applications. Methods Mol Biol 2011;698:3–8.

20. Beyer Nardi N, da Silva Meirelles L. Mesenchymal stem cells: isolation, in vitro expansion and characterization. Handb Exp Pharmacol 2006;(174):249–82.
21. Bakopoulou A, Leyhausen G, Volk J, et al. Assessment of the impact of two different isolation methods on the osteo/odontogenic differentiation potential of human dental stem cells derived from deciduous teeth. Calcif Tissue Int 2011; 88:130–41.
22. Lin NH, Gronthos S, Bartold PM. Stem cells and periodontal regeneration. Aust Dent J 2008;53:108–21.
23. Gronthos S, Mankani M, Brahim J, et al. Postnatal human dental pulp stem cells (DPSCs) in vitro and in vivo. Proc Natl Acad Sci U S A 2000;97:13625–30.
24. Shi S, Bartold PM, Miura M, et al. The efficacy of mesenchymal stem cells to regenerate and repair dental structures. Orthod Craniofac Res 2005;8:191–9.
25. Miura M, Gronthos S, Zhao M, et al. SHED: stem cells from human exfoliated deciduous teeth. Proc Natl Acad Sci U S A 2003;100:5807–12.
26. Guo W, Gong K, Shi H, et al. Dental follicle cells and treated dentin matrix scaffold for tissue engineering the tooth root. Biomaterials 2012;33:1291–302.
27. Sonoyama W, Liu Y, Fang D, et al. Mesenchymal stem cell-mediated functional tooth regeneration in swine. PLoS One 2006;1:e79.
28. Kim JK, Shukla R, Casagrande L, et al. Differentiating dental pulp cells via RGD-dendrimer conjugates. J Dent Res 2010;89:1433–8.
29. Alge DL, Zhou D, Adams LL, et al. Donor-matched comparison of dental pulp stem cells and bone marrow-derived mesenchymal stem cells in a rat model. J Tissue Eng Regen Med 2010;4:73–81.
30. Dissanayaka WL, Zhan X, Zhang C, et al. Coculture of dental pulp stem cells with endothelial cells enhances osteo-/odontogenic and angiogenic potential in vitro. J Endod 2012;38:454–63.
31. Gronthos S, Brahim J, Li W, et al. Stem cell properties of human dental pulp stem cells. J Dent Res 2002;81:531–5.
32. Huang GT, Yamaza T, Shea LD, et al. Stem/progenitor cell-mediated de novo regeneration of dental pulp with newly deposited continuous layer of dentin in an in vivo model. Tissue Eng Part A 2010;16:605–15.
33. Sakai VT, Zhang Z, Dong Z, et al. SHED differentiate into functional odontoblasts and endothelium. J Dent Res 2010;89:791–6.
34. Cordeiro MM, Dong Z, Kaneko T, et al. Dental pulp tissue engineering with stem cells from exfoliated deciduous teeth. J Endod 2008;34:962–9.
35. Mimeault M, Batra SK. Great promise of tissue-resident adult stem/progenitor cells in transplantation and cancer therapies. Adv Exp Med Biol 2012;741:171–86.
36. Zhang W, Walboomers XF, Shi S, et al. Multilineage differentiation potential of stem cells derived from human dental pulp after cryopreservation. Tissue Eng 2006;12:2813–23.
37. Seo BM, Miura M, Sonoyama W, et al. Recovery of stem cells from cryopreserved periodontal ligament. J Dent Res 2005;84:907–12.
38. Chen YK, Huang AH, Chan AW, et al. Human dental pulp stem cells derived from different cryopreservation methods of human dental pulp tissues of diseased teeth. J Oral Pathol Med 2011;40:793–800.
39. Lee SY, Chiang PC, Tsai YH, et al. Effects of cryopreservation of intact teeth on the isolated dental pulp stem cells. J Endod 2010;36:1336–40.
40. Seo BM, Miura M, Gronthos S, et al. Investigation of multipotent postnatal stem cells from human periodontal ligament. Lancet 2004;364:149–55.
41. Morsczeck C, Gotz W, Schierholz J, et al. Isolation of precursor cells (PCs) from human dental follicle of wisdom teeth. Matrix Biol 2005;24:155–65.

42. Srisuwan T, Tilkorn DJ, Al-Benna S, et al. Revascularization and tissue regeneration of an empty root canal space is enhanced by a direct blood supply and stem cells. Dent Traumatol 2012. http://dx.doi.org/10.1111/j.600–9657.2012.01136.x.

43. Hargreaves KM, Giesler T, Henry M, et al. Regeneration potential of the young permanent tooth: what does the future hold? J Endod 2008;34:S51–6.

44. Yu J, He H, Tang C, et al. Differentiation potential of STRO-1+ dental pulp stem cells changes during cell passaging. BMC Cell Biol 2010;11:32.

45. Zhang W, Walboomers XF, Van Kuppevelt TH, et al. In vivo evaluation of human dental pulp stem cells differentiated towards multiple lineages. J Tissue Eng Regen Med 2008;2:117–25.

46. About I, Bottero MJ, de Denato P, et al. Human dentin production in vitro. Exp Cell Res 2000;258:33–41.

47. Leprince JG, Zeitlin BD, Tolar M, et al. Interactions between immune system and mesenchymal stem cells in dental pulp and periapical tissues. Int Endod J 2012. http://dx.doi.org/10.1111/j.365-2591.012.02028.x.

48. Yamagishi VT, Torneck CD, Friedman S, et al. Blockade of TLR2 inhibits Porphyromonas gingivalis suppression of mineralized matrix formation by human dental pulp stem cells. J Endod 2011;37:812–8.

49. Cooper PR, Takahashi Y, Graham LW, et al. Inflammation-regeneration interplay in the dentine-pulp complex. J Dent (Tehran) 2010;38:687–97.

50. McLachlan JL, Smith AJ, Sloan AJ, et al. Gene expression analysis in cells of the dentine-pulp complex in healthy and carious teeth. Arch Oral Biol 2003;48:273–83.

51. Simon SR, Berdal A, Cooper PR, et al. Dentin-pulp complex regeneration: from lab to clinic. Adv Dent Res 2011;23:340–5.

52. Arthur A, Koblar S, Shi S, et al. Eph/ephrinB mediate dental pulp stem cell mobilization and function. J Dent Res 2009;88:829–34.

53. Mathieu S, El-Battari A, Dejou J, et al. Role of injured endothelial cells in the recruitment of human pulp cells. Arch Oral Biol 2005;50:109–13.

54. Rosa V, Botero TM, Nor JE. Regenerative endodontics in light of the stem cell paradigm. Int Dent J 2011;61(Suppl 1):23–8.

55. Alongi DJ, Yamaza T, Song Y, et al. Stem/progenitor cells from inflamed human dental pulp retain tissue regeneration potential. Regen Med 2010;5:617–31.

56. Galler KM, D'Souza RN, Federlin M, et al. Dentin conditioning codetermines cell fate in regenerative endodontics. J Endod 2011;37:1536–41.

57. Nakamura S, Yamada Y, Katagiri W, et al. Stem cell proliferation pathways comparison between human exfoliated deciduous teeth and dental pulp stem cells by gene expression profile from promising dental pulp. J Endod 2009;35:1536–42.

58. Casagrande L, Demarco FF, Zhang Z, et al. Dentin-derived BMP-2 and odontoblast differentiation. J Dent Res 2010;89:603–8.

59. Ring KC, Murray PE, Namerow KN, et al. The comparison of the effect of endodontic irrigation on cell adherence to root canal dentin. J Endod 2008;34:1474–9.

60. Huang GT, Sonoyama W, Liu Y, et al. The hidden treasure in apical papilla: the potential role in pulp/dentin regeneration and bioroot engineering. J Endod 2008;34:645–51.

61. Sonoyama W, Liu Y, Yamaza T, et al. Characterization of the apical papilla and its residing stem cells from human immature permanent teeth: a pilot study. J Endod 2008;34:166–71.

62. Bakopoulou A, Leyhausen G, Volk J, et al. Comparative analysis of in vitro osteo/odontogenic differentiation potential of human dental pulp stem cells (DPSCs) and stem cells from the apical papilla (SCAP). Arch Oral Biol 2011;56:709–21.

63. Trevino EG, Patwardhan AN, Henry MA, et al. Effect of irrigants on the survival of human stem cells of the apical papilla in a platelet-rich plasma scaffold in human root tips. J Endod 2011;37:1109–15.

64. McCulloch CA. Progenitor cell populations in the periodontal ligament of mice. Anat Rec 1985;211:258–62.

65. Sonoyama W, Seo BM, Yamaza T, et al. Human Hertwig's epithelial root sheath cells play crucial roles in cementum formation. J Dent Res 2007;86:594–9.

66. Gronthos S, Mrozik K, Shi S, et al. Ovine periodontal ligament stem cells: isolation, characterization, and differentiation potential. Calcif Tissue Int 2006;79:310–7.

67. Gay IC, Chen S, MacDougall M. Isolation and characterization of multipotent human periodontal ligament stem cells. Orthod Craniofac Res 2007;10:149–60.

68. Techawattanawisal W, Nakahama K, Komaki M, et al. Isolation of multipotent stem cells from adult rat periodontal ligament by neurosphere-forming culture system. Biochem Biophys Res Commun 2007;357:917–23.

69. Feng F, Akiyama K, Liu Y, et al. Utility of PDL progenitors for in vivo tissue regeneration: a report of 3 cases. Oral Dis 2010;16:20–8.

70. Volponi AA, Pang Y, Sharpe PT. Stem cell-based biological tooth repair and regeneration. Trends Cell Biol 2010;20:715–22.

71. Luan X, Ito Y, Dangaria S, et al. Dental follicle progenitor cell heterogeneity in the developing mouse periodontium. Stem Cells Dev 2006;15:595–608.

72. Handa K, Saito M, Tsunoda A, et al. Progenitor cells from dental follicle are able to form cementum matrix in vivo. Connect Tissue Res 2002;43:406–8.

73. Handa K, Saito M, Yamauchi M, et al. Cementum matrix formation in vivo by cultured dental follicle cells. Bone 2002;31:606–11.

74. Honda MJ, Imaizumi M, Suzuki H, et al. Stem cells isolated from human dental follicles have osteogenic potential. Oral Surg Oral Med Oral Pathol Oral Radiol Endod 2011;111:700–8.

75. Angiero F, Rossi C, Ferri A, et al. Stromal phenotype of dental follicle stem cells. Front Biosci (Elite Ed) 2012;4:1009–14.

76. Guo W, He Y, Zhang X, et al. The use of dentin matrix scaffold and dental follicle cells for dentin regeneration. Biomaterials 2009;30:6708–23.

77. Morsczeck C, Vollner F, Saugspier M, et al. Comparison of human dental follicle cells (DFCs) and stem cells from human exfoliated deciduous teeth (SHED) after neural differentiation in vitro. Clin Oral Investig 2010;14:433–40.

78. Takahashi K, Yamanaka S. Induction of pluripotent stem cells from mouse embryonic and adult fibroblast cultures by defined factors. Cell 2006;126:663–76.

79. Takahashi K, Tanabe K, Ohnuki M, et al. Induction of pluripotent stem cells from adult human fibroblasts by defined factors. Cell 2007;131:861–72.

80. Yu J, Vodyanik MA, Smuga-Otto K, et al. Induced pluripotent stem cell lines derived from human somatic cells. Science 2007;318:1917–20.

81. O'Connor MD, Kardel MD, Iosfina I, et al. Alkaline phosphatase-positive colony formation is a sensitive, specific, and quantitative indicator of undifferentiated human embryonic stem cells. Stem Cells 2008;26:1109–16.

82. O'Connor MD, Kardel MD, Eaves CJ. Functional assays for human embryonic stem cell pluripotency. Methods Mol Biol 2011;690:67–80.

83. Okita K, Ichisaka T, Yamanaka S. Generation of germline-competent induced pluripotent stem cells. Nature 2007;448:313–7.

84. Oda Y, Yoshimura Y, Ohnishi H, et al. Induction of pluripotent stem cells from human third molar mesenchymal stromal cells. J Biol Chem 2010;285:29270–8.

85. Atari M, Gil-Recio C, Fabregat M, et al. Dental pulp of the third molar: a new source of pluripotent-like stem cells. J Cell Sci 2012. http://dx.doi.org/10.1242/jcs.096537.
86. Hussein SM, Batada NN, Vuoristo S, et al. Copy number variation and selection during reprogramming to pluripotency. Nature 2011;471:58–62.
87. Kim K, Doi A, Wen B, et al. Epigenetic memory in induced pluripotent stem cells. Nature 2010;467:285–90.
88. Robinton DA, Daley GQ. The promise of induced pluripotent stem cells in research and therapy. Nature 2012;481:295–305.
89. Park IH, Arora N, Huo H, et al. Disease-specific induced pluripotent stem cells. Cell 2008;134:877–86.
90. Itzhaki I, Maizels L, Huber I, et al. Modelling the long QT syndrome with induced pluripotent stem cells. Nature 2011;471:225–9.
91. Stephens N, Atkinson P, Glasner P. Documenting the doable and doing the documented: bridging strategies at the UK Stem Cell Bank. Soc Stud Sci 2011;41:791–813.
92. Huang YH, Yang JC, Wang CW, et al. Dental stem cells and tooth banking for regenerative medicine. J Exp Clin Med 2010;2:111–7.

Effects of Growth Factors on Dental Stem/Progenitor Cells

Sahng G. Kim, DDS, MS[a,b], Jian Zhou, DDS, PhD[a],
Charles Solomon, DDS[b], Ying Zheng, DDS, PhD[a],
Takahiro Suzuki, DDS, PhD[a], Mo Chen, PhD[a], Songhee Song, DDS[a],
Nan Jiang, DDS[a], Shoko Cho, PhD[a], Jeremy J. Mao, DDS, PhD[a,*]

KEYWORDS

- Growth factors • Dentin • Dental pulp • Dental pulp cells • Regeneration • Repair

KEY POINTS

- The goal of regenerative endodontics is to regain the vitality and functions of dental pulp–dentin complex. Dental pulp is the only vascularized tissue in mature, functional teeth in humans, and maintains homeostasis of the dentin.
- Current root canal therapy ends up with a devitalized tooth, therefore predisposing endodontically treated teeth to reinfections and fractures. Recent work showing regeneration of dental pulp-dentin–like tissues by cell homing that is orchestrated by growth factor delivery, without cell transplantation, provides one of the tangible pathways toward clinical translation.
- Growth factors regulate either transplanted cells or endogenously homed cells in dental pulp–dentin regeneration. Further understanding of the actions of growth factors is pivotal for dental pulp–dentin regeneration.

INTRODUCTION

Regenerative endodontics aims to restore the vitality and functions of the pulp–dentin complex that has been lost to trauma or infections (**Table 1**). Several recent reports have shown that dental pulp–like tissues can regenerate in vivo following the delivery of dental or nondental stem/progenitor cells.[1–3] An alternative approach is to orchestrate dental pulp–dentin regeneration by the homing of host endogenous cells relies on growth factor delivery, instead of cell delivery.[4] Regardless of cell transplantation or

Funding: The work for composition of this article is supported by NIH grants R01DE018248, R01EB009663 and RC2DE020767 (to J.J.M.).
Conflict of interest: Columbia University is the owner of patents for several regenerative endodontic agents and methods on behalf of Dr Jeremy Mao's laboratory.
[a] Center for Craniofacial Regeneration, Columbia University, 630 West 168 Street, PH7E, New York, NY 10032, USA; [b] Division of Endodontics, College of Dental Medicine, Columbia University, 630 West 168 Street, PH7Stem #128, New York, NY 10032, USA
* Corresponding author.
E-mail address: jmao@columbia.edu

Table 1
Primary effects and interactions of signaling molecules for regenerative endodontics

Signaling Molecules	Target Cells	Primary Effects	Interactions
Growth Factors			
PDGF	Dental pulp cells	Cell proliferation[22,25,26]	Combined with IGF-1 or dexamethasone, increased cell proliferation[22]
		Dentin matrix synthesis[22,25,26]	Combined with PDGF, increased cell proliferation[25]
		Odontoblastic differentiation[24]	
		Dentinogenesis	
TGFβ1	Dental pulp cells	Cell proliferation[40]	
		Extracellular matrix synthesis[40]	
		Odontoblastic differentiation[41]	
		Dentinogenesis[42]	
	Dental pulp stem cells	Chemotaxis[43]	Combined with FGF2, increased odontoblastic differentiation[41]
BMP2	Dental pulp cells	Odontoblastic differentiation[51–55]	
		Dentinogenesis[54–56]	
BMP4	Dental pulp cells	Odontoblastic differentiation[55]	
		Dentinogenesis[54–56]	
BMP7 (OP-1)	Dental pulp cells	Dentinogenesis[5,57–60]	
BMP11 (GDF11)	Dental pulp stem cells	Odontoblastic differentiation[61,62]	
		Dentinogenesis[61,62]	
VEGF	Dental pulp stem cells	Odontoblastic differentiation[67]	Under osteogenic conditions, increased osteogenic differentiation[68]
		Cell proliferation[68]	
FGF2 (bFGF)	Dental pulp stem cells	Chemotaxis[7]	Combined with TGFβ1, increased odontoblastic differentiation[41]
		Cell proliferation[41]	
	Dental pulp cells	Cell proliferation[76–78]	
		Dentinogenesis[76–78]	
IGF	Dental pulp cells	Cell proliferation[84]	Combined with PDGF, increased cell proliferation[25]
		Odontoblastic differentiation[84]	
NGF	Dental papilla cells	Odontoblastic differentiation[92]	
Cytokine			
SDF-1	Dental pulp cells (CD31⁻/CD146⁻ SP cells)	Chemotaxis[97,98]	
		Cell proliferation[97,98]	

cell homing approaches in dental pulp regeneration, a multitude of growth factors has been shown to have effects on dental pulp cells.[5–7]

The dental pulp is a unique, specialized loose connective tissue that contains mainly interstitial fibroblasts in a cell-rich zone in the center of the pulp[8] and odontoblasts that align dentin surface in the periphery (the odontoblast layer).[9] Stem/progenitor cells reside among interstitial fibroblasts and, perhaps, adjacent to blood vessels.[10] When dental pulp cells are isolated and studied in vitro, some of the mononucleated and adherent cells, but certainly not all and not even the majority, have stem/progenitor cell properties including clonogenicity, self-renewal, and multipotentiality.[11] Clonogenicity refers to the ability of a single cell to yield a progeny. Self-renewal refers to the ability of cells to multiply themselves, with the offspring cells possessing the same properties as the parent cells. Multipotentiality is the capacity of a cell to differentiate into multiple, dissimilar cell lineages.[12,13]

Fundamental to our understanding of regenerative endodontics is the knowledge of growth factors that affect a broad range of cellular activities including migration, proliferation, differentiation, and apoptosis of all dental pulp cells, including stem/progenitor cells (**Fig. 1**). Growth factors and cytokines may act as signaling molecules that modulate cell behavior by mediating intracellular communication. Growth factors are polypeptides or proteins that bind to specific receptors on the surface of target

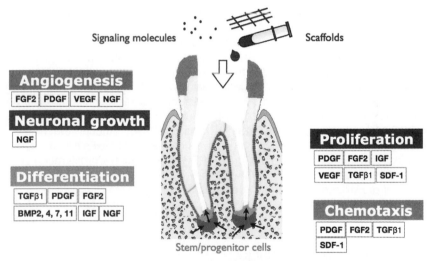

Fig. 1. Signaling molecules: hypothetical mechanisms of action and pulp-dentin complex regeneration. If the injury extends to the entire pulp tissue and no vital pulp tissue remains, the cells residing near the root apex of a tooth serve as a source of cells. Bioactive cues that recruit the proper cells will be critical in pulp regeneration. Examples of the signaling molecules that play a role in cell mobilization and homing include PDGF,[17,18] TGFβ,[43] bFGF,[7] and SDF-1.[94–98] The recruited stem/progenitor cells proliferate in the area of injury and differentiate into a specific cell phenotype to replace the damaged cells. The replacement cells are stimulated to produce extracellular matrix that is essential for tissue to function biologically. These events of repair and regeneration can be coordinated and modulated by growth factors such as PDGF,[22,24–26] TGF,[40,41] BMP,[5,51–62] VEGF,[68] FGF,[41,76–78] and IGF.[84–87] Angiogenesis and neuronal growth also can be stimulated by growth factors such as FGF2, PDGF, VEGF and NGF. Angiogenesis is stimulated by growth factors such as FGF2[75] PDGF,[19,20] VEGF,[66] and the survival and growth of neuron is regulated by NGF.[91] These signaling molecules are exemplary and not meant to be exclusive.

cells.[14] Growth factors can initiate a cascade of intracellular signaling, and act in either an autocrine or paracrine manner.[15] Cytokines are typically referred to as immuno-modulatory proteins or polypeptides.[16] Cytokines are often used interchangeably with growth factors because many cytokines share similar actions with growth factors. As opposed to systemic effects by hormones on target cells, growth factors or cyto-kines typically act locally on target cells. This review first discusses the effects of various growth factors on dental pulp cells, and then explores how some of the growth factors may participate in dental pulp–dentin regeneration.

PLATELET-DERIVED GROWTH FACTOR

Platelet-derived growth factor (PDGF) is released by platelets, and has potency in promoting angiogenesis and cell proliferation.[17–22] PDGF has 4 isoform homodimers AA, BB, CC, and DD, in addition to a heterodimer, PDGF-AB. PDGF dimers bind to 2 cell-surface receptors known as PDGFRα and PDGFRβ.[23] The receptors form dimers before binding to different isoforms of PDGF. PDGF-AA, -BB, and -CC bind to PDGFR α/α, whereas PDGF-AB, -BB, -CC, and -DD bind to PDGFR α/β.[23] PDGF-BB and -DD bind to PDGFR β/β.[23] Therefore, the biological effect of PDGF depends on the expression level of PDGFR dimer on target cells.

The chemotaxis and proliferation of mesenchymal stem/progenitor cells can be induced by PDGF in the injury site. In trauma, hemorrhage is followed by blood-clot formation in dental pulp. Platelets in the blood clot release α-granules containing PDGFs and attract neutrophils and macrophages.[18] These cells play key roles in early wound healing by producing other signaling molecules for the formation of granulation tissues. However, PDGFs appear to have little effect on the formation of the dentinlike nodule in dental pulp cells isolated from rat lower incisors, although PDGF-AB and -BB isoforms stimulate the expression of dentin sialoprotein (DSP).[24] PDGFs stimulate cell proliferation and dentin matrix protein synthesis, but appear to inhibit alkaline phos-phatase (ALP) activity in dental pulp cells in culture.[22,25,26] DSP expression is inhibited by PDGF-AA but is enhanced by PDGF-AB and PDGF-BB, although the mineralized tissue formation is inhibited, suggesting diverging effects of PDGFs on odontoblastic differentiation depending on dimeric form.[24] PDGFs enhance the proliferation of fibro-blasts in human dental pulp.[22] PDGF-BB may increase the expression of vascular endothelial growth factor (VEGF) in osteoblasts and promotes angiogenesis at the site of dental pulp injury.[20] In vivo, PDGF promotes de novo formation of dental pulp–like tissues in endodontically treated human teeth that are implanted in rats.[4]

TRANSFORMING GROWTH FACTOR β

The transforming growth factor β (TGFβ) family comprises a group of diverse growth factors including TGFβ, bone morphogenetic proteins (BMPs), growth/differentiation factors (GDFs), anti-Mullerian hormone (AMH), activin, and nodal.[27–30] TGFβ is composed of approximately 390 amino acids, which are released mainly from plate-lets, macrophages, and bone.[30] This inactive polypeptide undergoes proteolytic cleavage to create the active C-terminal 112-amino-acid form. The active form of TGFβ dimerizes to form 25-kDa homodimers.[31] The 3 isoforms present in mammals, TGFβ1, TGFβ2, and TGFβ3, are detected in human dentin.[32] Inactive TGFβ exists as a large latent complex.[33] After proteolytic cleavage, the active TGFβ binds to the type II receptor (TGFβRII) and recruits type I receptor (TGFβRI) to dimerize. TGFβRI, in turn, phosphorylates the intracellular proteins SMAD (homologues of Drosophila proteins including Caenorhabditis elegans protein [SMA] and mothers against decapentaplegic

[MAD]), in particular, SMAD2 and SMAD3.[34,35] The activated SMAD complex translocates to the nucleus and activates downstream TGFβ gene transcription.

The effect of TGFβ is highly variable and dependent on the type of cells and tissues. TGFβ1 regulates a wide range of cellular activities, such as cell migration, cell proliferation, cell differentiation, and extracellular matrix synthesis.[36–40] TGFβ1has been shown to increase cell proliferation and production of the extracellular matrix in dental pulp tissue culture,[40] and promotes odontoblastic differentiation of dental pulp cells.[41] The effect of TGFβ1 can be synergistically upregulated by fibroblast growth factor 2 (FGF2), as evidenced by the increased ALP activity, the formation of mineralized nodule, and the expression of DSP and dentin matrix protein 1.[41] The dentinogenic ability of dental pulp cells in the mechanically exposed dental pulp of dog teeth is shown to be induced by exogenous TGFβ1.[42] TGFβ is chemotactic on dental pulp cells in vitro.[43] TGFβ1 also plays an important role in the immune response during dental pulp injury.[44,45]

BONE MORPHOGENETIC PROTEIN

BMPs comprise a subgroup of the TGFβ superfamily and are involved in many biological activities including cell proliferation, differentiation, and apoptosis.[46] BMPs have strong osteoinductive and chondrogenic effects. BMP2 was discovered by Urist,[47] who showed ectopic bone formation in connective tissues by transplanted dimineralized bone. Later some of BMPs were identified, purified and sequenced from proteins extracted from bone.[48] To date, more than 20 BMPs have been identified and characterized, among which GDFs are included.[46] Unlike TGFβ, BMPs are secreted as an active form of 30- to 38-kDa homodimers after proteolytic cleavage of a synthesized form composed of 400 to 525 amino acids.[46] Two TGFβ receptors (type I and type II) are known to be involved in the BMP signaling pathway.[46] The activity of BMPs is regulated by the antagonists of BMPs such as noggin and chordin.[49] This modulation of BMP activity by the BMP antagonists may have a critical role in tooth development.[50]

BMP2, BMP4, BMP7. and BMP11 are of clinical significance because of their role in inducing mineralization.[5,51–62] Human recombinant BMP2 stimulates the differentiation of dental pulp cells into odontoblasts,[51] inducing mRNA expression of dentin sialophosphoproteins (DSPPs) and higher ALP activity on BMP2 application, but has no effect on cell proliferation. DSPP expression and odontoblastic differentiation are regulated likely via BMP2-induced signaling by nuclear transcription factor Y.[52] BMP2 also stimulates the differentiation of dental pulp stem/progenitor cells into odontoblasts in vivo and in vitro.[53] Human recombinant BMP2 or BMP4 induces dentin formation when used in capping materials over amputated canine pulp.[54,55] Osteodentin formation occurs in amputated canine pulps treated with BMPs in collagen matrix.[56] Bovine dental pulp cells treated with BMP2 and BMP4 differentiate into preodontoblasts.[55] BMP7, also known as osteogenic protein 1, promotes dentin formation when placed over amputated dental pulp in macaque teeth.[57,58] The dentinogenic effect of BMP7 on amputated dental pulp has been shown in several animal models including rats,[59] ferrets,[5] and miniature swine.[60] Dental pulp cells transfected with BMP11, also known as GDF11, yields mineralization.[61] Dentin matrix protein 1, ALP, DSPP, enamelysin, and phosphate-regulating gene are highly expressed in BMP11-transfected cells.[61] Transplantation of BMP11-transfected cell pellets induces formation of dentinlike tissue on amputated dental pulp in dogs.[61] Ultrasound-mediated gene delivery of BMP11 stimulates odontoblastic differentiation of dental pulp stem/progenitor cells in vitro and reparative dentin formation in vivo.[62]

VASCULAR ENDOTHELIAL GROWTH FACTOR

VEGF is a heparin-binding protein with specific affinity to endothelial cells, and plays a key role in angiogenesis.[63] The functions of VEGF involve the proliferation of endothelial cells and their enhanced survival,[64] stimulating neovascularization in the area of injury. The VEGF family includes VEGF-A, VEGF-B, VEGF-C, VEGF-D, and placenta growth factor.[65] Among these isoforms, VEGF-A is the most versatile in function. VEGF-A, also known as vascular permeability factor, promotes cell migration, cell proliferation, vasodilatation, and vascular permeability by binding to 2 tyrosine kinases receptors, VEGFR1 and VEGFR2.[65] VEGF increases microvessel density of the dental pulp when tooth slices containing severed dental pulp were treated with VEGF and implanted into subcutaneous tissues of severely combined immunodeficiency (SCID) mice.[66]

VEGF appears to induce the differentiation of human dental pulp cells into endothelial cells.[67] Dental pulp cells become positive for CD29, CD44, CD73, CD105, and CD166, but negative for CD14, CD34, and CD45 after VEGF treatment.[67] VEGF increases the expression of VEGFR1 (fms-like tyrosine kinase, Flt-1) and VEGFR2 (kinase-insert domain containing receptor, KDR) and microvessel formation in a 3-dimensional fibrin mesh seeded with dental pulp cells.[67] However, VEGF treatment does not appear to promote CD31, CD34, and CD144 positivity in dental pulp cells that are positive for CD29, CD90, CD105, CD166, CD146, and STRO-1.[68] Of note, VEGF increases the proliferation and osteogenic differentiation of dental pulp cells under osteogenic conditions, suggesting a possible stimulatory role of VEGF in osteogenesis.[68]

FIBROBLAST GROWTH FACTOR

Fibroblast growth factor (FGF) plays key roles in cell migration, proliferation, and differentiation during embryonic development[69] and wound healing.[70] To date 22 members have been identified in humans,[71] of which FGF2 appears to be significant in regeneration of the pulp–dentin complex. Four FGF receptors, FGFR1 through FGFR4, are expressed in humans.[72] Signal transduction is mediated by interaction between FGFs with the ability to bind to heparan sulfate and heparan sulfate proteoglycans on cell surface.[73] FGF2 is a basic FGF, whereas FGF1 is acidic. FGF2 regulates tooth morphogenesis by controlling cell proliferation and differentiation.[74] FGF2 is a potent angiogenic factor that stimulates formation of new blood vessels in the dental pulp[75] along with PDGF[19,20] and VEGF.[66] Given its role in cell proliferation and angiogenesis, FGF2 acts as an early stimulating factor in formation of granulation tissue during wound healing.[75]

FGF2 induces the migration of dental pulp cells.[7] Using a transwell migration assay, significantly more dental pulp cells are recruited by basic FGF (FGF2) into a 3-dimensional collagen gel than compared with controls without cytokines and BMP7.[7] FGF2 also stimulates the proliferation of dental pulp cells without differentiation, whereas FGF2 combined with TGFβ1 induces differentiation of dental pulp cells into odontoblast-like cells, and synergistically upregulates the effect of TGFβ1 on odontoblast differentiation.[41] The FGF2 on exposed dental pulp in rat molars induces vascular invasion and cell proliferation early in wound healing.[76–78] Also, FGF2 stimulates reparative dentin formation or dentin particles in the exposed pulp.[76–78]

INSULIN-LIKE GROWTH FACTOR

Insulin-like growth factors (IGFs) are single-chain polypeptides that have high sequence similarity to proinsulin.[79] IGFs, comprising IGF-1 and IGF-2, contribute to odontogenesis and dental tissue repair by cell proliferation and differentiation.[80] There are 2 known IGF receptors, of which IGF-1R has tyrosine kinase activity that phosphorylates the insulin receptor substrates and activates MAP kinase and the phosphatidylinositol-3-kinase (PI3K) cascades.[81] However, IGF-2R has no intrinsic kinase activity. IGF-1R binds to both isoforms of IGFs, but IGF-2R binds only to IGF-2.[82,83]

Of the 2 isoforms, IGF-1, also known as somatomedin C, has potency in growth and differentiation of dental pulp cells.[84] IGF-1 induces proliferation and differentiation of dog dental pulp cells into odontoblast-like cells in serum-free medium.[84] IGF-1 with PDGF-BB has a synergistic effect on the proliferation of dental pulp cells in vitro.[25] IGF-1 and IGF-1R have a higher level of expression in dental pulp tissue from teeth with complete root development than from teeth with incomplete root formation, suggesting that IGF-1 stimulates mineralization and cell differentiation.[85–87]

NERVE GROWTH FACTOR

Nerve growth factors (NGFs), also known as neutrophins, promote the survival and maintenance of sympathetic and sensory neurons. NGFs bind to 2 receptors, a p75 low-affinity neutrophin receptor (p75 LANR) and a high-affinity tyrosine kinase receptor (trk).[88] NGFs are involved in the survival and differentiation of neuronal and nonneuronal cells through high-affinity trkA, but NGFs regulates apoptosis through p75 LANR.[89] The expression of NGF and p75 LANR increases in dental pulp cells at the injury site.[90] NGFs play a role in regulating tooth morphogenesis and tooth innervation in rat tooth development.[91] NGFs induce the differentiation of immortalized dental papilla cells into odontoblasts in vitro, suggesting that NGF acts as a stimulant for mineralization.[92]

STROMAL CELL–DERIVED FACTOR 1

Stromal cell–derived factor 1 (SDF-1), also known as chemokine (C-X-C motif) ligand 12 (CXCL12), is a chemoattractant involved in cell mobilization and homing by binding to the chemokine receptor CXCR4.[93] SDF-1 functions as a chemokine for hematopoietic stem cells,[94] mesenchymal stromal cells,[95] and immune cells.[96] SDF-1 stimulates the migration and proliferation of CD31$^-$/CD146$^-$ side population (SP) cells isolated from porcine tooth germ that are positive for CXCR4 and negative for hematopoietic markers.[97] Furthermore, the CD31$^-$/CD146$^-$ SP cells have strong migration and proliferation activity with localized SDF-1 expression in amputated canine dental pulp.[98] Dental pulp–like tissue with capillaries and nerves regenerate in dog teeth following pulp extirpation and autologous transplantation of the CD31$^-$/CD146$^-$ SP cells or CD105$^+$ cells with SDF-1 into root canals.[99]

DENTAL PULP–DENTIN REGENERATION BY CELL HOMING

Previous work on dental pulp–dentin regeneration has followed typical approaches of tissue engineering by delivering cells in biomaterial scaffolds. Moreover, previous work has typically relied on tooth slices or fragments for in vivo implantation.[100–102] In a recent study, a cell-homing approach was used to regenerate the pulp–dentin complex by the delivery of growth factors rather than cells in entire human teeth following root canal treatment.[4] Several growth factors, including FGF2, VEGF, NGF, PDGF, and BMP7, were delivered singularly or in combination into root canal spaces of endodontically treated human teeth (without gutta percha filling).[4] Basic FGF was chosen for chemotaxis and angiogenesis; VEGF for chemotaxis, mitogenesis, and angiogenesis; PDGF for angiogenesis; NGF for survival and growth of nerve fibers; and BMP-7 for mineralized tissue formation. Dental pulp-dentin–like tissues regenerated with new blood vessels, representing the first study showing that dental pulp-dentin–like tissues can regenerate without cell transplantation.[4] The cell-homing approach for dental pulp–dentin regeneration by using multiple growth factors may accelerate clinical translation (see **Fig. 1**).

SUMMARY

The goal of regenerative endodontics is to regain the vitality and functions of the dental pulp–dentin complex. Dental pulp is the only vascularized tissue in mature, functional teeth in humans, and maintains homeostasis of the dentin. Current root canal therapy ends up with a devitalized tooth, therefore predisposing endodontically treated teeth to reinfections and fractures. Recent work showing regeneration of dental pulp-dentin–like tissues by cell homing that is orchestrated by growth factor delivery, without cell transplantation, provides one of the tangible pathways toward clinical translation. Growth factors regulate either transplanted cells or endogenously homed cells in dental pulp–dentin regeneration. Further understanding of the actions of growth factors is pivotal for dental pulp–dentin regeneration.

ACKNOWLEDGMENTS

The authors thank F. Guo and J. Melendez for technical and administrative assistance.

REFERENCES

1. Huang GT, Yamaza T, Shea LD, et al. Stem/progenitor cell-mediated de novo regeneration of dental pulp with newly deposited continuous layer of dentin in an in vivo model. Tissue Eng Part A 2010;16(2):605–15.
2. Cordeiro MM, Dong Z, Kaneko T, et al. Dental pulp tissue engineering with stem cells from exfoliated deciduous teeth. J Endod 2008;34(8):962–9.
3. Ishizaka R, Iohara K, Murakami M, et al. Regeneration of dental pulp following pulpectomy by fractionated stem/progenitor cells from bone marrow and adipose tissue. Biomaterials 2012;33(7):2109–18.
4. Kim JY, Xin X, Moioli EK, et al. Regeneration of dental-pulp-like tissue by chemotaxis-induced cell homing. Tissue Eng Part A 2010;16(10):3023–31.
5. Rutherford RB, Gu K. Treatment of inflamed ferret dental pulps with recombinant bone morphogenetic protein-7. Eur J Oral Sci 2000;108(3):202–6.
6. Jiang L, Zhu YQ, Du R, et al. The expression and role of stromal cell-derived factor-1alpha-CXCR4 axis in human dental pulp. J Endod 2008;34(8):939–44.
7. Suzuki T, Lee CH, Chen M, et al. Induced migration of dental pulp stem cells for in vivo pulp regeneration. J Dent Res 2011;90(8):1013–8.
8. Jo YY, Lee HJ, Kook SY, et al. Isolation and characterization of postnatal stem cells from human dental tissues. Tissue Eng 2007;13(4):767–73.
9. Goldberg M, Smith AJ. Cells and extracellular matrices of dentin and pulp: a biological basis for repair and tissue engineering. Crit Rev Oral Biol Med 2004; 15(1):13–27.
10. Feng J, Mantesso A, De Bari C, et al. Dual origin of mesenchymal stem cells contributing to organ growth and repair. Proc Natl Acad Sci U S A 2011; 108(16):6503–8.
11. Kajstura J, Rota M, Hall SR, et al. Evidence for human lung stem cells. N Engl J Med 2011;364(19):1795–806.

12. Gronthos S, Brahim J, Li W, et al. Stem cell properties of human dental pulp stem cells. J Dent Res 2002;81(8):531–5.
13. Ruch JV. Patterned distribution of differentiating dental cells: facts and hypotheses. J Biol Buccale 1990;18(2):91–8.
14. Lind M. Growth factors: possible new clinical tools. A review. Acta Orthop Scand 1996;67(4):407–17.
15. Lázár-Molnár E, Hegyesi H, Tóth S, et al. Autocrine and paracrine regulation by cytokines and growth factors in melanoma. Cytokine 2000;12(6):547–54.
16. Nicholas C, Lesinski GB. Immunomodulatory cytokines as therapeutic agents for melanoma. Immunotherapy 2011;3(5):673–90.
17. Seppä H, Grotendorst G, Seppä S, et al. Platelet-derived growth factor in chemotactic for fibroblasts. J Cell Biol 1982;92(2):584–8.
18. Deuel TF, Senior RM, Huang JS, et al. Chemotaxis of monocytes and neutrophils to platelet-derived growth factor. J Clin Invest 1982;69(4):1046–9.
19. Hellberg C, Ostman A, Heldin CH. PDGF and vessel maturation. Recent Results Cancer Res 2010;180:103–14.
20. Bouletreau PJ, Warren SM, Spector JA, et al. Factors in the fracture microenvironment induce primary osteoblast angiogenic cytokine production. Plast Reconstr Surg 2002;110(1):139–48.
21. Heldin CH, Westermark B. Mechanism of action and in vivo role of platelet-derived growth factor. Physiol Rev 1999;79(4):1283–316.
22. Rutherford RB, Trail Smith MD, Ryan MF, et al. Synergistic effects of dexamethasone on platelet-derived growth factor mitogenesis in vitro. Arch Oral Biol 1992;37(2):139–45.
23. Alvarez RH, Kantarjian HM, Cortes JE. Biology of platelet-derived growth factor and its involvement in disease. Mayo Clin Proc 2006;81(9):1241–57.
24. Yokose S, Kadokura H, Tajima N, et al. Platelet-derived growth factor exerts disparate effects on odontoblast differentiation depending on the dimers in rat dental pulp cells. Cell Tissue Res 2004;315(3):375–84.
25. Denholm IA, Moule AJ, Bartold PM. The behaviour and proliferation of human dental pulp cell strains in vitro, and their response to the application of platelet-derived growth factor-BB and insulin-like growth factor-1. Int Endod J 1998;31(4):251–8.
26. Nakashima M. The effects of growth factors on DNA synthesis, proteoglycan synthesis and alkaline phosphatase activity in bovine dental pulp cells. Arch Oral Biol 1992;37(3):231–6.
27. Watabe T, Miyazono K. Roles of TGF-beta family signaling in stem cell renewal and differentiation. Cell Res 2009;19(1):103–15.
28. Burt DW, Law AS. Evolution of the transforming growth factor-beta superfamily. Prog Growth Factor Res 1994;5(1):99–118.
29. Kingsley DM. The TGF-beta superfamily: new members, new receptors, and new genetic tests of function in different organisms. Genes Dev 1994;8(2):133–46.
30. Wahl SM. Transforming growth factor beta (TGF-beta) in inflammation: a cause and a cure. J Clin Immunol 1992;12(2):61–74.
31. Derynck R, Jarrett JA, Chen EY, et al. Human transforming growth factor-beta complementary DNA sequence and expression in normal and transformed cells. Nature 1985;316(6030):701–5.
32. Cassidy N, Fahey M, Prime SS, et al. Comparative analysis of transforming growth factor-beta isoforms 1-3 in human and rabbit dentine matrices. Arch Oral Biol 1997;42(3):219–23.

33. Javelaud D, Mauviel A. Mammalian transforming growth factor-betas: Smad signaling and physio-pathological roles. Int J Biochem Cell Biol 2004;36(7):1161–5.
34. Lan HY, Chung AC. Transforming growth factor-β and Smads. Contrib Nephrol 2011;170:75–82.
35. Gold LI, Sung JJ, Siebert JW, et al. Type I (RI) and type II (RII) receptors for transforming growth factor-beta isoforms are expressed subsequent to transforming growth factor-beta ligands during excisional wound repair. Am J Pathol 1997;150(1):209–22.
36. Lambert KE, Huang H, Mythreye K, et al. The type III transforming growth factor-β receptor inhibits proliferation, migration, and adhesion in human myeloma cells. Mol Biol Cell 2011;22(9):1463–72.
37. Verrecchia F, Mauviel A. Transforming growth factor-beta signaling through the Smad pathway: role in extracellular matrix gene expression and regulation. J Invest Dermatol 2002;118(2):211–5.
38. Massagué J, Blain SW, Lo RS. TGFbeta signaling in growth control, cancer, and heritable disorders. Cell 2000;103(2):295–309.
39. Moses HL, Serra R. Regulation of differentiation by TGF-beta. Curr Opin Genet Dev 1996;6(5):581–6.
40. Melin M, Joffre-Romeas A, Farges JC, et al. Effects of TGFbeta1 on dental pulp cells in cultured human tooth slices. J Dent Res 2000;79(9):1689–96.
41. He H, Yu J, Liu Y, et al. Effects of FGF2 and TGFbeta1 on the differentiation of human dental pulp stem cells in vitro. Cell Biol Int 2008;32(7):827–34.
42. Tziafas D, Papadimitriou S. Role of exogenous TGF-beta in induction of reparative dentinogenesis in vivo. Eur J Oral Sci 1998;106(Suppl 1):192–6.
43. Howard C, Murray PE, Namerow KN. Dental pulp stem cell migration. J Endod 2010;36(12):1963–6.
44. Wahl SM. TGF-beta in the evolution and resolution of inflammatory and immune processes. Introduction. Microbes Infect 1999;1(15):1247–9.
45. Farges JC, Romeas A, Melin M, et al. TGF-beta1 induces accumulation of dendritic cells in the odontoblast layer. J Dent Res 2003;82(8):652–6.
46. Chen D, Zhao M, Mundy GR. Bone morphogenetic proteins. Growth Factors 2004;22(4):233–41.
47. Urist MR. Bone: formation by autoinduction. Science 1965;150(3698):893–9.
48. Wozney JM, Rosen V, Celeste AJ, et al. Novel regulators of bone formation: molecular clones and activities. Science 1988;242(4885):1528–34.
49. Gazzerro E, Canalis E. Bone morphogenetic proteins and their antagonists. Rev Endocr Metab Disord 2006;7(1–2):51–65.
50. Hu X, Wang Y, He F, et al. Noggin is required for early development of murine upper incisors. J Dent Res 2012;91(4):394–400.
51. Saito T, Ogawa M, Hata Y, et al. Acceleration effect of human recombinant bone morphogenetic protein-2 on differentiation of human pulp cells into odontoblasts. J Endod 2004;30(4):205–8.
52. Chen S, Gluhak-Heinrich J, Martinez M, et al. Bone morphogenetic protein 2 mediates dentin sialophosphoprotein expression and odontoblast differentiation via NF-Y signaling. J Biol Chem 2008;283(28):19359–70.
53. Iohara K, Nakashima M, Ito M, et al. Dentin regeneration by dental pulp stem cell therapy with recombinant human bone morphogenetic protein 2. J Dent Res 2004;83(8):590–5.
54. Nakashima M. Induction of dentin formation on canine amputated pulp by recombinant human bone morphogenetic proteins (BMP)-2 and -4. J Dent Res 1994;73(9):1515–22.

55. Nakashima M, Nagasawa H, Yamada Y, et al. Regulatory role of transforming growth factor-beta, bone morphogenetic protein-2, and protein-4 on gene expression of extracellular matrix proteins and differentiation of dental pulp cells. Dev Biol 1994;162(1):18–28.
56. Nakashima M. Induction of dentine in amputated pulp of dogs by recombinant human bone morphogenetic proteins-2 and -4 with collagen matrix. Arch Oral Biol 1994;39(12):1085–9.
57. Rutherford RB, Spångberg L, Tucker M, et al. The time-course of the induction of reparative dentine formation in monkeys by recombinant human osteogenic protein-1. Arch Oral Biol 1994;39(10):833–8.
58. Rutherford RB, Wahle J, Tucker M, et al. Induction of reparative dentine formation in monkeys by recombinant human osteogenic protein-1. Arch Oral Biol 1993;38(7):571–6.
59. Six N, Lasfargues JJ, Goldberg M. Differential repair responses in the coronal and radicular areas of the exposed rat molar pulp induced by recombinant human bone morphogenetic protein 7 (osteogenic protein 1). Arch Oral Biol 2002;47(3):177–87.
60. Jepsen S, Albers HK, Fleiner B, et al. Recombinant human osteogenic protein-1 induces dentin formation: an experimental study in miniature swine. J Endod 1997;23(6):378–82.
61. Nakashima M, Iohara K, Ishikawa M, et al. Stimulation of reparative dentin formation by ex vivo gene therapy using dental pulp stem cells electrotransfected with growth/differentiation factor 11 (Gdf11). Hum Gene Ther 2004; 15(11):1045–53.
62. Nakashima M, Tachibana K, Iohara K, et al. Induction of reparative dentin formation by ultrasound-mediated gene delivery of growth/differentiation factor 11. Hum Gene Ther 2003;14(6):591–7.
63. Leung DW, Cachianes G, Kuang WJ, et al. Vascular endothelial growth factor is a secreted angiogenic mitogen. Science 1989;246(4935):1306–9.
64. Nör JE, Christensen J, Mooney DJ, et al. Vascular endothelial growth factor (VEGF)-mediated angiogenesis is associated with enhanced endothelial cell survival and induction of Bcl-2 expression. Am J Pathol 1999;154(2):375–84.
65. Ferrara N. Vascular endothelial growth factor: basic science and clinical progress. Endocr Rev 2004;25(4):581–611.
66. Mullane EM, Dong Z, Sedgley CM, et al. Effects of VEGF and FGF2 on the revascularization of severed human dental pulps. J Dent Res 2008;87(12):1144–8.
67. Marchionni C, Bonsi L, Alviano F, et al. Angiogenic potential of human dental pulp stromal (stem) cells. Int J Immunopathol Pharmacol 2009;22(3):699–706.
68. D'Alimonte I, Nargi E, Mastrangelo F, et al. Vascular endothelial growth factor enhances in vitro proliferation and osteogenic differentiation of human dental pulp stem cells. J Biol Regul Homeost Agents 2011;25(1):57–69.
69. Metzger RJ, Krasnow MA. Genetic control of branching morphogenesis. Science 1999;284(5420):1635–9.
70. DiMario J, Buffinger N, Yamada S, et al. Fibroblast growth factor in the extracellular matrix of dystrophic (mdx) mouse muscle. Science 1989;244(4905):688–90.
71. Itoh N, Ornitz DM. Fibroblast growth factors: from molecular evolution to roles in development, metabolism and disease. J Biochem 2011;149(2):121–30.
72. Walsh S, Jefferiss C, Stewart K, et al. Expression of the developmental markers STRO-1 and alkaline phosphatase in cultures of human marrow stromal cells: regulation by fibroblast growth factor (FGF)-2 and relationship to the expression of FGF receptors 1-4. Bone 2000;27(2):185–95.

73. Brown KJ, Hendry IA, Parish CR. Acidic and basic fibroblast growth factor bind with differing affinity to the same heparan sulfate proteoglycan on BALB/c 3T3 cells: implications for potentiation of growth factor action by heparin. J Cell Biochem 1995;58(1):6–14.

74. Tsuboi T, Mizutani S, Nakano M, et al. Fgf-2 regulates enamel and dentine formation in mouse tooth germ. Calcif Tissue Int 2003;73(5):496–501.

75. Tran-Hung L, Mathieu S, About I. Role of human pulp fibroblasts in angiogenesis. J Dent Res 2006;85(9):819–23.

76. Kitamura C, Nishihara T, Terashita M, et al. Local regeneration of dentin-pulp complex using controlled release of fgf-2 and naturally derived sponge-like scaffolds. Int J Dent 2012;2012:190561.

77. Ishimatsu H, Kitamura C, Morotomi T, et al. Formation of dentinal bridge on surface of regenerated dental pulp in dentin defects by controlled release of fibroblast growth factor-2 from gelatin hydrogels. J Endod 2009;35(6):858–65.

78. Kikuchi N, Kitamura C, Morotomi T, et al. Formation of dentin-like particles in dentin defects above exposed pulp by controlled release of fibroblast growth factor 2 from gelatin hydrogels. J Endod 2007;33(10):1198–202.

79. Humbel RE. Insulin-like growth factors I and II. Eur J Biochem 1990;190(3):445–62.

80. Joseph BK, Savage NW, Young WG, et al. Expression and regulation of insulin-like growth factor-I in the rat incisor. Growth Factors 1993;8(4):267–75.

81. Melmed S, Yamashita S, Yamasaki H, et al. IGF-I receptor signalling: lessons from the somatotroph. Recent Prog Horm Res 1996;51:189–215 [discussion: 215–6].

82. Siddle K, Ursø B, Niesler CA, et al. Specificity in ligand binding and intracellular signalling by insulin and insulin-like growth factor receptors. Biochem Soc Trans 2001;29(Pt 4):513–25.

83. Braulke T. Type-2 IGF receptor: a multi-ligand binding protein. Horm Metab Res 1999;31(2–3):242–6.

84. Onishi T, Kinoshita S, Shintani S, et al. Stimulation of proliferation and differentiation of dog dental pulp cells in serum-free culture medium by insulin-like growth factor. Arch Oral Biol 1999;44(4):361–71.

85. Caviedes-Bucheli J, Canales-Sánchez P, Castrillón-Sarria N, et al. Expression of insulin-like growth factor-1 and proliferating cell nuclear antigen in human pulp cells of teeth with complete and incomplete root development. Int Endod J 2009;42(8):686–93.

86. Caviedes-Bucheli J, Angel-Londoño P, Díaz-Perez A, et al. Variation in the expression of insulin-like growth factor-1 in human pulp tissue according to the root-development stage. J Endod 2007;33(11):1293–5.

87. Caviedes-Bucheli J, Muñoz HR, Rodríguez CE, et al. Expression of insulin-like growth factor-1 receptor in human pulp tissue. J Endod 2004;30(11):767–9.

88. Davidson B, Reich R, Lazarovici P, et al. Expression of the nerve growth factor receptors TrkA and p75 in malignant mesothelioma. Lung Cancer 2004;44(2):159–65.

89. Woodnutt DA, Wager-Miller J, O'Neill PC, et al. Neurotrophin receptors and nerve growth factor are differentially expressed in adjacent nonneuronal cells of normal and injured tooth pulp. Cell Tissue Res 2000;299(2):225–36.

90. Byers MR, Wheeler EF, Bothwell M. Altered expression of NGF and P75 NGF-receptor by fibroblasts of injured teeth precedes sensory nerve sprouting. Growth Factors 1992;6(1):41–52.

91. Luukko K, Moshnyakov M, Sainio K, et al. Expression of neurotrophin receptors during rat tooth development is developmentally regulated, independent of

innervation, and suggests functions in the regulation of morphogenesis and innervation. Dev Dyn 1996;206(1):87–99.

92. Arany S, Koyota S, Sugiyama T. Nerve growth factor promotes differentiation of odontoblast-like cells. J Cell Biochem 2009;106(4):539–45.

93. Mizoguchi T, Verkade H, Heath JK, et al. Sdf1/Cxcr4 signaling controls the dorsal migration of endodermal cells during zebrafish gastrulation. Development 2008;135(15):2521–9.

94. Wright DE, Bowman EP, Wagers AJ, et al. Hematopoietic stem cells are uniquely selective in their migratory response to chemokines. J Exp Med 2002;195(9): 1145–54.

95. Dar A, Kollet O, Lapidot T. Mutual, reciprocal SDF-1/CXCR4 interactions between hematopoietic and bone marrow stromal cells regulate human stem cell migration and development in NOD/SCID chimeric mice. Exp Hematol 2006;34(8):967–75.

96. Wright N, Hidalgo A, Rodríguez-Frade JM, et al. The chemokine stromal cell-derived factor-1 alpha modulates alpha 4 beta 7 integrin-mediated lymphocyte adhesion to mucosal address in cell adhesion molecule-1 and fibronectin. J Immunol 2002;168(10):5268–77.

97. Iohara K, Zheng L, Wake H, et al. A novel stem cell source for vasculogenesis in ischemia: subfraction of side population cells from dental pulp. Stem Cells 2008; 26(9):2408–18.

98. Iohara K, Zheng L, Ito M, et al. Regeneration of dental pulp after pulpotomy by transplantation of CD31(-)/CD146(-) side population cells from a canine tooth. Regen Med 2009;4(3):377–85.

99. Nakashima M, Iohara K. Regeneration of dental pulp by stem cells. Adv Dent Res 2011;23(3):313–9

100. Hargreaves KM, Giesler T, Henry M, et al. Regeneration potential of the young permanent tooth: what does the future hold? J Endod 2008;34(Suppl 7):S51–6.

101. Murray PE, Garcia-Godoy F, Hargreaves KM. Regenerative endodontics: a review of current status and a call for action. J Endod 2007;33(4):377–90.

102. Sloan AJ, Smith AJ. Stem cells and the dental pulp: potential roles in dentine regeneration and repair. Oral Dis 2007;13(2):151–7.

Constructs and Scaffolds Employed to Regenerate Dental Tissue

Peter E. Murray, PhD

KEYWORDS

- Constructs • Scaffolds • Dental tissue • Tissue grafting

KEY POINTS

- There are 8 key elements that are needed to create tissue constructs for dental regeneration.
- The creation of tissue constructs requires scaffolds to be seeded with stem cells in a controlled environment with growth factors.
- The type of stem cells and selection of scaffolds are based on the need to regenerate mucosa, gingiva, pulp or other dental tissue.

Dental tissue Injury and regeneration affects the daily lives of almost everyone. People who have missing teeth and dental tissues have difficulty eating[1] and speaking,[2] suffer a lower health-related quality of life,[3] are less likely to be employed,[4] more likely to be depressed,[5] and can suffer emotional problems because of their unhealthy appearance.[6] Dental implants and dentures can be aesthetically and functionally effective and also satisfy patients.[7] But dental implants are not able to completely replace all the functions of natural teeth.[8] Gingiva, skin, and bone can be replaced by transplanting donor tissues, but these therapies are limited by donor shortage,[9] or sometimes the limited regenerative ability of donated tissues.[10] Tissue engineering is emerging as a promising therapy to regenerate missing teeth and dental tissues.[10] A key element of tissue engineering is to generate a functional tissue construct, to replace lost or damaged tissues. Most dentists believe that regenerative dental treatments involving the delivery of stem cells and tissue constructs will become common within the next 10 to 20 years.[11] Most dentists are willing to receive training to be able to provide regenerative endodontic procedures for their patients.[12] Half of dentists already use membranes, scaffolds, or bioactive materials.[12] It was surprising that 55% of dentists were unsure whether regenerative procedures would be successful. The surveys[11,12] indicate broad support among dentists for using scaffolds and

Department of Endodontics, College of Dental Medicine, Nova Southeastern University, 3200 South University Drive, Fort Lauderdale, FL 33328-2018, USA
E-mail address: petemurr@nova.edu

Dent Clin N Am 56 (2012) 577–588
doi:10.1016/j.cden.2012.05.008
0011-8532/12/$ – see front matter © 2012 Elsevier Inc. All rights reserved.

dental.theclinics.com

constructs to regenerate tissues, but also the need for strong evidence that demonstrates the reliability of using these new therapies.

REGENERATION OF DENTAL TISSUE

The aim of regenerative dental therapies is to restore patients to full oral health. This means restoring normal function to tissue that has been damaged or missing due to trauma, disease, cancer, or a congenital condition. Greenwood and colleagues[13] described regenerative medicine as the "emerging interdisciplinary field of research and clinical applications focused on the repair, replacement, and regeneration of cells, tissues, or organs to restore impaired function resulting from any cause, including congenital defects, disease, trauma, and aging." Regeneration approaches use a combination of scaffolds, stem cells, growth factors, tissue engineering, organ tissue culture, transplantation, and tissue grafting. There are 8 key elements to create and use tissue constructs for tissue regeneration.

>   Step #1. The size, shape, functions, and aesthetics of the missing or defective tissue, such as a bone defect, needs to be assessed using cone beam micro-computer tomography[14] and radiographs.
>   Step #2. Stem cells, such as dental pulp stem cells from an exfoliated baby tooth,[15] need to be obtained from the host patient or a donor to serve as the building blocks for tissue regeneration.[15]
>   Step #3. Stem cells account for a very small percentage of the cells within tissues. The stem cells must be identified using surface markers and be isolated from all the donated cells using fluorescent cell sorting.[16]
>   Step #4. Millions of stem cells are needed to create functional tissues; this requires that they be expanded using cell culture.[17]
>   Step #5. The activity of the stem cells must be controlled by growth factors during cell culture to ensure that the stem cells differentiate into a useful cell type (eg, bone or periodontal ligament).[18]
>   Step #6. Cells grown in culture lack a 3-dimensional scaffold necessary to function and have the correct size and shape to generate a tissue; therefore the cells need to be seeded onto a scaffold to form a tissue construct that gives the cells the characteristics of a tissue, such as dental pulp stem cells seeded onto polymer and collagen scaffolds to generate replacement pulp tissue.[19,20]
>   Step #7. The tissue construct is maintained in cell culture until a functional tissue is generated.[21]
>   Step #8. The tissue construct is grafted or implanted into the donor site,[21] where the regenerated tissue is required.

These steps to create and use tissue constructs are shown in **Fig. 1**.

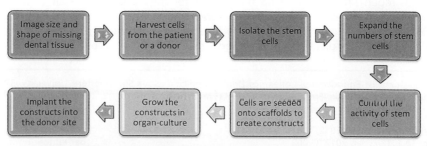

Fig. 1. Steps to create and use constructs to for tissue regeneration.

DENTAL REGENERATION

Dental regeneration can be defined as the process in people by which specialized dental tissues are replaced by the recruitment, proliferation, migration, and differentiation of dental stem cells.[22] It is important that the newly regenerated tissues recapitulate the architecture and function of the missing or damaged dental tissue. However, ideal reconstructive goals, such as a complete return to original clinical form and function, are frequently not completely achieved.[23] Regeneration can occur more readily in some tissue types compared with others (eg, the oral mucosa can readily regenerate without scarring, while most other dental tissues heal by granulation tissue, which can eventually form fibrous scar tissue).[24] Dental tissue regeneration depends on the activity of progenitor cells or stem cells to be seeded within a scaffold to generate a new tissue construct[25] (eg, artificial skin that can serve as a scaffold for the regrowth of dermal tissue using the hosts own cells).[26] Another example is freeze-dried bone, which provides a scaffold for the host's own osteoblasts to regenerate bone defects.[27] By combining different types of stem cells with different types of scaffolds and controlling the cell culture and tissue engineering conditions, the outcome of the construct can be altered to create various types of dental tissues, from teeth to salivary glands, shown in **Fig. 2**.

HISTORY OF DENTAL REGENERATION

From the beginnings of dentistry in Egypt almost 5000 years ago,[28] dentists have been seeking improved procedures to generate replacement teeth, and to regenerate dental tissues for their patients. In 1952, BW Hermann[29] was reported to have made one of the first attempts at dental tissue regeneration. Herman used calcium hydroxide (calxyl) to promote dentin bridge formation for vital pulp therapy following partial pulp amputation.[29] In 1961, Nygaard-Ostby[30] established a blood clot to use as a scaffold to revascularize tissue within the root canals of teeth (**Fig. 3**). During recent decades, many more dental procedures and scaffolds have been developed to promote dental tissue regeneration, especially in the field of periodontics to guide bone and tissue regeneration. The concepts of guided tissue and bone regeneration (GTR/GBR) were first published by Melcher in 1976,[31] who outlined the necessity of using barrier membranes to exclude unwanted cell lines from healing sites to allow tissue growth. The first clinical case reports of GTR/GBR were presented by Nyman and colleagues[32] through the intraoral application of *Millipore* bacterial filters composed of a cellulose acetate as the first barrier membranes used to achieve

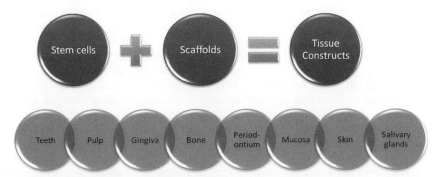

Fig. 2. Generation of dental tissue constructs.

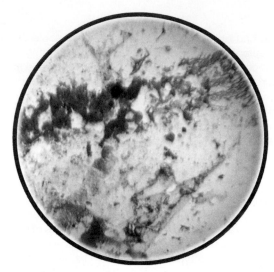

Fig. 3. Blood clot revascularization within the root canal of a tooth.

regeneration of periodontal tissues as a direct alternative to surgical resection procedures to reduce periodontal pocket depths.

Next came the introduction of platelet-rich plasma (PRP) to use as a natural fibrin scaffold as part of oral surgery by Whitman and colleagues[33] in 1997. PRP is thought to activate platelets and release growth factors to enhance wound healing.[33] PRP became more popular after Marx and colleagues[34] demonstrated that combining PRP with autogenous bone in mandibular continuity defects resulted in significantly faster radiographic maturation and histomorphometrically denser bone regeneration.[34] PRP has also been used in the field of regenerative endodontics, with the recent case report of Torabinejad and Turman,[35] which demonstrated the merits of PRP as a natural scaffold for pulp revascularization.[35]

SCAFFOLDS

People and animals have a natural scaffold that surrounds cells and provides structural support for the formation and maintenance of tissues and organs. The scaffold is mainly composed of extracellular matrix proteins (ECMPs). The key ECMPs are collagen, vitronectin, fibronectin, and laminin, which provide cells with anchorage, sequestration of growth factors, and signal cells to migrate, differentiate, and proliferate through integrin receptor-mediated signaling pathways.[36] ECMPs have important roles in dental regeneration. Laminin promotes odontoblast differentiation,[37] and a recent study by Howard and colleagues[38] demonstrated that it is an important factor in dental pulp stem cell migration. Fibronectin has been shown to increase ameloblast growth and differentiation, while vitronectin provides a structural framework.[39] Collagen is the predominant structural component of all tissues and has been observed to immobilize growth factors to regulate cell proliferation and differentiation.[40]

Natural ECMP scaffolds have varying chemical and physical characteristics which contribute to the specific functions of the tissue in which they reside. Scaffolds for tissue engineering have been created with a range of physical properties; these include porosity, pore size, weight, and hydration capacity, as shown in **Table 1**. A

Table 1 Physical properties of 3-dimensional tissue engineering scaffolds					
Scaffold Type	Average Dimensions	Hydration Capacity	Porosity (Pores Per Linear Inch)	Average Pore Size	Weight/Wet Weight
Polymer	5 × 4 mm 0.039 cm³	30 mL	120−/+20	100–200 mm	5.2 mg/32 mg
Collagen	4.5 × 4.2 mm 0.039 cm³	25 mL	120−/+20	100–200 mm	3.5 mg/45 mg
Calcium Phosphate	5 × 3 mm 0.058 cm³	30 mL	60−/+10	200–400 mm	45 mg/99 mg

high porosity and sufficient pore size are necessary to facilitate cell seeding and diffusion of cells and nutrients throughout scaffold.[41] The other important properties are biocompatibility and biodegradability. Some scaffolds are permanent, while for other scaffolds, they need to be absorbed by the surrounding tissues to avoid interfering with the regenerated tissue. The rate of degradation should coincide with the rate of tissue formation.[42] The latest generations of scaffolds have been engineered to have ideal properties and functional customization: injectability, synthetic manufacture, biocompatibility, nonimmunogenicity, transparency, nano-scale fibers, low concentration, and high resorption rates.[43] Scaffolds for tissue engineering can be created from synthetic materials such as polymers, similar to absorbable surgical sutures,[44] or by collagen, a natural ECMP scaffold material,[45] or by calcium phosphate.[46] The architecture of these scaffolds is shown in **Fig. 4**.

Scaffolds for dental tissue regeneration are comprised of a very diverse group of natural tissues such as skin and bone sourced from human donors, to synthetic materials designed to be used as skin and bone scaffolds. Some scaffolds are injectible, which makes them easy to deliver; however these hydrogel and nanofiber scaffolds are often not able to maintain good cell survival. Spongy scaffolds include absorbable collagen and polymers, which can maintain good stem cell survival, but which lack the structural strength needed for load bearing and muscle movement. The advantages and limitations of the common types of scaffolds for dental regeneration are summarized in **Table 2**.

DENTAL TISSUE CONSTRUCTS

Dental pulp and periodontal tissue constructs have been created by seeding dental stem cells onto scaffolds made from bovine collagen, open polylactic acid (polymer), and calcium phosphate, followed by cell culture and tissue engineering.[20] Tissue engineered dental pulp constructs can be created by seeding stem cells from human exfoliated deciduous (SHED) teeth onto scaffolds, which are then implanted into human teeth (**Fig. 5**).[19] Tissue-engineered periodontal constructs can be created by seeding periodontal stem cells onto several different types of scaffolds. The most successful scaffolds for maintaining periodontal ligament stem cell (PDLSC) survival appear to be the spongy scaffolds, particularly scaffolds created from polymer or collagen, as shown in **Figs. 6** and **7**. Calcium phosphate scaffolds appear to be less effective at maintaining periodontal stem cell survival (see **Figs. 6** and **7**). The injectible scaffolds are comprised of a hydrogel, Pepgen P15, or DBX are the easiest to apply in the mouth, but unfortunately appear to be the least effective for maintaining the survival of the periodontal stem cells (see **Figs. 6** and **7**). The survival of stem cells within scaffolds is essential for the success of regenerating functional dental tissues.

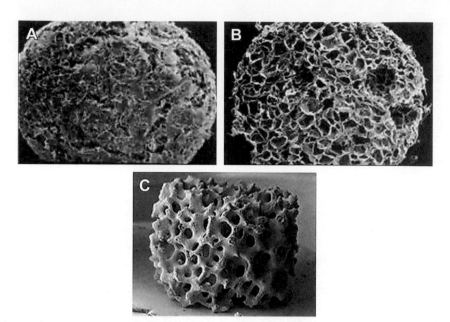

Fig. 4. Photomicrograph of scaffold structures. (*A*) Photomicrograph of the collagen scaffold structure. The 3-dimensional collagen composite scaffold is a natural scaffold manufactured from a mixture of collagens that are derived from bovine hide. Overall, this material exhibits collagen fibrillar architecture, which is representative of the structure of collagen within the interstitial matrix. (*B*) Photomicrograph of the polymer scaffold structure. The 3D OPLA (Open-Cell Polylactic Acid) scaffold is a synthetic polymer scaffold that is synthesized from D,D-L,L polylactic acid. This material has a facetted architecture, which is effective for culturing high density cell suspensions. (*C*) Photomicrograph of the calcium phosphate scaffold structure. The 3-dimensional calcium phosphate scaffold is a proprietary mineralized calcium phosphate bioceramic that is ideal for in vitro analysis of bone metabolism and cartilage regeneration.

PERIODONTAL LIGAMENT CONSTRUCTS

The regeneration of severe periodontal bone defects used to require bone grafts. Today, several types of injectable, cement, ceramic, and spongy scaffold materials are available as an alternative to bone grafts; these scaffolds provide a framework for the patient's own osteoblasts and stem cells to repair bone defects.[47,48] The scaffolds can also be seeded with autologous PDLSCs to create a tissue construct that can enhance periodontal regeneration in animals.[49] Periodontal and bone regeneration can be accelerated by using bioactive materials containing enamel matrix proteins such as Emdogain[50] (Straumann USA, Andover, MA, USA) and growth factors such as platelet-derived growth factor,[51] insulin-derived growth factor,[52] and platelet-rich plasma.[53]

PDLSCs were isolated and characterized by Seo and colleagues[54]; these stem cells were found to be capable of forming all components of the periodontal apparatus including cementoblasts, osteoblasts, and fibroblasts.[54] PDLSCs readily attach to the root surface of teeth, even in the absence of growth factors.[55] The seeding of PDLSCs onto the root surfaces of teeth can be used to bioengineer functional periodontal ligament in rodents.[56] This demonstrates that the success of bioactive materials for the regeneration of small bone defects may be supplemented in the future by seeding PDLSCs onto scaffolds and the roots of teeth to regenerate large bone defects.

Table 2
Common types of scaffolds for dental regeneration

Scaffold Type	Properties	Advantages	Limitations
Hydrogel	A colloid jelly-like scaffold	Injectable, biocompatible, and absorbed by body	Low stem cell survival, lacks functional strength, variable outcomes
Nanofiber	Self-assembling peptides often mixed with hydrogel		
Collagen Polymer	Sponge	Easy to handle, clinically effective absorbed by body	Lacks functional strength to support tissues or muscle movement
Calcium Phosphate	Brittle		
Silk	Fibers		
Fibrin	Centrifuged from peripheral blood	Easily made scaffold from host peripheral blood	
Bone	Sourced from donor and freeze-dried into a powder	Bone grafts are clinically very effective	Expensive and requires a donor, risk of contamination
Synthetic bone	Bone defect filling material	Clinically effective and safe	Not as effective as natural bone
Skin	Sourced from a cadaver or host	Clinically effective	Need cadavers or donor skin, risk of contamination
Synthetic skin	Wound dressing material	Clinically useful and safe	Temporary fix, patient will still need skin grafts

DENTAL PULP CONSTRUCTS

The seeding of polymer scaffolds with dental pulp stem cells (DPSCs) to create dental pulp constructs, which were implanted subcutaneously into a New Zealand rabbit, was able to regenerate dentin/pulp-like tissues including and osteodentin.[57] The seeding of DPSCs on polymer scaffolds inside tooth slices, which have been

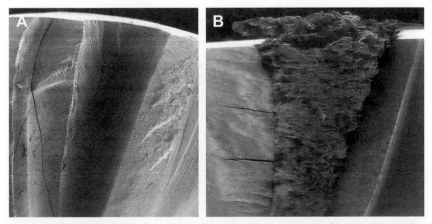

Fig. 5. Tissue engineered dental pulp constructs in the root canal of teeth. (*A*) Tooth with a cleaned and shaped root canal. (*B*) Tooth with a dental pulp construct.

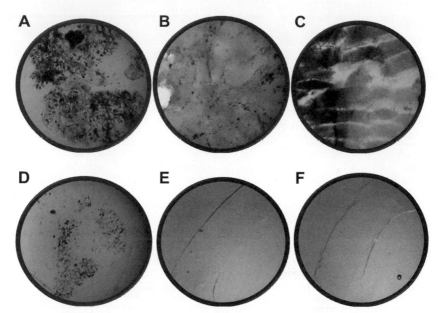

Fig. 6. Periodontal stem cell survival in scaffolds to create tissue engineered periodontal constructs: (*A*) Polymer scaffold. (*B*) Collagen scaffold. (*C*) Calcium phosphate scaffold. (*D*) Hydrogel scaffold. (*E*) Pepgen P15 scaffold. (*F*) DBX scaffold.

implanted subcutaneously in mice, has been successful at angiogenesis[58] and for regenerating odontoblast-like cells and dental pulp tissues.[59] The roots of teeth were regenerated by seeding stem cells onto scaffolds that were then implanted into tooth sockets in minipigs.[60] After 3 months, the construct, called a bioroot, had a post inserted and porcelain crown cemented.[60] This demonstrated the potential to bioengineer replacement teeth.

The regeneration of pulpal tissue can potentially revitalize already-existing end-odontically treated teeth; the prospect of regenerating entire teeth or bio-roots may one day provide an alternative to dentures, fixed prosthetics, and dental implants to replace missing teeth.

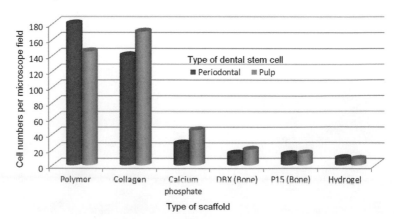

Fig. 7. Bar chart of periodontal and dental pulp stem cell survival in tissue engineered constructs.

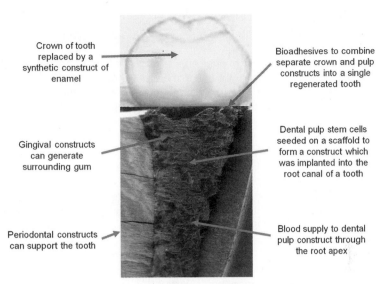

Crown of tooth replaced by a synthetic construct of enamel

Bioadhesives to combine separate crown and pulp constructs into a single regenerated tooth

Gingival constructs can generate surrounding gum

Dental pulp stem cells seeded on a scaffold to form a construct which was implanted into the root canal of a tooth

Periodontal constructs can support the tooth

Blood supply to dental pulp construct through the root apex

Fig. 8. The role of tissue engineered constructs in future dental treatment.

Autologous cell homing is an underrecognized approach in tissue regeneration[61] that offers an alternative to the allotransplantation of stem cells from a donor. Promoting a patient's own stem cells to home to a scaffold and regenerate tissue could help avoid the time-consuming and expensive steps of ex vivo stem cell isolation, harvesting, and manipulation and expansion. Simplifying tissue regeneration by promoting patient stem cell homing may accelerate regulatory, commercial, and clinical processes. Stem cell homing has been demonstrated to generate new pulp tissue in human molars that have been implanted into mice.[61] In another rodent study, the grafting of scaffolds was able to create teeth and periodontal ligament by cell homing.[62]

SUMMARY

Dental regenerative treatments and guided tissue regeneration already save millions of teeth each year. Synthetic bone regeneration materials are routinely used to regenerate the bone defects of dental patients. Researchers are aiming to develop enhanced regenerative therapies that have the capability to regenerate teeth and tissues beyond current limits. This will require the development of new protocols using stem cells, scaffolds, and growth factors.[63] Several bioengineering approaches involving stem cells, scaffolds, and growth factors can be combined to regenerate the different tissues needed to generate a tooth and its supporting tissues. The role of tissue engineered constructs in future dental treatment is shown in **Fig. 8**.

REFERENCES

1. Rodrigues HL Jr, Scelza MF, Boaventura GT, et al. Relation between oral health and nutritional condition in the elderly. J Appl Oral Sci 2012;20:38–44.
2. Foerster U, Gilbert GH, Duncan RP. Oral functional limitation among dentate adults. J Public Health Dent 1998;58:202–9.
3. Albaker AM. The oral health-related quality of life in edentulous patients treated with conventional complete dentures. Gerodontology 2012. [Epub ahead of print].
4. Williams C. Good teeth improves the job corps image. Dent Stud 1972;50:30–42.

5. Okoro CA, Strine TW, Eke PI, et al. The association between depression and anxiety and use of oral health services and tooth loss. Community Dent Oral Epidemiol 2012;40:134–44.

6. McMillan AS, Wong MC. Emotional effects of tooth loss in community-dwelling elderly people in Hong Kong. Int J Prosthodont 2004;17:172–6.

7. Pjetursson BE, Karoussis I, Bürgin W, et al. Patients' satisfaction following implant therapy. A 10-year prospective cohort study. Clin Oral Implants Res 2005;16:185–93.

8. Lekholm U, Gröndahl K, Jemt T. Outcome of oral implant treatment in partially edentulous jaws followed 20 years in clinical function. Clin Implant Dent Relat Res 2006;8:178–86.

9. Clayton M, Parker A, Willis S. Developments in addressing the organ donor shortage. Nurs Times 2005;101:25–6.

10. Murray PE, García-Godoy F. The outlook for implants and endodontics: a review of the tissue engineering strategies to create replacement teeth for patients. Dent Clin North Am 2006;50:299–315.

11. Epelman I, Murray PE, Garcia-Godoy F, et al. A practitioner survey of opinions toward regenerative endodontics. J Endod 2009;35:1204–10.

12. Manguno C, Murray PE, Howard C, et al. A survey of dental residents' expectations for regenerative endodontics. J Endod 2012;38:137–43.

13. Greenwood HL, Thorsteinsdottir H, Perry G, et al. Regenerative medicine: new opportunities for developing countries. Int J Biotechnol 2006;8:60–77.

14. Sohn DS, Heo JU, Kwak DH, et al. Bone regeneration in the maxillary sinus using an autologous fibrin-rich block with concentrated growth factors alone. Implant Dent 2011;20:389–95.

15. Bakopoulou A, Leyhausen G, Volk J, et al. Assessment of the impact of two different isolation methods on the osteo/odontogenic differentiation potential of human dental stem cells derived from deciduous teeth. Calcif Tissue Int 2011; 88:130–41.

16. Shi S, Gronthos S. Perivascular niche of postnatal mesenchymal stem cells in human bone marrow and dental pulp. J Bone Miner Res 2003;18:696–704.

17. Govindasamy V, Ronald VS, Abdullah AN, et al. Human platelet lysate permits scale-up of dental pulp stromal cells for clinical applications. Cytotherapy 2011;13:1221–33.

18. Chadipiralla K, Yochim JM, Bahuleyan B, et al. Osteogenic differentiation of stem cells derived from human periodontal ligaments and pulp of human exfoliated deciduous teeth. Cell Tissue Res 2010;340:323–33.

19. Gotlieb EL, Murray PE, Namerow KN, et al. An ultrastructural investigation of tissue-engineered pulp constructs implanted within endodontically treated teeth. J Am Dent Assoc 2008;139:457–65.

20. Gebhardt M, Murray PE, Namerow KN, et al. Cell survival within pulp and periodontal constructs. J Endod 2009;35:63–6.

21. Abukawa H, Terai H, Hannouche D, et al. Formation of a mandibular condyle in vitro by tissue engineering. J Oral Maxillofac Surg 2003;61:94–100.

22. Mathieu S, El-Battari A, Dejou J, et al. Role of injured endothelial cells in the recruitment of human pulp cells. Arch Oral Biol 2005;50:109–13.

23. Costello BJ, Shah G, Kumta P, et al. Regenerative medicine for craniomaxillofacial surgery. Oral Maxillofac Surg Clin North Am 2010;22:33–42.

24. Yannas IV. Tissue and organ regeneration in adults. New York (NY): Springer Publishing; 2007.

25. Garcia-Godoy F, Murray P. Regenerative dentistry: translating advancements in basic science research to the dental practice. J Tenn Dent Assoc 2010;90:12–8.

26. Scuderi N, Anniboletti T, Carlesimo B, et al. Clinical application of autologous three-cellular cultured skin substitutes based on esterified hyaluronic acid scaffold: our experience. In Vivo 2009;23:991–1003.
27. Mishra S, Singh RK, Mohammad S, et al. A comparative evaluation of decalcified freeze dried bone allograft, hydroxyapatite and their combination in osseous defects of the jaws. J Maxillofac Oral Surg 2010;9:236–40.
28. Leek FF. The practice of dentistry in ancient Egypt. J Egypt Archaeol 1967;53: 51–8.
29. Herman BW. On the reaction of the dental pulp to vital amputation and calxyl capping. Dtsch Zahnarztl Z 1952;7:1446–7 [in German].
30. Ostby BN. The role of the blood clot in endodontic therapy. An experimental histologic study. Acta Odontol Scand 1961;19:324–53.
31. Melcher AH. On the repair potential of periodontal tissues. J Periodontol 1976;47: 256–60.
32. Nyman S, Lindhe J, Karring T, et al. New attachment following surgical treatment of human periodontal disease. J Clin Periodontol 1982;9:290–6.
33. Whitman DH, Berry RL, Green DM. Platelet gel: an autologous alternative to fibrin glue with applications in oral and maxillofacial surgery. J Oral Maxillofac Surg 1997;55:1294–9.
34. Marx RE, Carlson ER, Eichstaedt RM, et al. Platelet-rich plasma: growth factor enhancement for bone grafts. Oral Surg Oral Med Oral Pathol Oral Radiol Endod 1998;85:638 46.
35. Torabinejad M, Turman M. Revitalization of tooth with necrotic pulp and open apex by using platelet-rich plasma: a case report. J Endod 2011;37:265–8.
36. Kim SH, Turnbull J, Guimond S. Extracellular matrix and cell signalling: the dynamic cooperation of integrin, proteoglycan and growth factor receptor. J Endocrinol 2011;209:139–51.
37. Yamashiro T, Zheng L, Shitaku Y, et al. Wnt10a regulates dentin sialophosphoprotein mRNA expression and possibly links odontoblast differentiation and tooth morphogenesis. Differentiation 2007;75:452–62.
38. Howard C, Murray PE, Namerow KN. Dental pulp stem cell migration. J Endod 2010;36:1963–6.
39. Tabata MJ, Matsumura T, Fujii T, et al. Fibronectin accelerates the growth and differentiation of ameloblast lineage cells in vitro. J Histochem Cytochem 2003; 51:1673–9.
40. Paralkar VM, Vukicevic S, Reddi AH. Transforming growth factor beta type 1 binds to collagen IV of basement membrane matrix: implications for development. Dev Biol 1991;143:303–8.
41. Sachlos E, Czernuszka JT. Making tissue engineering scaffolds work. Review: the application of solid freeform fabrication technology to the production of tissue engineering scaffolds. Eur Cell Mater 2003;30:29–39.
42. Freed LE, Vunjak-Novakovic G, Biron RJ, et al. Biodegradable polymer scaffolds for tissue engineering. Biotechnology (N Y) 1994;12:689–93.
43. Almeida HA, Bártolo PJ. Structural and vascular analysis of tissue engineering scaffolds, part 2: topology optimisation. Methods Mol Biol 2012;868:209–36.
44. Ge Z, Wang L, Heng BC, et al. Proliferation and differentiation of human osteoblasts within 3D printed poly-lactic-co-glycolic acid scaffolds. J Biomater Appl 2009;23:533–47.
45. Yannas IV, Tzeranis DS, Harley BA, et al. Biologically active collagen-based scaffolds: advances in processing and characterization. Philos Transact A Math Phys Eng Sci 2010;368:2123–39.

46. Bose S, Tarafder S. Calcium phosphate ceramic systems in growth factor and drug delivery for bone tissue engineering: a review. Acta Biomater 2012;8: 1401–21.
47. Aichelmann-Reidy ME, Yukna RA. Bone replacement grafts. The bone substitutes. Dent Clin North Am 1998;42:491–503.
48. Singh VP, Nayak DG, Uppoor AS, et al. Clinical and radiographic evaluation of nano-crystalline hydroxyapatite bone graft (Sybograf) in combination with bioresorbable collagen membrane (Periocol) in periodontal intrabony defects. Dent Res J (Isfahan) 2012;9:60–7.
49. Suaid FF, Ribeiro FV, Rodrigues TL, et al. Autologous periodontal ligament cells in the treatment of class II furcation defects: a study in dogs. J Clin Periodontol 2011;38:491–8.
50. Kadonishi Y, Deie M, Takata T, et al. Acceleration of tendon-bone healing in anterior cruciate ligament reconstruction using an enamel matrix derivative in a rat model. J Bone Joint Surg Br 2012;94:205–9.
51. McGuire MK, Kao RT, Nevins M, et al. rhPDGF-BB promotes healing of periodontal defects: 24-month clinical and radiographic observations. Int J Periodontics Restorative Dent 2006;26:223–31.
52. Howell TH, Fiorellini JP, Paquette DW, et al. A phase I/II clinical trial to evaluate a combination of recombinant human platelet-derived growth factor-BB and recombinant human insulin-like growth factor-I in patients with periodontal disease. J Periodontol 1997;68:1186–93.
53. Tozum TF, Demiralp B. Platelet-rich plasma: a promising innovation in dentistry. J Can Dent Assoc 2003;69:664.
54. Seo BM, Miura M, Gronthos S, et al. Investigation of multipotent postnatal stem cells from human periodontal ligament. Lancet 2004;364:149–55.
55. Elseed MA, Murray PE, Garcia-Godoy F, et al. Assessment of bioactive and bioadhesive therapies to enhance stem cell attachment to root surface dentine. Int Endod J 2009;42:576–83.
56. Dangaria SJ, Ito Y, Luan X, et al. Successful periodontal ligament regeneration by periodontal progenitor preseeding on natural tooth root surfaces. Stem Cells Dev 2011;20:1659–68.
57. El-Backly RM, Massoud AG, El-Badry AM, et al. Regeneration of dentine/pulp-like tissue using a dental pulp stem cell/poly(lactic-co-glycolic) acid scaffold construct in New Zealand white rabbits. Aust Endod J 2008;34:52–67.
58. Goncalves SB, Dong Z, Bramante CM, et al. Tooth slice-based models for the study of human dental pulp angiogenesis. J Endod 2007;33:811–4.
59. Demarco FF, Casagrande L, Zhang Z, et al. Effects of morphogen and scaffold porogen on the differentiation of dental pulp stem cells. J Endod 2010;36: 1805–11.
60. Sonoyama W, Liu Y, Fang D, et al. Mesenchymal stem cell-mediated functional tooth regeneration in swine. PLoS One 2006;1:e79.
61. Kim JY, Xin X, Moioli EK, et al. Regeneration of dental-pulp-like tissue by chemotaxis-induced cell homing. Tissue Eng Part A 2010;16:3023–31.
62. Kim K, Lee CH, Kim BK, et al. Anatomically shaped tooth and periodontal regeneration by cell homing. J Dent Res 2010;89(8):842–7.
63. Murray PE, Garcia-Godoy F, Hargreaves KM. Regenerative endodontics: a review of current status and a call for action. J Endod 2007;33:377–90.

Harnessing the Natural Regenerative Potential of the Dental Pulp

Anthony J. Smith, PhD*, James G. Smith, BMedSc,
Richard M. Shelton, BDS, PhD, Paul R. Cooper, PhD

KEYWORDS

- Dentin • Pulp • Regeneration • Stem cells • Tissue engineering • Injury
- Wound healing

KEY POINTS

- Biological solutions to the repair and regeneration of the dental tissues offer significant potential for improved clinical treatment outcomes.
- Translation of dental tissue-engineering approaches to the clinic will make considerable contributions to these outcomes in the future, but exploiting the natural regenerative potential of dentin-pulp to enhance wound-healing responses offers solutions for maintaining pulp vitality now.
- Strategies to harness the natural regenerative potential of the pulp must be based on a sound biological understanding of the cellular and molecular events taking place, and require careful consideration of the interplay of infection, inflammation, and regeneration.

Regenerative medicine offers many advantages for the treatment of disease with its aim of "replacing or regenerating human cells, tissues or organs to restore or establish normal function,"[1] and within dentistry there is exciting future potential for engineering whole teeth.[2–8] Nevertheless, several challenges still exist before such tooth-replacement therapies can be clinically implemented in dental practice. Paramount among these challenges is programmed development of appropriate crown and cuspal morphology for occlusal function and engineering of the tooth/periodontium interface to allow normal oral function. Use of scaffolds of defined morphology may assist with overcoming some of the morphologic challenges. Recently the authors generated a mineralized tissue construct, retaining the morphology of the human tooth

Financial Disclosure and Conflict of Interest: The authors declare no conflict of interest or financial interest with any commercial company in relation to the content of this article. The University of Birmingham was the only body/organization that provided funding support for the preparation of this article.
School of Dentistry, University of Birmingham, St Chads Queensway, Birmingham B4 6NN, UK
* Corresponding author.
E-mail address: a.j.smith@bham.ac.uk

Dent Clin N Am 56 (2012) 589–601
doi:10.1016/j.cden.2012.05.011
0011-8532/12/$ – see front matter © 2012 Elsevier Inc. All rights reserved.

dental.theclinics.com

used as a mold for production of an alginate scaffold within which dental pulp cells were seeded (**Fig. 1**). Such approaches may contribute to realization of the engineering of whole teeth, although this remains a future goal for dentistry.

Considerable recent interest in the concept of regenerative endodontics has led to reports of engineering of individual dental component tissues, which provides a more achievable goal in the shorter term. Seeding of pulp cells isolated from exfoliated primary teeth in a simple polylactic acid scaffold within a dentin slice before subcutaneous implantation in vivo has allowed engineering of tissue with the same appearance and structure as normal pulp.[9] A scaffold of collagen I gel containing isolated dental pulp cells and angiogenic growth factors within a pulpless tooth chamber

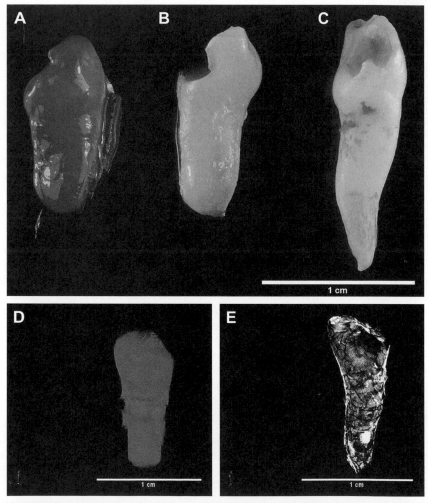

Fig. 1. (*A*) Encapsulated pulp cells in tooth-shaped alginate construct after 5 weeks in control medium, (*B*) encapsulated pulp cells in tooth-shaped alginate construct after 5 weeks in dentinogenic medium, and (*C*) human deciduous tooth used for production of alginate gel mold. (*D*, *E*) Image analysis of micro–computed tomography scanned tooth-shaped alginate gels after 5 weeks in (*D*) control medium, and (*E*) dentinogenic medium (image thresholded to pixel intensity above average level of control).

showed evidence of revascularization and tissue generation after in vivo implantation.[10] Although these tissue-engineering approaches may ultimately provide shorter-term solutions to the management of gross dental disease than whole tooth replacement, there are already viable regenerative endodontic techniques available to the clinician. Dentistry has long been a pioneer in regenerative medicine with the use of direct pulp-capping techniques for vital pulp therapy. Agents such as calcium hydroxide have been used for more than 90 years to stimulate natural pulp wound healing,[11,12] although lack of understanding of the mechanistic basis of such treatments has perhaps led to their somewhat empiric application. Newer pulp-capping materials such as mineral trioxide aggregate (MTA) have demonstrated considerable clinical merit[13] and, with appropriate strategic planning with regard to their clinical application, these agents can offer regenerative therapies to the practitioner now. However, opportunities exist to improve and optimize the use of such agents, and this will be important in bringing a more regenerative philosophy to the endodontics arena.

Natural wound healing essentially represents one end of the spectrum of tissue regeneration, and promotion of vital pulp therapy relies on principles applicable to healing of any of the body's tissues. Promoting wound cleansing to enable the body's natural defense responses of inflammation and immune reactions to take place in a controlled manner and not to become self perpetuating, however, can be particularly challenging in the tooth where the tissues are exposed to significant bacterial infection. Furthermore, the low-compliance nature of the dentin-pulp complex encased by rigid mineralized tissues followed by the introduction of dental restorative materials, sometimes possessing cytotoxic properties, may inhibit natural tissue-repair responses. It is perhaps not surprising that the prognosis for long-term survival of dental restorations corresponds poorly with desired health care outcomes, and mean survival rates of the order of 50% to 60% after 5 to 10 years have been reported.[14] Together, such findings highlight the opportunities for development of new approaches to management of dental disease, whose success will be significantly enhanced by using new treatment modalities based on the cellular and molecular events associated with the healing responses of the dentin-pulp complex following injury.

These healing responses will be very dependent on the tissue environment resulting from the injury to the tooth and will often guide treatment-management decisions. For instance, it has been recommended that vital pulp therapy should only be attempted in primary and young permanent teeth where there is a good prognosis for pulp regeneration, and not in teeth with irreversible pulpitis or a necrotic pulp.[15] Of course, this belies a fundamental issue of accurately diagnosing the status of the pulp with a limited armory of clinical tools, which do not necessarily correlate well with more biological measures. Nevertheless, it is well recognized that caries can present as a broad spectrum of disease activity, with consequent influence on the pulp and dental hard tissues and their regenerative potential. A regenerative response in the form of tertiary dentin secretion can be observed during slowly progressing caries but not rapidly progressing caries,[16,17] highlighting the influence of microbial challenges to regeneration. However, it is not only the direct effects of the bacteria that are responsible for these responses, but also their indirect effects on various other events contributing to the overall regenerative picture. Of particular importance is the role of bacteria in triggering inflammatory and immune responses in the pulp, which in turn will affect pulpal regeneration. It is now apparent that the dentin matrix contains a heterogeneous cocktail of growth factors and cytokines, which may be released during bacterial acid demineralization of the matrix during caries, and these molecules will significantly contribute to the regenerative responses taking place. Surgical intervention to remove and restore carious hard tissue from the tooth may further contribute to tissue injury and cellular responses, in view of the intimate relationship between odontoblasts and their extracellular matrix. The extensive network of odontoblast processes and their lateral extensions[18] in dentin permeates the whole tissue, and any surgical intervention to dentin is likely to provoke a cellular response. This premise is corroborated by data on odontoblast viability beneath cavities prepared to different depths through dentin, which indicate that survival is compromised in deeper cavities.[19] Thus, there is a complex interplay between factors determining the environment within which regeneration may occur (**Fig. 2**).

For regeneration to occur in the dentin-pulp complex, there is both a requirement for cells to secrete new tissue and for appropriate molecular and cellular signaling to occur, to enable cells to secrete the newly regenerated tissue. One can therefore envisage regeneration being determined by the following:

- A permissive environment in which regeneration can occur
- Cells capable of secreting the extracellular matrices of the dentin-pulp complex
- Secretion of molecular signals and cell-cell interactions to occur for upregulation of cellular synthesis and secretion of new dentin-pulp tissue.

CREATING A CONDUCIVE ENVIRONMENT FOR REGENERATION
Microbial Challenges

The diverse microflora and variable intensity of infection in dentin caries[20] provide significant clinical challenges for both assessment of the level of disease activity and control of the infection. The clinical picture for dentin caries largely provides evidence of previous rather than current disease activity, and without longitudinal review it can be difficult to assess current disease status. Such information can easily lead to greater clinical intervention than is either required or desirable. The traditional approach of removing as much infected, and at-risk, tissue as possible (Black's "extension for

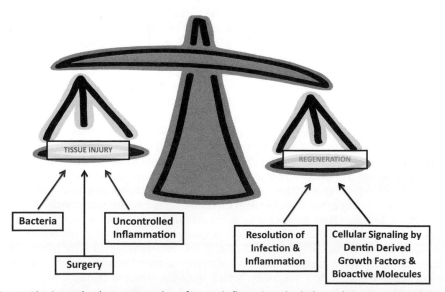

Fig. 2. The interplay between various factors influencing the balance between tissue injury and regeneration.

prevention" philosophy) has possibly led to increased tissue injury with consequent effects on preservation of pulp vitality in the battle to control infection. Modern approaches of minimally invasive dentistry[21] have helped to moderate the effects of surgical intervention but to increase the risk for restoration failure caused by secondary (recurrent) caries,[22] whereby incomplete removal of residual caries during restoration can be a contributory factor. It is clear, however, that good clinical outcomes can be achieved using minimally invasive techniques despite the increased chance of incomplete removal of infected tissue. This outcome may well reflect the antibacterial effects of the agents and materials used in restorative procedures combined with the host's defense mechanisms. Several chemicals, including sodium hypochlorite, various acids, ethylenediaminetetraacetic acid (EDTA), chlorhexidine, and so forth, are commonly used during cavity preparation and as irrigants in endodontics, and will exert antibacterial effects to varying degrees. Within adhesive dentistry, antibacterial agents are already being incorporated within dentin primers.[23] Some materials, such as calcium hydroxide and Portland cement–like materials (eg, MTA), generate a strongly basic pH during setting, which will likely contribute to their antibacterial effects.[24] Constituents of the dentin matrix also demonstrate antibacterial effects[25] and, while these effects appear to derive from a heterogeneous mixture of molecules, including neuropeptides[26–29] and cytokines such as adrenomedullin,[30,31] there is still much to learn as regards the range of such molecules involved. These antibacterial activities may not necessarily be the prime functions for some of these molecules, but their release (and also their breakdown products) during carious demineralization of dentin will nevertheless expose such roles. It is thus clear that there is a need for a more focused therapeutic approach to microbial control in the carious tooth to promote regenerative activity.

Inflammatory and Immune Challenges

A complex range of inflammatory and immune responses can occur in the dental pulp in response to carious injury and subsequent clinical treatment involving many molecular mediators.[32–34] While recognized as a terminally differentiated matrix-secreting cell, the odontoblast can participate in expression of various inflammatory mediators, and together with the strategic position of this cell in relation to carious bacterial invasion it should be considered as a part of the tooth's cellular defense system.[34] The complexity of the repertoire of the odontoblast's responses, however, becomes apparent when considering the close interplay between inflammation and tissue regeneration within the dental pulp.[32,33] Identification and characterization of the molecular and cellular events associated with pulpal inflammation is crucial to the development of improved approaches to vital pulp therapy and regeneration of the tissues.

Initiation of inflammatory and immune responses in the pulp reflects the injurious challenge to the tissue, a major determinant of which will be bacterial infection, although chemicals and materials used in restorative dentistry may also contribute to these responses. The importance of bacteria in driving pulpal inflammation is reflected in its exacerbation when the bacterial challenge persists.[35] It has long been a significant challenge to correlate the clinical and histologic features of pulpal inflammation, which is of critical importance in determining when the step from reversible to irreversible pulpitis occurs with its consequent impact on clinical management of the tooth. The low-compliance environment of the dentin-pulp complex, which constrains tissue swelling, likely contributes to the control of the extent and intensity of the inflammatory response. Uncontrolled inflammatory responses associated with irreversible pulpitis severely compromise the opportunities for tissue regeneration within the dentin-pulp complex and drive treatment-planning decisions. There would thus be considerable merit in developing therapeutic strategies to control inflammatory/immune processes in the pulp, while recognizing that an inflammatory response of short-lived duration and intensity is a fundamental defense response for any tissue in the body. Microbial control in the carious tooth clearly provides a prime mode of dampening the inflammatory responses, but targeting signaling cascades, including the Toll-like receptors, nuclear factor κβ activation, and transcription pathways, such as those involving p38 MAP-kinase,[32,33] may also have merit. Proresolving lipid mediators, including lipoxins, resolvins, and protectins, are important in the suppression of inflammation[36] and may also provide valuable targets. The broad range of anti-inflammatory peptides and other molecules being developed within the pharmaceutical industry may have potential application in the diseased tooth and thereby provide more generic solutions to sourcing such drugs. Focus on the control of inflammation, and the associated challenge from carious bacteria, offers immense potential to significantly improve opportunities for successful vital pulp therapy and facilitate pulpal regeneration.

CELLULAR EVENTS IN DENTIN-PULP REGENERATION

Development of effective strategies for pulpal regeneration requires both consideration and understanding of the behavior of the cells of the pulp in health as well as disease. Many aspects of regeneration within the dentin-pulp complex seem to recapitulate developmental events, albeit with a lesser degree of regulatory control.[37] This aspect perhaps highlights the great adaptability of the dentin-pulp complex to respond to environmental changes and its strong regenerative potential. Fundamental to this responsiveness is the odontoblast, which can mediate defense as well as secretory roles. These cells represent a unique population of cells that survive for the life of a tooth in the absence of injury. Following terminal differentiation during tooth development, these cells become postmitotic in nature, and have an active synthetic and secretory role during primary dentinogenesis as the crown and root of the tooth are laid down. Subsequently, during secondary dentinogenesis their activity is significantly downregulated and they become largely quiescent, slowly secreting secondary dentin. However, odontoblasts may become upregulated in response to injury, secreting a tertiary dentin matrix to repair and regenerate the tissue and thereby restoring the tooth's structural integrity. This adaptability of the odontoblast makes it an excellent candidate target for regenerative strategies in the treatment of dental disease.

Tertiary dentinogenesis in fact represents a range of cellular responses, which are dependent on the severity of the injury to the tooth (**Fig. 3**). For injury of lesser intensity,

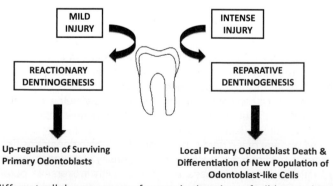

Fig. 3. The different cellular sequences of events in situations of mild versus intense injury to the tooth.

such as during early caries, tooth wear, and so forth, a response of reactionary dentinogenesis may be seen. In such situations, the primary odontoblasts responsible for dentin formation during tooth development will survive, their activity being upregulated to secrete a reactionary tertiary dentin matrix. This matrix increases the distance between the cells and the injurious challenge, and protects the pulp from greater injury. As the injury intensifies, however, the survival of the odontoblasts beneath the site of injury is increasingly compromised, and eventually cellular death can occur. If the tissue environment is conducive in terms of control of the microbial and inflammatory challenges, a new generation of odontoblast-like cells may differentiate from stem/progenitor cells from within the pulp and secrete a reparative tertiary dentin matrix. A specific example of such reparative dentinogenesis is the dentin-bridge formation seen at sites of pulpal exposure after direct pulp-capping interventions. The complexity of cellular events differs significantly between reactionary and reparative dentinogenesis.[38] Reactionary dentinogenesis simply represents the upregulation of existing primary odontoblasts from their quiescent state following primary dentinogenesis, whereas reparative dentinogenesis is more complex and requires the recruitment and differentiation of stem/progenitor cells before upregulation of the newly differentiated odontoblast-like cells for reparative dentine secretion.

Reparative dentinogenesis clearly is important in both providing a barrier to further injurious cellular challenge and helping to restore the tooth's structural integrity. As the matrix is secreted by a new generation of odontoblast-like cells, there will commonly not be tubular continuity with the dentinal tubules of the primary dentin, thereby increasing the role of this matrix as a protective barrier. In fact, the morphology of reparative dentin can be very variable in terms of its degree of tubularity,[39] which has consequences for the permeability of the tissue and perhaps also reflects the pathologic nature of the secretion. The tight control of events leading to odontoblast differentiation during tooth development will not necessarily be replicated during reparative dentinogenesis and, importantly, the cells differentiating to odontoblast-like cells may not all be of the same embryonic origin or developmental state as those giving rise to primary odontoblasts. Over the last decade there has been considerable interest in the presence of stem cells in pulp and their potential application to regenerative medicine, in both the tooth and other tissues of the body. Several populations of stem cells have been reported in the pulp, including dental pulp stem cells, stem cells from the apical part of the papilla, and stem cells from human exfoliated deciduous teeth, and there is still much to learn about these various populations in terms of their homogeneity, derivation, and responses.[40] An important question to address is whether these represent mesenchymal stem cells recruited through the circulation from sites outside the tooth and if their exposure to the niche environment within the pulp provides their phenotypic characteristics. Recent evidence supports such an origin for some cells involved in odontoblast-like cell differentiation,[41] which has significant implications for tissue-engineering strategies in the dentin-pulp complex. It is possible that the neural-crest origin of odontoblasts[42] may not be critical to the differentiation of odontoblast-like cells and the reparative dentin matrix they secrete. Pulp tissue engineering clearly has immense potential to have an impact on the future direction of endodontics, but unlike regenerative approaches exploiting the presence of cells in residual pulp tissue, tissue engineering requires identification of suitable stem-cell sources for the engineering of tissue constructs. SHED cells provide a source of autologous cells that may be harvested noninvasively, and their seeding in a polylactic acid polymeric scaffold within a tooth slice has allowed engineering of pulp tissue resembling that seen physiologically.[9] Isolated dental pulp cells seeded with angiogenic growth factors in a collagen scaffold within a pulpless tooth chamber have been reported to allow tissue generation, with evidence of revascularization after in vivo implantation.[10] Such tissue-engineering approaches offer exciting potential for the future of endodontics, but regenerative strategies based on the concept of pulpotomy provide significant potential for many patients if the management of cases can be better targeted in terms of controlling the pulpal environment to be more conducive to regeneration.

MOLECULAR EVENTS IN DENTIN-PULP REGENERATION

The signaling of cellular differentiation and secretory regulation for dentinogenesis is closely controlled in temporospatial terms through epithelial-mesenchymal interactions between the cells of the tooth germ. These interactions, many of which are recapitulated during repair and regeneration in the mature tooth, have a molecular basis.[37] Understanding these molecular signaling events is crucial to not only initiating pulpal regeneration but also to controlling subsequent cellular activity in the tissue, where overall tooth architecture must be maintained if pulp-canal obliteration is to be avoided. Several aspects of molecular signaling of cellular events are of critical importance:

- Recruitment of stem/progenitor cells
- Induction of odontoblast-like cell differentiation
- Upregulation of odontoblast-like cell synthetic and secretory activity
- Stimulation of pulpal revascularization
- Control of odontoblast-like cell activity to preserve crown and root architecture.

It seems likely that several molecules can provide a stimulus for cellular migration in the pulp, including various growth factors, cytokines,[43] and extracellular matrix molecules.[44] There is still much to learn about how these molecules may be directed for cellular recruitment to injury sites in a controlled manner, but their identification provides a first step to achieving this goal. Once recruited, the differentiation of these cells perhaps shows close parallels to tooth development whereby signals from the inner-enamel epithelium induce odontoblast differentiation in cells at the periphery of the dental papilla through the intermediary action of the dental basement membrane. Growth factors, particularly those of the transforming growth factor-β (TGF-β) family, are important in signaling odontoblast differentiation during tooth development.[45,46] Although an epithelial-derived source of signaling is absent in the mature tooth, an alternative source can be found within the dentin matrix. Isolated dentin-matrix components have been demonstrated to induce reparative dentinogenesis in a pulp-capping situation,[47] which reflects a long-recognized observation that dentin chips have similar effects.[48] Dentin matrix, in fact, contains a plethora of noncollagenous components[49] in addition to the collagen and mineral generally recognized to comprise this matrix. Many of these noncollagenous components have significant biological activities, and dentin should therefore be considered as a bioactive matrix[50] rather than the more traditional view of it as an inert tissue with primarily a mechanical role. Many growth factors and cytokines are reported as sequestered within dentin matrix during its secretion,[31,51,52] and it is probable that many others will be identified too. Of particular note is the presence of members of the TGF-β family,[51] which have been implicated in the signaling of odontoblast differentiation during tooth development.[45] Release of these growth factors during carious demineralization of the tissue may signal odontoblast-like cell differentiation for dentin-pulp regeneration in a parallel manner to the role of enamel organ signaling during tooth development. The presence of angiogenic growth factors in dentin[52] and the demonstration of the action of these matrix-derived molecules in signaling angiogenic events[53] suggest ways by which pulpal revascularization may be promoted, which will be of fundamental importance to pulpal regeneration.

Regulation of odontoblast or odontoblast-like cell secretion during reactionary and reparative dentinogenesis, respectively, is critical to maintenance of the tooth's normal architecture and avoidance of pulp-canal obliteration. The latter event represents a significant challenge in endodontic treatment and is not uncommon,[54] highlighting the importance of understanding the control of odontoblast secretory activity and the need to address this issue in developing new regenerative approaches for the dentin-pulp complex. The ability to switch odontoblast secretion on or off would represent a powerful clinical tool in the management of the diseased tooth. Odontoblast secretion can be upregulated by growth factors of the TGF-β family,[55] but downregulation of secretion may not be achieved in the necessary time frame by simply limiting the supply of this ligand. However, targeting of the intracellular signaling pathways for these ligands may provide a suitable approach to control these events. Indeed, the MAP-kinase pathway activated via p38 phosphorylation may provide the molecular switch in the odontoblast to turn secretion on and off.[56] Pharmaceutical inhibitors of this pathway are available, and offer exciting potential for clinical control of odontoblast secretion in endodontics.

TRANSLATIONAL OPPORTUNITIES FOR DENTIN-PULP REGENERATION

Our understanding of the biology of the dentin-pulp complex in both health and disease has improved significantly over the last 2 decades, and has positioned endodontics to be able to respond as a specialty to the opportunities for introduction of novel regenerative strategies for disease management. In the future, as pulp tissue-engineering therapies become a part of routine clinical practice, they will have significant impact on endodontic root canal treatment. Stimulation of regeneration in the inflamed pulp following caries, however, provides the opportunity to make significant contributions to preservation of pulp vitality and improvements to the currently unsatisfactory long-term survival rates for many dental restorations. The challenge, however, perhaps lies in assessing the disease status of each individual case and tailoring treatment planning to reflect this. There is commonly an assumption that pulp regeneration should only be attempted in immature teeth with open apices, and there may be merit in being a little more ambitious than this in case selection. More focused control of bacteria and inflammation may also aid in the realization of such a goal.

Cavity irrigants/etchants and disinfectants have considerable potential to improve treatment outcomes, and may only require more minor changes to daily practice. Use of these agents has been targeted mainly in cavity cleansing and smear-layer removal, to promote better bonding of restorations and to minimize the bacterial load at the tissue-restoration interface where marginal leakage can compromise retention of restorations. To date, there has been only limited consideration given as to how these agents might be used to biological advantage and also how to avoid further tissue damage. This aspect is highlighted by sodium hypochlorite and EDTA, commonly used for disinfection and irrigation, whereby the manner of their use has important implications for preservation of tissue structure.[57] Based on scanning electron microscopic observations, sodium hypochlorite followed by EDTA treatment of an instrumented canal allows preservation of dentin structure morphologically, but EDTA followed by sodium hypochlorite treatment results in considerable dentin damage. This finding perhaps reflects protection of the dentin from the oxidizing action of sodium hypochlorite when still mineralized while still allowing its antibacterial action to be exerted. However, etching with EDTA appears to remove this protective effect. These agents may also have significant potential to locally release the bioactive growth factors and other molecules sequestered within dentin, which can signal regenerative events. Several studies have demonstrated the capacity of cavity etchants and irrigants to release and expose growth factors in dentin,[58–60] and their potential to directly stimulate reactionary dentinogenesis[61] highlights the opportunities to exploit their use to promote regenerative events.

Restorative materials also offer potential for promotion of regenerative events in dentin-pulp. Direct pulp capping with calcium hydroxide has long been used to stimulate healing in the exposed pulp, although in the absence of mechanistic understanding its use has been perhaps somewhat empiric, with consequent implications for treatment outcomes. A possible mechanism for the action of this agent is its ability to give rise to limited dissolution of the dentin surface with which it make contact, thereby releasing bioactive constituents such as growth factors from the dentin.[62] Release of TGF-β and other bioactive constituents of dentin may be important in signaling regenerative events responsible for reparative dentinogenesis, giving rise to dentin-bridge formation. Similar actions for MTA in the dissolution of growth factors and bioactive molecules from dentin[30] imply parallel mechanisms of action. The relative proportions of these molecules dissolved from dentin differ for white and gray variants of MTA,[30] although the reasons for this are unclear. Nevertheless, if these mechanisms of action for calcium hydroxide and MTA prove important, there is considerable opportunity to optimize their effects by modification of the formulations, setting characteristics and associated mechanical properties. Undoubtedly other restorative materials will be found to also have pro-regenerative effects, and development of materials with antimicrobial and anti-inflammatory properties offers significant potential benefits.

SUMMARY

Significant opportunities exist to improve on clinical treatment outcomes for dental disease with more focused attention on the biological processes taking place in the tissues. Harnessing the natural regenerative potential of dentin-pulp can improve opportunities for maintenance of a vital pulp and tooth survival following injury. However, the close interplay between infection, inflammation, and regeneration requires careful consideration of the cellular and molecular events occurring in the tissues and treatment strategies that tip the balance toward regeneration. Such approaches can be exploited now, and will help to underpin the clinical translation of dental tissue-engineering therapies in the future.

REFERENCES

1. Mason C, Dunnill P. A brief definition of regenerative medicine. Regen Med 2006; 3:1–5.
2. Ohazama A, Modino SA, Miletich I, et al. Stem-cell-based tissue engineering of murine teeth. J Dent Res 2004;83:518–22.
3. Duailibi MT, Duailibi SE, Young CS, et al. Bioengineered teeth from cultured rat tooth bud cells. J Dent Res 2004;83:523–8.
4. Hu B, Nadiri A, Bopp-Küchler S, et al. Dental epithelial histomorphogenesis in vitro. J Dent Res 2005;84:521–5.
5. Hu B, Unda F, Bopp-Kuchler S, et al. Bone marrow cells can give rise to ameloblast-like cells. J Dent Res 2006;85:416–21.

6. Honda MJ, Tsuchiya S, Sumita Y, et al. The sequential seeding of epithelial and mesenchymal cells for tissue-engineered tooth regeneration. Biomaterials 2007; 28:80–689.
7. Smith AJ, Sharpe PT. Biological tooth replacement and repair. In: Lanza R, Langer R, Vacanti J, editors. Principles of tissue engineering. 3rd edition. Amsterdam: Elsevier; 2007. p. 1067–79.
8. Ikeda E, Morita R, Nakao K, et al. Fully functional bioengineered tooth replacement as an organ replacement therapy. Proc Natl Acad Sci U S A 2009;106:13475–80.
9. Cordeiro MM, Dong Z, Kaneko T, et al. Dental pulp tissue engineering with stem cells from exfoliated deciduous teeth. J Endod 2008;34:962–9.
10. Srisuwan T, Tilkorn DJ, Al-Benna S, et al. Revascularization and tissue regeneration of an empty root canal space is enhanced by a direct blood supply and stem cells. Dent Traumatol 2012. DOI: 10.1111/j.1600-9657.2012.01136.x.
11. Hermann BW. Calcium hydroxyd als mitten zum behandeln und füllen von wurzelkanällen [dissertation]. University of Wursburg: 1920. [reprinted in: Malo PRT, Kessler Nieto F, Vadillo MVM. Hidroxido de calcio y apicoformacio. Revista Española de Endodoncia 1987;5:41–61].
12. Zander HA. Reaction of the dental pulp to calcium hydroxide. J Dent Res 1939; 181:373–9.
13. Nair PN, Duncan HF, Pitt Ford TR, et al. Histological, ultrastructural and quantitative investigations on the response of healthy human pulps to experimental capping with mineral trioxide aggregate: a randomized controlled trial. Int Endod J 2008;41:128–50.
14. Lucarotti PS, Holder RL, Burke FJ. Analysis of an administrative database of half a million restorations over 11 years. J Dent 2005;33:791–803.
15. Guideline on pulp therapy for primary and immature permanent teeth. American Academy of pediatric Dentistry (AAPD) Reference manual. Available at: http://www.aapd.org/media/policies_guidelines/g_pulp.pdf. Accessed May 14, 2012.
16. Bjorndal L, Darvann T, Thylstrup A. A quantitative light microscopic study of the odontoblast and subdontoblastic reactions to active and arrested enamel caries without cavitation. Caries Res 1998;31:59–69.
17. Bjorndal L, Darvann T. A light microscopic study of odontoblastic and non-odontoblastic cells involved in tertiary dentinogenesis in well-defined cavitated carious lesions. Caries Res 1999;33:50–60.
18. Lu Y, Xie Y, Zhang S, et al. DMP1-targeted Cre expression in odontoblasts and osteocytes. J Dent Res 2007;86:320–5.
19. Murray PE, Hafez A, Smith AJ, et al. Hierarchy of pulp capping and repair activities responsible for dentin bridge formation. Am J Dent 2002;15:236–43.
20. Love RM, Jenkinson HF. Invasion of dentinal tubules by oral bacteria. Crit Rev Oral Biol Med 2002;13:171–83.
21. Murdoch-Kinch CA, Mclean ME. Minimally invasive dentistry. J Am Dent Assoc 2003;134:87–95.
22. Mjor IA. Clinical diagnosis of recurrent caries. J Am Dent Assoc 2005;136: 1426–33.
23. Imazato S, Kinomoto Y, Tarumi H, et al. Incorporation of antibacterial monomer MDPB into dentin primer. J Dent Res 1997;76:768–72.
24. Desai S, Chandler N. Calcium hydroxide-based root canal sealers: a review. J Endod 2009;35:475–80.
25. Smith JS, Smith AJ, Shelton RM, et al. Antibacterial activity of dentine and pulp extracellular matrix extracts. Int Endod J 2012. DOI: 10.1111/j.1365-2591.2012.02031.x.

26. Awawdeh LA, Lundy FT, Linden GJ, et al. Quantitative analysis of substance P, neurokinin A and calcitonin gene-related peptide in gingival crevicular fluid associated with painful human teeth. Eur J Oral Sci 2002;110:185–91.

27. El Karim I, Lundy FT, Linden GJ, et al. Extraction and radioimmunoassay quantitation of neuropeptide Y (NPY) and vasoactive intestinal polypeptide (VIP) from human dental pulp tissue. Arch Oral Biol 2003;48:249–54.

28. El Karim IA, Lamey PJ, Ardill J, et al. Vasoactive intestinal polypeptide (VIP) and VPAC1 receptor in adult human dental pulp in relation to caries. Arch Oral Biol 2006;51:849–55.

29. El Karim IA, Linden GJ, Orr DF, et al. Antimicrobial activity of neuropeptides against a range of micro-organisms from skin, oral, respiratory and gastrointestinal tract sites. J Neuroimmunol 2008;200:11–6.

30. Tomson PL, Grover LM, Lumley PJ, et al. Dissolution of bio-active dentine matrix components by mineral trioxide aggregate. J Dent 2007;35:636–42.

31. Musson DS, McLachlan JL, Sloan AJ, et al. Adrenomedullin is expressed during rodent dental tissue development and promotes cell growth and mineralisation. Biol Cell 2010;102:145–57.

32. Cooper PR, Takahashi Y, Graham LW, et al. Inflammation-regeneration interplay in the dentine-pulp complex. J Dent 2010;38:687–97.

33. Cooper PR, McLachlan JL, Simon S, et al. Mediators of inflammation and regeneration. Adv Dent Res 2011;23:290–5.

34. Fouad AF. Molecular mediators of pulp inflammation. In: Hargreaves KM, Goodis HE, Tay FR, editors. Seltzer and Bender's dental pulp. 2nd edition. Chicago: Quintessence Pub Co Inc; 2012. p. 241–76.

35. Murray PE, Smith AJ. Saving pulps—a biological basis. Prim Dent Care 2002;9: 21–6.

36. Serhan CN. The resolution of inflammation: the devil in the flask and in the details. FASEB J 2011;25:1441–8.

37. Smith AJ, Lesot H. Induction and regulation of crown dentinogenesis—embryonic events as a template for dental tissue repair. Crit Rev Oral Biol Med 2001;12: 425–37.

38. Smith AJ, Cassidy N, Perry H, et al. Reactionary dentinogenesis. Int J Dev Biol 1995;39:273–80.

39. Smith AJ. Formation and repair of dentin in the adult. In: Hargreaves KM, Goodis HE, Tay FR, editors. Seltzer and Bender's dental pulp. 2nd edition. Chicago: Quintessence Pub Co Inc; 2012. p. 27–46.

40. Sloan AJ, Smith AJ. Stem cells and the dental pulp: potential roles in tissue regeneration. Oral Dis 2007;13:151–7.

41. Feng J, Mantesso A, De Bari C, et al. Dual origin of mesenchymal stem cells contributing to organ growth and repair. Proc Natl Acad Sci U S A 2011;108: 6503–8.

42. Chai Y, Jiang X, Ito Y, et al. Fate of the mammalian cranial neural crest during tooth and mandibular morphogenesis. Development 2000;127:1671–9.

43. Suzuki T, Lee CH, Chen M, et al. Induced migration of dental pulp stem cells for in vivo pulp regeneration. J Dent Res 2011;90:1013–8.

44. Smith JG, Smith AJ, Shelton RM, et al. The effects of pulp and dentine ECM components and their breakdown products on dental pulp cell recruitment. Int Endod J 2012, in press.

45. Begue-Kirn C, Smith AJ, Ruch JV, et al. Effects of dentin proteins, transforming growth factor β1 (TGFβ1) and bone morphogenetic protein 2 (BMP2) on the differentiation of odontoblasts in vitro. Int J Dev Biol 1992;36:491–503.

46. Begue-Kirn C, Smith AJ, Loriot M, et al. Comparative analysis of TGFβs, BMPs, IGF, msxs, fibronectin, osteonectin and bone sialoprotein gene expressions during normal and in vitro induced odontoblast differentiation. Int J Dev Biol 1994;38:405–20.

47. Smith AJ, Tobias RS, Plant CG, et al. In vivo morphogenetic activity of dentine matrix proteins. J Biol Buccale 1990;18:123–9.

48. Anneroth G, Bang G. The effect of allogeneic demineralized dentin as a pulp capping agent in Java monkeys. Odontol Revy 1972;23:315–28.

49. Goldberg M, Smith AJ. Cells and extracellular matrices of dentin and pulp: a biological basis for repair and tissue engineering. Crit Rev Oral Biol Med 2004;15:13–27.

50. Smith AJ, Scheven BA, Takahashi Y, et al. Dentine as a bioactive extracellular matrix. Arch Oral Biol 2012;57:109–21.

51. Cassidy N, Fahey M, Prime SS, et al. Comparative analysis of transforming growth factor-beta (TGF-β) isoforms 1-3 in human and rabbit dentine matrices. Arch Oral Biol 1997;42:219–23.

52. Roberts-Clark D, Smith AJ. Angiogenic growth factors in human dentine matrix. Arch Oral Biol 2000;45:1013–6.

53. Zhang R, Cooper PR, Smith G, et al. Angiogenic activity of dentin matrix components. J Endod 2011;34:26–30.

54. McCabe PS, Dummer PM. Pulp canal obliteration: an endodontic diagnosis and treatment challenge. Int Endod J 2012;45:177–97.

55. Sloan AJ, Smith AJ. Stimulation of the dentine-pulp complex of rat incisor teeth by transforming growth factor-β isoforms 1-3 in vitro. Arch Oral Biol 1999;44:149–56.

56. Simon S, Smith AJ, Berdal A, et al. The MAPK pathway is involved in odontoblast stimulation via p38 phosphorylation. J Endod 2010;36:256–9.

57. Haapasalo M, Shen Y, Qian W, et al. Irrigation in endodontics. Dent Clin North Am 2010;54:291–312.

58. Smith AJ, Smith G. Solubilisation of TGF-β1 by dentine conditioning agents. J Dent Res 1998;77:1034.

59. Zhao S, Sloan AJ, Murray PE, et al. Ultrastructural localisation of TGF-β exposure in dentine by chemical treatment. Histochem J 2000;32:489–94.

60. Galler KM, D'Souza RN, Federlin M, et al. Dentin conditioning codetermines cell fate in regenerative endodontics. J Endod 2011;37:1536–41.

61. Murray PE, Smith AJ, Garcia-Godoy F, et al. Comparison of operative procedure variables on pulpal viability in an ex vivo model. Int Endod J 2008;41:389–400.

62. Graham L, Cooper PR, Cassidy N, et al. The effect of calcium hydroxide on solubilisation of bio-active dentine matrix components. Biomaterials 2006;27:2865–73.

Clinical Considerations for Regenerative Endodontic Procedures

Todd M. Geisler, DDS

KEYWORDS

- Revascularization • Regeneration • Immature teeth • Open apex • Stem cells • MTA
- Dental pulp • Tissue engineering

KEY POINTS

- Case reports have indicated that biologically based endodontic therapies can result in the elimination of apical periodontitis. There is no question that regenerative endodontics procedures can be successful. The present issue is how to develop safe, effective and consistent methods for regenerating a functional pulp-dentin complex in patients.
- There are obvious benefits of regenerative endodontic procedures for the immature root; however, mature teeth may also benefit from the regeneration of a vital pulp-dentin complex. If the treatment plan of a tooth with extensive caries could be altered from certain extraction to being properly restored as a result of the regeneration of dentinal tooth structure, endodontists would have engineered a more desirable outcome.
- The reestablishment of vitality and a functional immune response may allow the body to better fight the presence of any remaining bacteria within the canal system. Thus, future efforts must focus on a more biologic and scientific approach to these endodontic procedures.
- Randomized prospective multicenter trials offer the potential to develop evidenced-based methodologies for these pioneering regenerative endodontic procedures.

INTRODUCTION

Regenerative endodontic procedures (REPs) can be defined as biologically based procedures designed to replace damaged structures including dentin and cells of the pulp-dentin complex.[1] Case studies have presented clinically successful regenerative endodontic procedures in vivo (**Table 1**), but the present information remains inadequate to define a single regenerative protocol. Despite published outcomes, clinicians continue to question the predictability of the procedure. Anecdotal evidence suggests moderate success rates and a need for more reliable protocols.

Author is President and Co-founder of BioMatRx. BioMatRx, LLC is a Minnesota-based biotech company that supplies tissue engineering products, equipment and information to the dental industry. Specifically, BioMatRx products focus on the regeneration of the dental pulp. BioMatRx, LLC, 5775 Wayzata Boulevard, Suite 700, Minneapolis, MN 55416, USA
E-mail address: geislerendo@me.com

Dent Clin N Am 56 (2012) 603–626
http://dx.doi.org/10.1016/j.cden.2012.05.010
0011-8532/12/$ – see front matter © 2012 Elsevier Inc. All rights reserved.

Table 1
Human in vivo case reports. The table organizes multiple factors that may be related to specific outcomes such as age, teeth treated, periapical diagnosis (at time of presentation to endodontic clinic), irrigant, depth/technique of irrigation, antimicrobial, antimicrobial placement method, duration of antimicrobial tissue in canal, creation of blood clot scaffold, pulp space barrier/restoration

	Age (y)	Tooth No. Treated	Periapical Diagnosis (at Time of Presentation to Endodontic Clinic)	Irrigant(s)	Depth/ Technique of Irrigation	Antimicrobial	Antimicrobial Placement Method	Duration of Antimicrobial	Tissue in Canal?	Evoke Blood Clot-Scaffold?	Pulp Space Barrier/ Restoration
Iwaya et al,[2] 2001	13	29	Chronic apical abscess	5% NaOCl; 3% hydrogen peroxide (weekly for 5 wk)	Coronal portion of root	Metronidazole; ciprofloxacin (weekly for 5 wk)	No indication	4 wk	Yes	Smooth broach inserted to vital tissue; no report of bleeding	Ca(OH)$_2$; glass ionomer; composite resin
Banchs and Trope,[3] 2004	11	29	Chronic apical abscess	5.25% NaOCl; Peridex	Within 1 mm of apex	Metronidazole; ciprofloxacin; minocycline	Lentulo	26 d	Yes	Endodontic explorer used to create bleeding 3 mm below CEJ	MTA; composite resin
Chueh and Huang,[4] 2006	10	20	Chronic apical abscess	2.5% NaOCl	Pulp chamber	Ca(OH)$_2$	No indication	3 mo	Hard tissue barrier	None	Ca(OH)$_2$; Cavit; amalgam
	10	29	Acute apical abscess	2.5% NaOCl	Pulp chamber	Ca(OH)$_2$	No indication	8 wk	Hard tissue barrier	Hemorrhage observed	Ca(OH)$_2$; Cavit; Ketac Silver
	10	20	Chronic apical abscess	2.5% NaOCl	Canal irrigated	Formocresol (before referral) Ca(OH)$_2$	No indication	1 mo	Hard tissue barrier	None	Ca(OH)$_2$; Cavit; glass ionomer; removed at 18.5 mo and amalgam placed
	9	29	Acute apical abscess	2.5% NaOCl	Canal irrigated	Ca(OH)$_2$	No indication	5 wk	Hard tissue barrier	None	Ca(OH)$_2$; IRM; removed at 3y and amalgam placed

Study			Diagnosis	Irrigant	Placement	Medicament	Delivery	Time	Apical barrier	Bleeding induction	Material
Petrino[5] 2007	8	8	Chronic apical abscess	5.25% NaOCl; Peridex	Within 1 mm of apex	Metronidazole; ciprofloxacin; minocycine	No indication	No indication	Yes; vital tissue felt	Endodontic explorer used to create bleeding 3 mm below CEJ	MTA; composite resin
Thibodeau and Trope,[6,7] 2007 and 2009	9	8	Acute apical abscess	1.25% NaOCl	Canal irrigated	Metronidazole; ciprofloxacin; cefaclor	Lentulo and tamped down with sterile paper points	11 wk	No	Endodontic file to create bleeding	wMTA; composite resin
Jung et al,[8] 2008	10	29	Chronic apical abscess	5.25% NaOCl	Canal irrigated	(1) Metronidazole; ciprofloxacin; minocycine. (2) Erythromycin and Ca(OH)$_2$. (3) Ca(OH)$_2$	Lentulo	88 d	Hard tissue barrier	None	Gutta-percha; composite resin
		28	Chronic apical abscess	5.25% NaOCl	Canal irrigated	Metronidazole; ciprofloxacin; minocycine	Lentulo	67 d	Hard tissue barrier	None	Gutta-percha; composite resin
	10	29	Chronic apical abscess	5.25% NaOCl	Canal irrigated	Metronidazole; ciprofloxacin; minocycine	Lentulo	11 d	Yes	None	MTA; composite resin
	10	20	Asymptomatic apical periodontitis (left open)	5.25% NaOCl	Canal irrigated	(1) Metronidazole; ciprofloxacin; minocycine (2) Ca(OH)$_2$	Lentulo	(1) 30 d (2) 40 d	Yes	Hemorrhage observed after 30 d	MTA; composite resin
	13	20	Symptomatic apical periodontitis	5.25% NaOCl	Canal irrigated	Metronidazole; ciprofloxacin; minocycine	Lentulo	2 wk	Yes	None	MTA; IRM
	10	20	Asymptomatic apical periodontitis (left open)	2.5% NaOCl	Canal irrigated	Metronidazole; ciprofloxacin; minocycline	No indication	1 wk	No	Endodontic file to create bleeding	MTA; composite resin
	9	20	Chronic apical abscess	2.5% NaOCl	Canal irrigated	Metronidazole; ciprofloxacin; minocycline	Lentulo	1 wk	Yes	Endodontic file to create bleeding	MTA; composite resin

(continued on next page)

Table 1
(continued)

	Age (y)	Tooth No. Treated	Periapical Diagnosis (at Time of Presentation to Endodontic Clinic)	Irrigant(s)	Depth/Technique of Irrigation	Antimicrobial	Antimicrobial Placement Method	Duration of Antimicrobial	Tissue in Canal?	Evoke Blood Clot-Scaffold?	Pulp Space Barrier/Restoration
	14	29	Chronic apical abscess	2.5% NaOCl	Canal irrigated	Ca(OH)$_2$ (aqueous)	No indication	1 wk	No	Endodontic file to create bleeding	MTA; composite resin
	10	29	Asymptomatic apical periodontitis (left open)	2.5% NaOCl	Canal irrigated	Metronidazole; ciprofloxacin; minocycline	No indication	3 wk	No	Endodontic file to create bleeding	Collatape; MTA; composite resin
Cotti et al,[9] 2008	9	8	Chronic apical abscess	5% NaOCl; 3% hydrogen peroxide	Coronal portion of root	Ca(OH)$_2$ powder	Plugger	2 wk	Yes	Endodontic file to create bleeding	MTA; glass ionomer; composite resin
Shah et al,[10] 2008	9–18	14 teeth	Chronic apical abscess; asymptomatic apical periodontitis	2.5% NaOCl; 3% hydrogen peroxide	Canal irrigated	Formocresol	Cotton pellet	Subsequent appointment	No	Needle to create bleeding	Glass ionomer
Chueh et al,[11] 2009	6–14	23 teeth	Chronic apical abscess; asymptomatic apical periodontitis; acute apical abscess	2.5% NaOCl	Canal irrigated	Ca(OH)$_2$	Loosely placed	1–25 mo	Hard tissue barrier	No instrumentation OR Endodontic instrument to create bleeding	(1) Gutta-percha/composite or Amal. (2) MTA/gutta-percha/composite or amalgam. (3) Amalgam
Ding et al,[12] 2009	8–11	3 (available for analysis)	Chronic apical abscess; acute apical abscess	5.25% NaOCl	Gently flushed	Metronidazole; ciprofloxacin; minocycline	No indication	1 wk	No indication	Endodontic file to create bleeding	MTA; composite
Shin et al,[13] 2009	12	29	Chronic apical abscess	6% NaOCl/Saline/2% chlorhexidine	Coronal portion of root	None (1-step procedure)	N/A	N/A	Yes	Endodontic file to create bleeding	wMTA; composite

Reynolds et al,[14] 2009	11	2 teeth	Chronic apical abscess	6% NaOCl/Saline/2% chlorhexidine	2 mm from apex	Metronidazole; ciprofloxacin; minocycline (composite bonding/no staining)	Needle 2 mm short of apex	4 wk	No indication	Endodontic file to create bleeding	gMTA/composite
Kim et al,[15] 2010	7	8	Symptomatic apical periodontitis	3% NaOCl	Canal irrigated	Metronidazole; ciprofloxacin; minocycline (staining/bleached)	Lentulo	6 wk	No indication	Paper points to create bleeding	MTA/glass ionomer/composite
Petrino et al,[16] 2010	6–13	5 teeth	Chronic apical abscess; asymptomatic apical periodontitis	5.25% NaOCl/saline/Peridex	Canal irrigated	Metronidazole; ciprofloxacin; minocycline	No indication	3 wk	No	Endodontic file to create bleeding and CollaPlug (2 teeth)	MTA/composite
Thomson and Kahler,[17] 2010	12	20	Chronic apical abscess	1% NaOCl (with ultrasonic activation)	2 mm from apex	Metronidazole; ciprofloxacin; minocycline	Lentu o	6 wk	No indication	Endodontic explorer used to create bleeding 3 mm below CEJ	wMTA/glass ionomer/composite
Nosrat et al,[18] 2011	9	30	Symptomatic apical periodontitis	5.25% NaOCl	Canal irrigated	Metronidazole; ciprofloxacin; minocycline	Placed with K file	3 wk	Necrotic tissue	Endodontic file to create bleeding	CEM cement (calcium-enriched mixture)/glass ionomer/amalgam
	8	30	Chronic apical abscess	5.25% NaOCl	Canal irrigated	Metronidazole; ciprofloxacin; minocycline	Placed with K file	3 wk	No indication	Endodontic file to create bleeding	CEM cement (calcium-enriched mixture)/glass ionomer/SSC

(continued on next page)

Table 1
(continued)

Age (y)	Tooth No. Treated	Periapical Diagnosis (at Time of Presentation to Endodontic Clinic)	Irrigant(s)	Depth/ Technique of Irrigation	Antimicrobial	Antimicrobial Placement Method	Duration of Antimicrobial	Tissue in Canal?	Evoke Blood Clot-Scaffold?	Pulp Space Barrier/ Restoration
Lenzi and Trope,[19] 2012	3	8	Inconclusive	2.5% NaOCl	Canal irrigated	Metronidazole; ciprofloxacin; minocycline	Lentulo	35 d	No indication	Endodontic file to create bleeding	MTA Angelus/ composite
		9	Asymptomatic apical periodontitis	2.5% NaOCl	Canal irrigated	Metronidazole; ciprofloxacin; minocycline	Lentulo	35 d	No indication	Endodontic file to create bleed ng	MTA Angelus/ composite
Cehreli et al,[20] 2011	3–11	6 teeth	Asymptomatic apical periodontitis	2.5% NaOCl	1–2 mm below orifice	Ca(OH)$_2$	Loosely placed	3 wk	No indication	Endodontic file to create bleeding	MTA; glass ionomer; composite or amalgam
Torabinejad and Turman,[21] 2011	11	4	Symptomatic apical periodontitis	5.25% NaOCl	Canal irrigated	Metronidazole; ciprofloxacin; minocycline	Amalgam carrier and endodontic pluggers	22 d	No indication	No creation of bleeding; PRP placed	MTA/Cavit/ amalgam
Iwaya et al,[22] 2011	7	24	Acute apical abscess	5% NaOCl; 3% hydrogen peroxide	Coronal portion of root (×5)	Ca(OH)$_2$		6 wk	Hard tissue barrier	None	Gutta-percha/ composite resin

Abbreviations: CEJ, cement-enamel junction; gMTA, gray mineral trioxide aggregate; IRM, immediate restorative material; N/A, not available; SSC, stainless steel crown; wMTA, white mineral trioxide aggregate.

Tissue Engineering

The ability to predictably regenerate natural tissues and create new tissues is the objective of the emerging field of tissue engineering. Nakashima[23] described 3 essential components of tissue engineering: stem/progenitor cells, morphogenetic signals and three-dimensional (3D) scaffolds. Stem cells, morphogens/growth factors, and biomimetic scaffolds all play essential roles in the restoration of previously damaged structures. By addressing the 3 elements of tissue engineering in future clinical guidelines, it is hoped to provide a microenvironment that is conducive to regeneration of pulplike tissues in patients.

COMMITMENT TO REGENERATIVE ENDODONTICS

Regenerative endodontics is a high priority for the specialty of endodontics. The number of publications in peer-reviewed journals related to regenerative endodontics has increased greatly in recent years (**Fig. 1**). Organized endodontics is committed to identifying evidence-based methodologies for these procedures. The next logical phase of regenerative endodontic research will be prospective randomized clinical trials.

The American Association of Endodontists (AAE) and the AAE Foundation recently released a request for proposals for clinical research into regenerative endodontic treatment with up to $2.5 million in funding for the project. Aside from these future high-level studies, the current case studies offer the benefit of being performed in patients and thus provide a higher level of evidence than animal studies or in vitro studies.

TRAUMA LITERATURE

Much of the basis for these case studies has rudiments in the trauma literature. Revascularization can occur but requires a particular set of circumstances that, until recently, were thought to be exclusive to the avulsed immature permanent tooth.[24] First, the exclusion of bacteria is the key factor in the success of this process. Second,

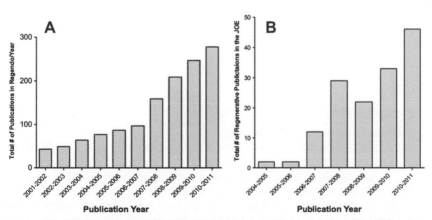

Fig. 1. (*A*) An OVID/Medline search was performed with the key words revascularization or regenerative or stem cells, and dental pulp or endodontics. Peer-reviewed publication number in each year since 2001 is presented. (*B*) A search was performed on www. jendodon.com with the key words revascu or regen or stem cell. Publication number in each year is presented. (*Courtesy of* A. Diogenes.)

the combination of an open apex and a short root allows the ingrowth of well-vascularized tissue. Third, the devitalized uninfected pulp is also thought to act as a scaffold for the ingress of apical tissue.[25] Successful revascularization of the pulp leads to the maturation of the root and deposition of hard tissue within the root, both of which improve the probability of long-term retention of the tooth.[26]

The notion then emerged that, if the pulp could be adequately disinfected, a blood clot matrix induced, and a bacteria-tight seal restored in a necrotic infected immature tooth, then, by extrapolation, revascularization should be expected to occur as in the devitalized, uninfected, avulsed, immature permanent tooth.[3,27–29]

Terminology

Revascularization, revitalization, and regeneration have all been used to describe the outcome of these procedures. There remains some disagreement in the terminology.[30,31] In vivo evidence suggests that it is unlikely that a functional pulp-dentin complex is being regenerating with current protocols. Wang and colleagues[32] noted that the tissue that is responsible for increased root thickness in their study was cementum and not dentin. As more is learned about the tissues that are present through both molecular methods and human histology, it will become possible to better define what it is being accomplished. This article unifies all 3 terms under the broader category of REPs and regenerative endodontic outcomes.

Goals of REPs

The goal of regenerative therapies is to regenerate a fully functional pulp-dentin complex that fosters continued root development for immature teeth, and prevents or resolves apical periodontitis.[33] As in traditional endodontic therapy, outcomes have various criteria for success. The degree of success of REPs is largely measured by the extent to which it is possible to attain primary, secondary, and tertiary goals.

The primary goals are the elimination of symptoms and the evidence of bony healing. Secondary goals (which are desirable but perhaps not essential) include increased root wall thickness and/or increased root length. A tertiary goal (which, if achieved, indicates a high level of success) is a positive response to vitality testing. Histologic confirmation of dental pulp with an intact odontoblastic layer and restoration of a functional pulp is the pinnacle of regenerative treatment goals.[34]

Regardless of this ultimate outcome, it is often beneficial to consider REPs if only to have a tooth act as a space maintainer until a suitable restorative option is available. In some cases, the achievement of the primary goals is all that is necessary to deem the procedure a success. REPs may provide hope for those teeth with unfavorable prognoses (**Fig. 2**).

Early Case Study Protocols

Nygaard-Østby and colleagues: pioneers

Attempts to pioneer regenerative procedures date as far back as the 1960s. In 1971, Nygaard-Østby and Hjortdal[35] evaluated the role of the blood clot in healing. They showed great foresight when they discussed the use of "growth promoting substances" to aid in healing after this partial root canal filling. The basic protocol was to aseptically access, extirpate the pulp, overinstrument the apex to evoke bleeding, and obturate the canals short of full length with Kloroperka and a gutta-percha point. They reported that the blood clot seemed to be essential for the connective tissue healing at the apex of an immature tooth. This finding was supported recently by an animal study[36] that indicated that it was the presence of the blood clot that was crucial for healing. In addition, Nygaard-Østby and Hjortdal[35] reported

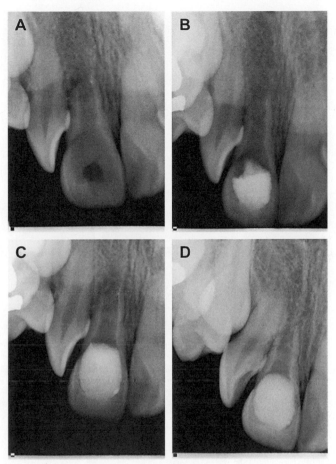

Fig. 2. Hope for the hopeless. (*A*) A 10-year-old patient presents with extensive caries, +2 mobility, and sinus tract. (*B*) 1:1 by volume of ciprofloxacin/metronidazole placed in canal. (*C*) At the 3-week visit for finalization of REP. Sinus tract resolved. (*D*) At the 20-month recall. The tooth does not respond to vitality testing but the tooth is asymptomatic with no mobility and there is radiographic evidence of healing.

that the blood clot in the root canal seemed to be organized by the granulation tissue growing in from the periapical area and not from the blood cells originally contained in the clot.

Although these were encouraging findings, histologic analysis was unable to confirm the regeneration of a pulp-dentin complex. In retrospect, these results are to be expected considering the availability of instruments, medications, and biomaterials at the time. Subsequent researchers[37,38] reported attempts to revitalize teeth with necrotic pulp with moderate success. Regenerative procedures then went largely ignored until an interest in these treatments was piqued by a case report by Iwaya and colleagues.[22]

Iwaya and colleagues: a renewed interest
In 2001, Iwaya and colleagues[2] showed the revascularization potential of an immature permanent tooth. A summary of the case report (**Fig. 3**) is as follows: a 13-year-old girl presented with a diagnosis of necrosis and chronic apical abscess on tooth 29. The

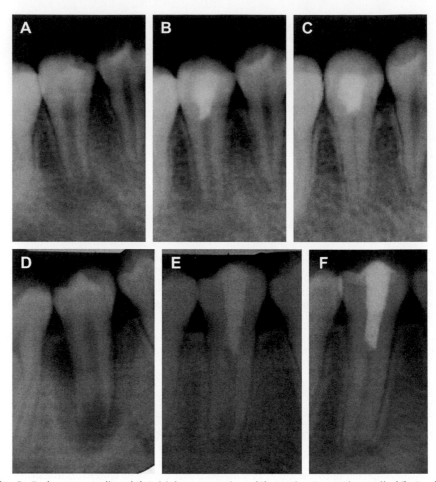

Fig. 3. Early case studies. (*A*) Initial presentation. (*B*) At the 5-month recall. (*C*) At the 30-month recall. (*D*) Initial presentation. (*E*) At the 7-month recall. (*F*) At the 24-month recall. (*From* Iwaya SI, Ikawa M, Kubota M. Revascularization of an immature permanent tooth with apical periodontitis and sinus tract. Dent Traumatol 2001;17:186; with permission; and (*C*) *From* Banchs F, Trope M. Revascularization of immature permanent teeth with apical periodontitis: new treatment protocol? J Endod 2004;30(4):197–9; with permission.)

tooth was accessed and allowed to drain. The patient returned and the sinus tract had healed. The coronal portion of the root was irrigated with 5% NaOCl and 3% hydrogen peroxide over a 4-week period. No instrumentation was performed. Metronidazole and ciprofloxacin were placed in canals for disinfection and the tooth was temporized. At the final visit, calcium hydroxide was placed and the access restored with glass ionomer and composite. Root development continued (see **Fig. 3**B) and the tooth was fully formed at 30 months (see **Fig. 3**C). Vitality testing revealed that the tooth responded to electric pulp testing (EPT).

Banchs and Trope: a new protocol
Borrowing on the basic principles of the trauma literature and the 2001 case report, Banchs and Trope[3] reported a case in 2004 and suggested a new protocol for

revascularization of a tooth with an immature root and apical periodontitis (see **Fig. 3**). The following 3 goals for REPs are based on emulating the conditions present in cases of successful revascularization of an immature avulsed permanent tooth. The first requirement is elimination of bacteria by effective canal disinfection. The second condition is the creation of a scaffold for the ingrowth of new tissue. The third prerequisite is the prevention of bacterial reinfection with creation of a bacteria-tight seal.

The case report was that of an 11-year-old child with a diagnosis of necrosis and chronic apical abscess on tooth 29 (see **Fig. 3**A). The canal was disinfected without mechanical instrumentation but with irrigation using 5.25% sodium hypochlorite and Peridex by placing a needle within 1 mm of the apex. This was followed by the placement of 3Mix paste containing metronidazole, ciprofloxacin, and minocycline[39] with a lentulo. The patient returned 26 days after the initial appointment and it was noted that the sinus tract had resolved. After irrigation of the canal, bleeding was stimulated with an endodontic explorer and a blood clot was stopped below the level of the cementoenamel junction (CEJ) to provide a scaffold for the ingrowth of new tissue. An increment of mineral trioxide aggregate (MTA) and a bonded resin were placed coronally as a final restoration. Full radiographic healing was noted within 7 months (see **Fig. 3**E) and, at the 24th-month recall, the root walls were thickened and the root had attained a length similar to the adjacent teeth (see **Fig. 3**F). In addition, Banchs and Trope[3] reported that the tooth responded to vitality testing with cold.

Overview of Clinical Cases

In general, most of the in vivo cases (see **Table 1**) have shown consistent principles. First, most of the patients have been young (6–18 years old). Age may play a role in stem cell population and regenerative potential.[40] Kling and colleageus[29] suggested that the size of the apical opening has an effect on the successful revascularization of avulsed immature permanent teeth and, by extrapolation, it is thought that an open apex may be part of the age predilection of successful REPs. Not only is it generally accepted that a short and open root is more conducive to ingrowth of tissues but it is suggested that a short and open apex may indicate the increased presence and numbers of stem cells of the apical papilla (SCAP). Another principle, which is often counterintuitive to most clinicians, is the absence of instrumentation of the dentinal walls. In most cases, the disinfection approach was chemical (using either an antibiotic paste or calcium hydroxide) rather than chemomechanical. It is thought that the presence of the noninfected necrotic pulp as well as the induced blood clot scaffold may have been essential in providing a lattice for progenitor cell growth.[3,24] In addition, many of these cases have reported some vital tissue at the apical portion of the canal and most cases reported presence of a blood clot or other protein scaffold. There is some suggestion that outcomes may be significantly different between teeth that have some vital tissue in the apical portion of the canal versus those teeth in which the pulp has been lost. Huang[34] defines these 2 scenarios as (1) partial pulp regeneration and (2) de novo regeneration of the pulp. These 2 presentations may require separate protocols. The latter may require stem cells to be reseeded into the canal space with a scaffold that contains angiogenic growth factors to enhance the process of revascularization and, ultimately, regeneration of the dental pulp.

Current AAE Protocol Considerations

The following recommendations are based on the best available data and should be 1 possible source of information used to make treatment decisions (**Box 1**).

Box 1
Current considerations for REPs

Case selection:

- Tooth with necrotic pulp and an immature apex
- Pulp space not needed for post/core, final restoration
- Compliant patient

Informed consent:

- Two (or more) appointments
- Use of antimicrobial(s)
- Possible adverse effects: staining of crown/root, lack of response to treatment, pain/infection
- Alternatives: MTA apexification, no treatment, extraction (when deemed nonsalvageable)
- Permission to enter information into AAE database (optional)

First appointment:

- Local anesthesia, rubber dam isolation, access
- Copious, gentle irrigation with 20 mL NaOCl using an irrigation system that minimizes the possibility of extrusion of irrigants into the periapical space (eg, needle with closed end and side vents, or EndoVac). To minimize potential precipitate in the canal, use sterile water or saline between NaOCl; lower concentrations of NaOCl are advised, to minimize cytotoxicity to stem cells in the apical tissues.
- Dry canals
- Place antibiotic paste or calcium hydroxide. If the triple antibiotic paste is used: (1) consider sealing pulp chamber with a dentin bonding agent to minimize risk of staining, and (2) mix 1:1:1 ciprofloxacin/metronidazole/minocycline (or, if esthetics are crucial, then consider a 1:1 mixture of ciprofloxacin/metronidazole).
- Deliver into canal system via lentulo spiral, MAP system, or Centrix syringe
- If triple antibiotic paste is used, ensure that it remains below the CEJ (to minimize crown staining)
- Seal with 3 to 4 mm of Cavit, followed by immediate restorative material, glass ionomer cement, or another temporary material
- Dismiss patient for 3 to 4 weeks

Second appointment:

- Assess response to initial treatment. If there are signs/symptoms of persistent infection, consider additional treatment time with antimicrobial, or alternative antimicrobial.
- Anesthesia with 3% mepivacaine without vasoconstrictor, rubber dam, isolation
- Copious, gentle irrigation with 20 mL of ethylenediamine tetraacetic acid, followed by normal saline, using a similar closed-end needle
- Dry with paper points
- Create bleeding into canal system by overinstrumenting (endo file, endo explorer)
- Stop bleeding 3 mm from CEJ
- Place CollaPlug/CollaCote at the orifice, if necessary
- Place 3 to 4 mm of white MTA and reinforced glass ionomer and place permanent restoration

Follow-up:

Clinical and radiographic examination:

- No pain or soft tissue swelling (often observed between first and second appointments)
- Resolution of apical radiolucency (often observed 6–12 months after treatment)
- Increased width of root walls (this is generally observed before apparent increase in root length and often occurs 12–24 months after treatment)
- Increased root length

From American Association of Endodontics. Consideration for regenerative procedures. Available at: www.aae.org/Dental_Professionals/Considerations_for_Regenerative_Procedures.aspx; with permission.

Case selection
Future efforts must focus on a more biologic and scientific approach to REPs. Until standardized protocols have been developed, the AAE has made the following recommendations for case selection. Any tooth with necrotic pulp and an immature apex is a reasonable candidate for REPs, provided that the pulp space not needed for post/core and final restoration. As with most endodontic procedures, compliance is important but, because of the need for frequent follow-up, a compliant patient is essential for REPs.[5]

Informed consent
It is the clinician's duty to disclose all material information necessary to make an informed decision. Material information is defined as information a clinician knows or should know that would be regarded as significant by a reasonable person in the patient's position.[41] The AAE recommends that the clinician discuss with the patient and parent/guardian that treatment will take place over 2 or more appointments with the need for frequent follow-up.[16] It is also important that the clinician discuss the use of antimicrobials with regard to potential allergies/sensitivities. Although medications are placed with the intention of being confined to the root canal space, it is prudent that the clinician discuss the potential for adverse reactions to the medications. Other unfavorable side effects include staining of the crown/root and the potential for nonhealing, pain, and infection. Informed consent must also include viable alternatives to the recommended treatment, including 1-step apical barrier procedures (MTA apexification), no treatment, or extraction when the tooth is deemed nonsalvageable. In addition, because it is essential that insights are gained into both effective and ineffective treatment, the AAE suggests that the patient and parent/guardian consent to inclusion of their information in the AAE regenerative database.

First appointment: access and disinfection
It is recommended that the patient be anesthetized according to the clinician's standard protocol. The tooth is then isolated with a rubber dam and accessed. This stage is then followed by copious, gentle irrigation with 20 mL NaOCl using an irrigation system that minimizes the possibility of extrusion of irrigants into the periapical space (eg, needle with closed end and side vents, or EndoVac). Previous guidelines recommended the use 0.12% chlorhexidine; however, based on the work of Trevino and colleagues,[42] chlorhexidine is known to be cytotoxic to stem cells and thus should be avoided, particularly on a second appointment. If chlorhexidine is used, to minimize potential precipitate[43] in the canal it is suggested to use sterile water or saline between NaOCl and chlorhexidine. Lower concentrations of NaOCl are advised because higher concentrations of NaOCl seem to be harmful to stem cells.[42,44]

It is then recommended that the canals be dried with sterile paper points and an antibiotic paste or calcium hydroxide be placed below CEJ either by lentulo, MAP system, or syringe. Calcium hydroxide is effective as an antimicrobial in REPs,[45] but concerns have been raised that calcium hydroxide limits the possibility of increasing root canal wall thickness on the dentin surface in direct contact with this highly alkaline medicament (**Fig. 4**).[33]

Most investigators recommend a combination of antibiotics. Hoshino and colleagues[39] and Windley and colleagues[27] have shown the effectiveness of 3MIX or triple antibiotic paste both in vitro and in vivo. The original protocol indicates that pills are to be crushed with a mortar and pestle and mixed together as slurry with Macrogol ointment and propylene glycol (see www.Regenendo.com for video example). This process is inconvenient and the final paste contains filler found in the pill form of the

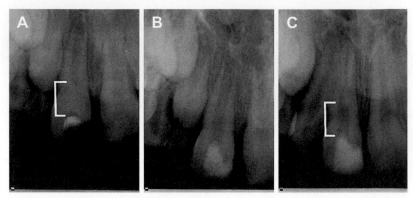

Fig. 4. Calcium hydroxide as antimicrobial agent. (*A*) Calcium hydroxide placed by referring doctor to the level of the CEJ. (*B*) Completion of REP; 3 weeks after initial appointment; (*C*) at the 24-month recall. Note that there is no thickening of walls in areas of previous placement of calcium hydroxide.

medication (eg, lactose). Pure United States Pharmacopeia–grade medications can be obtained and placed in a convenient capsule at a compounding pharmacy (**Fig. 5**).

There is some suggestion in recent work by Ruparel and colleagues[46] that undiluted slurry of antibiotics is cytotoxic to stem cells and that titrating the proper concentration

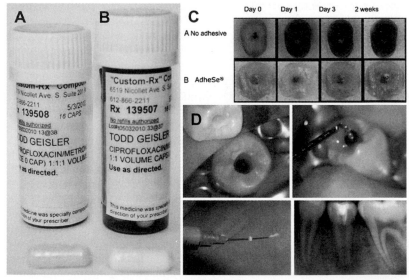

Fig. 5. Capsules obtained from a compounding pharmacy. (*A*) 1:1:1 by volume of ciprofloxacin/metronidazole/minocycline, and (*B*) 1:1 by volume of ciprofloxacin/metronidazole. Clinicians can contact the International Academy of Compounding Pharmacists at 1(800) 927-4227 to find their nearest compounding pharmacy, or visit www.iacprx.org. (*C*) Application of bonding agent in coronal chamber prevents staining. (*D*) Composite bonding in coronal chamber using Munce projectors. (Part [*C*] *From* Kim JH, Kim Y, Shin SJ, et al. Tooth discoloration of immature permanent incisor associated with triple antibiotic therapy: a case report. J Endod 2010;36:1089; with permission; [*D*] *From* Reynolds K, Johnson JD, Cohenca N. Pulp revascularization of necrotic bilateral bicuspids using a modified novel technique to eliminate potential coronal discoloration: a case report. Int Endod J 2009; 42:86; with permission.)

of antibiotic seems to be important. They found that a dilution of 1000 times (or 100 μg/mL) was necessary for stem cell survival and proliferation, which highlights that intracanal medicaments must be used at concentrations that are bactericidal but have minimal effects on stem cell viability.

There are other adverse effects using the triple antibiotic paste.[12,16] Minocycline has long been known to stain dentin. If the triple antibiotic paste mix (1:1:1 by volume of ciprofloxacin/metronidazole/minocycline) is used, avoid complications of dentinal staining by sealing the pulp chamber with a dentin bonding agent[15] or flowable composite.[14] If esthetics are crucial, consider eliminating the minocycline or exchanging with cefaclor.[36] In addition, seal with 3 to 4 mm of Cavit, followed by immediate restorative material, glass ionomer cement, or another temporary material and dismiss the patient for 2 to 4 weeks.

Second appointment: stimulate, scaffold, and seal

Assuming compliance, the patient will return at 2 to 4 weeks from the previous access and disinfection appointment. At this point, the clinician should assess how the patient has responded to the initial treatment. Depending on the diagnosis, there will be some indications that treatment is progressing. With an initial diagnosis of necrosis and chronic apical abscess, absence of a sinus tract often predicts effective disinfection and initial healing. If there are signs/symptoms of persistent infection, additional treatment time with the antimicrobial, or an alternative antimicrobial, would be considered.

Anesthetics containing epinephrine are to be avoided[16] because the objective is to stimulate bleeding to create a scaffold and epinephrine can significantly affect blood flow to the area. It is recommended that the clinician anesthetize with 3% mepivacaine without a vasoconstrictor. Isolation with a rubber dam is essential because strict attention to asepsis could affect outcome. In addition, external disinfection with chlorhexidine seems to be prudent but not necessary.

Next, it is recommended that there be copious, gentle irrigation with 20 mL ethylenediamine tetraacetic acid (EDTA). It is generally agreed that this process removes the smear layer, exposes dentinal tubules, and conditions the dentin to release growth factors such as transforming growth factor β (TGF-β).[47–49] This stage is then followed by normal saline or Hanks balanced salt solution, using a similar closed-end needle. The canal is then dried with sterile paper points.

It is suggested that the stimulation of a blood clot is essential to healing[36] and that this evoked-bleeding step in REPs leads to a significant increase in expression of undifferentiated mesenchymal stem cell markers in the root canal space (**Fig. 6**A).[50]

The next step is to create bleeding into canal system by overinstrumenting (endo file, endo explorer). Clinical tips include placing a small bend in the file and dipping the instrument in EDTA (a known anticoagulant) to aid in achieving a blood clot just below the CEJ.[3,28] This task of evoking bleeding into the coronal portion of the root has been a concern for clinicians.[12,16] An alternative is to draw blood (see **Fig. 6**B) and inject into the canal system. In a canal where a blood clot was not evoked, 1 case report[18] indicated that blood from adjacent canals was placed in the dry canal to create this clot.

A blood clot consists of network of fibrin, platelets, red blood cells, and white blood cells. A question that has been asked is whether clinicians can create a better 3D scaffold than a blood clot with an increased concentration of growth factors.[51–53] One of many advantages of using an autologous fibrin matrix (AFM) is that the level of clot can be controlled whether or not bleeding can be evoked. Autologous fibrin matrices also have the advantages of being easy to collect, providing a 3D scaffold, and supplying a concentrated source of growth factors such as TGF-β1 and VEGF (vascular

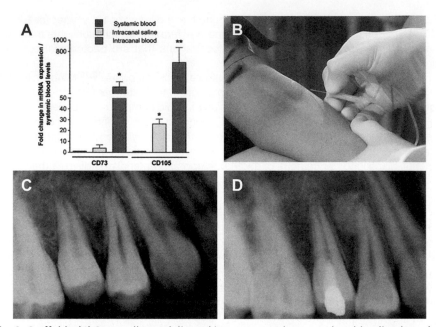

Fig. 6. Scaffolds. (*A*) Stem cells are delivered into root canal spaces when bleeding is evoked from the apical region of immature teeth. (*B*) Venipuncture from the Master Clinician Series 2011. (*C*) Preoperative radiograph showing lesion and immature apices. (*D*) Radiograph 5.5 months after REP shows resolution of periapical lesion, further root development, and continued apical closure of root apex. (Part [*A*] *From* Lovelace TW, Henry MA, Hargreaves KM. Evaluation of clinically delivered SCAP cells in regenerative endodontic procedures. J Endod 2010;36:136; with permission; and [*C, D*] *From* Torabinejad M, Turman M. Revitalization of tooth with necrotic pulp and open apex by using platelet-rich plasma: a case report. J Endod 2011;37:266; with permission.)

endothelial growth factor is a potent angiogenic factor shown to aid in revascularization).[54,55] Torabinejad and Turman[21] reported on a case (see **Fig. 6**C, D) in which no bleeding was evoked, but instead they hypothesized that the platelet-rich plasma (a form of AFM) injected into the canal attracted stem cells into the canal system. They concluded that whatever tissue was produced in the canal was result of the presence of AFM. Despite these favorable findings, some clinicians have raised concerns that performing venipuncture may be a barrier to this type of therapeutic adjunct (see **Fig. 6**B). Nonetheless, alternative protocols using AFM are beginning to be performed (**Figs. 7–9**).

Once bleeding has been evoked or AFM has been injected, it is recommended that a collagen matrix such as CollaPlug or CollaCote be placed at the orifice,[16] if deemed necessary. This matrix helps to prevent overextension of MTA or other restorative material. Numerous materials have been indicated for developing a bacteria-tight seal. MTA has been shown to provide an excellent bacteria-tight seal[56] is currently the material of choice in regenerative procedures.[3] An increment of 3 to 4 mm of MTA[57] seems to be sufficient to attain this seal. Thus, it is recommended that 3 to 4 mm of white MTA be placed and restoration performed with reinforced glass ionomer and composite or amalgam. It has been reported that white MTA stains dentin.[58,59] A side-by-side comparison (**Fig. 10**), suggests that staining of white

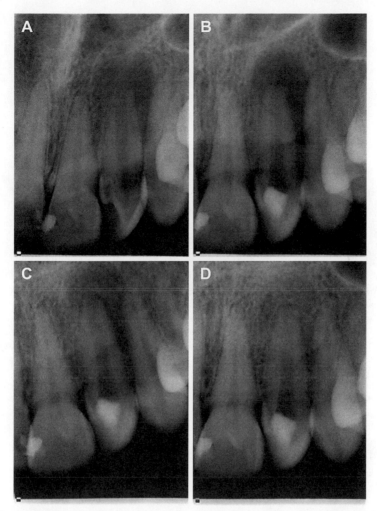

Fig. 7. A modified AFM or platelet-rich plasma (PRP) protocol (the same case as in **Fig. 8**). (*A*) Presence of periapical radiolucency (PARL) on tooth 10. Note the infolding of enamel on tooth 10 classified as an Oehlers 2 dens invaginatus. (*B*) Immediately after an REP. (*C*) At the 18-month recall (*D*) At the 27-month recall. Minimal increase of root wall thickness. Tooth now tests positive to EPT.

MTA is a real phenomenon. As an alternative, a different pulp space barrier (eg, glass ionomer)[2,10] may be indicated in areas where esthetics are crucial.

Follow-up

Follow-up for REPs includes both clinical and radiographic evaluation (see the article by Law elsewhere in this issue). Chueh and Huang[4] gave some general expectations for the progress of REPs. They observed radiographic evidence of bony healing in 3 to 21 months (mean 8 months), and radiographic evidence of root development in 10 to 29 months (mean 16 months). These results suggest that radiographic evidence of healing and root development should occur within 2 years. Signs and symptoms such as pain, soft tissue swelling, or increasing radiolucency indicate failure of

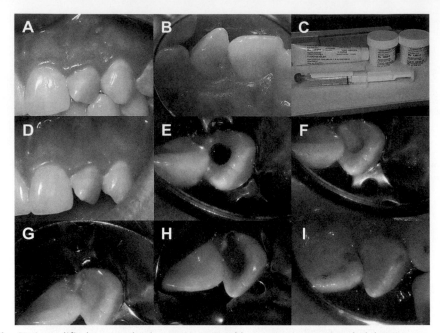

Fig. 8. A modified protocol using AFM or PRP (the same case as Fig. 7). (*A*) A 24-year-old patient presents with a diagnosis of necrosis with chronic apical abscess on tooth 10. Note presence of sinus tract. (*B*) The dens invaginatus can be appreciated on lingual aspect of tooth 10. (*C*) New antibiotic protocol in esthetic area using 2MIX or double antibiotic paste and the macrogol and propylene glycol carrier (MP) carrier (Macrogol ointment and propylene glycol) as described by Hoshino and colleagues.[39] (*D*) Absence of both sinus tract and coronal staining. (*E*) AFM or PRP placed in canal. (*F*) Collatape placed over PRP. (*G*) Resin-modified glass ionomer was placed over Collatape and the enamel was beveled, (*H*) etched, and (*I*) restored with composite.

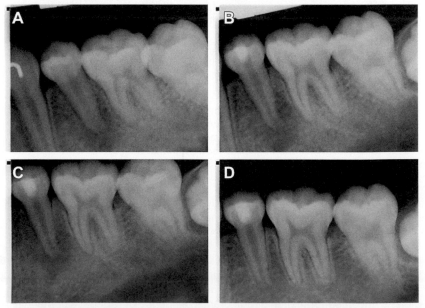

Fig. 9. A modified protocol using AFM or PRP. The patient was a 13-year-old girl with a diagnosis of necrosis and chronic apical abscess. (*A*) Presence of PARL on tooth 20. (*B*) 2MIX-saline paste placed with 18-gauge syringe. (*C*) At the 3-week appointment. Sinus tract resolution. Patient and parent consented to venipuncture. Immediately after an REP. (*D*) At the 5-month recall. Resolution of lesion and tooth now tests positive to EPT and cold.

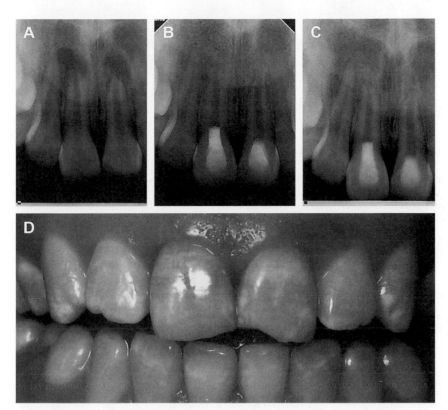

Fig. 10. Side-by-side comparison of 2 protocols. The case was performed at the 2011 Master Clinician Series. The patient is a 21-year-old woman. Both teeth received 2MIX or double antibiotic paste. The Banchs and Trope[3] (2004) protocol was used for tooth 8 (blood clot, antibiotic paste, white MTA, GI, and composite) and a modified protocol was incorporated for tooth 9 (AFM or PRP, antibiotic paste, Collatape, glass ionomer, and composite). (*A*) Preoperative radiolucency at time of initial visit 5 months before the Master Clinician Series. (*B*) Immediately after the Master Clinician Series. (*C*) At the 10-month recall. Note radiographic healing. (*D*) At the 10-month recall. Staining is attributed to white MTA. Tooth 8 was subsequently internally bleached with sodium perborate, with satisfactory results. For a video of the procedure visit the AAE Live Learning Center or www.regenendo.com.

procedure and will likely obviate alternative treatment such as artificial apical barrier with MTA or extraction.

Future Protocols

During the past 2 decades there has been a great expansion in knowledge and critical advancement of clinical tools. As endodontic treatment is approached with a beginner's mind, the limits of what is currently believed to be possible will be tested. Many researchers and clinicians are convinced that REPs will change endodontics much as surgical operating microscopes and nickel titanium files have done. REPs have the potential to increase the skill set of endodontists from not only master diagnostician and technician but cell biologist and tissue engineer as well. Although there is much to learn, new (albeit controversial) protocols are approaching, including

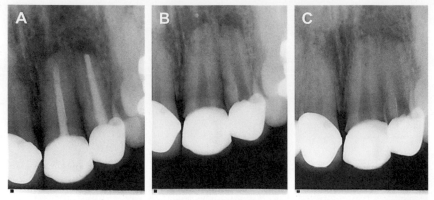

Fig. 11. Future protocol? REPs in older adults and previously treated teeth. (*A*) Failing endodontic treatment. (*B*) A modified protocol with removal of gutta-percha and placement of 3MIX antibiotic paste and subsequently an AFM scaffold. (*C*) At the 12-month recall, showing bony healing.

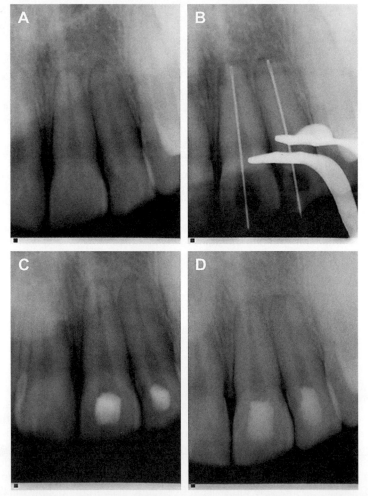

Fig. 12. Controversial protocol? Intentional apical opening. A 19-year-old patient (*A*) before surgery. (*B*) Intentional apical opening with Lightspeed LSX instrument to size 70. (*C*) 2MIX or double antibiotic paste placed. (*D*) After 6 weeks, a modified protocol using AFM was used.

procedures for older adults, previously treated teeth, and teeth with mature apices (**Figs. 11** and **12**).

Researchers are attempting to regenerate the pulp-dentin complex using a variety of approaches including autologous and synthetic scaffolds,[1] harvesting of various stem cell populations, use of gene therapy, and inclusion of various growth factors for their efficacy in REPs. Future efforts will focus the scientific approach to these endodontic procedures, and randomized prospective multicenter trials will develop evidenced-based methodologies for these pioneering REPs.

SUMMARY

There is a need for biologically based endodontic procedures that offer the potential to replace tissue lost because of trauma or disease. Although there are still significant scientific hurdles to overcome, it now seems more certain that, with the continued growth in the knowledge base and armamentarium, a regenerative endodontic concept that was once was only imagined will become reality: a fully functional regenerated pulp-dentin complex.

REFERENCES

1. Murray PE, Garcia-Godoy F, Hargreaves KM. Regenerative endodontics: a review of current status and a call for action. J Endod 2007;33:377–90.
2. Iwaya SI, Ikawa M, Kubota M. Revascularization of an immature permanent tooth with apical periodontitis and sinus tract. Dent Traumatol 2001;17:185–7.
3. Banchs F, Trope M. Revascularization of immature permanent teeth with apical periodontitis: new treatment protocol? J Endod 2004;30(4):196–200.
4. Chueh LH, Huang GT. Immature teeth with periradicular periodontitis or abscess undergoing apexogenesis: a paradigm shift. J Endod 2006;32:1205–13.
5. Petrino JA. Revascularization of necrotic pulp of immature teeth with apical periodontitis. Northwest Dent 2007;86:33–5.
6. Thibodeau B, Trope M. Pulp revascularization of a necrotic infected immature permanent tooth: case report and review of the literature. Pediatr Dent 2007; 29:47–50.
7. Thibodeau B. Case report: pulp revascularization of a necrotic, infected, immature, permanent tooth. Pediatr Dent 2009;31:145–8.
8. Jung IY, Lee SJ, Hargreaves KM. Biologically based treatment of immature permanent teeth with pulpal necrosis: a case series. J Endod 2008;34: 876–87.
9. Cotti E, Mereu M, Lusso D. Regenerative treatment of an immature, traumatized tooth with apical periodontitis: report of a case. J Endod 2008;34:611–6.
10. Shah N, Logani A, Bhaskar U, et al. Efficacy of revascularization to induce apexification/apexogensis in infected, nonvital, immature teeth: a pilot clinical study. J Endod 2008;34(8):919–25.
11. Chueh LH, Ho YC, Kuo TC, et al. Regenerative endodontic treatment for necrotic immature permanent teeth. J Endod 2009;35:160–4.
12. Ding RY, Cheung GS, Chen J, et al. Pulp revascularization of immature teeth with apical periodontitis: a clinical study. J Endod 2009;35:745–9.
13. Shin SY, Albert JS, Mortman RE. One step pulp revascularization treatment of an immature permanent tooth with chronic apical abscess: a case report. Int Endod J 2009;42:1118–26.

14. Reynolds K, Johnson JD, Cohenca N. Pulp revascularization of necrotic bilateral bicuspids using a modified novel technique to eliminate potential coronal discoloration: a case report. Int Endod J 2009;42:84–92.

15. Kim JH, Kim Y, Shin SJ, et al. Tooth discoloration of immature permanent incisor associated with triple antibiotic therapy: a case report. J Endod 2010;36: 1086–91.

16. Petrino JA, Boda KK, Shambarger S, et al. Challenges in regenerative endodontics: a case series. J Endod 2010;36:536–41.

17. Thomson A, Kahler B. Regenerative endodontics–biologically-based treatment for immature permanent teeth: a case report and review of the literature. Aust Dent J 2010;55:446–52.

18. Nosrat A, Seifi A, Asgary S. Regenerative endodontic treatment (revascularization) for necrotic immature permanent molars: a review and report of two cases with a new biomaterial. J Endod 2011;37:562–7.

19. Lenzi R, Trope M. Revitalization procedures in two traumatized incisors with different biological outcomes. J Endod 2012;38:411–4.

20. Cehreli ZC, Isbitiren B, Sara S, et al. Regenerative endodontic treatment (revascularization) of immature necrotic molars medicated with calcium hydroxide: a case series. J Endod 2011;37:1327–30.

21. Torabinejad M, Turman M. Revitalization of tooth with necrotic pulp and open apex by using platelet-rich plasma: a case report. J Endod 2011;37:265–8.

22. Iwaya S, Ikawa M, Kubota M. Revascularization of an immature permanent tooth with periradicular abscess after luxation. Dent Traumatol 2011;27(1):55–8.

23. Nakashima M, Akamine A. The application of tissue engineering to regeneration of pulp and dentin in endodontics. J Endod 2005;31:711–8.

24. Trope M, Blanco L, Chivan N, et al. The role of endodontics after dental traumatic injuries. In: Pathways of the pulp. 9th edition. St Louis (MO): Mosby; 2006. p. 610–49.

25. Skoglund A, Tronstad L. Pulpal changes in replanted and autotransplanted immature teeth of dogs. J Endod 1981;7:309–16.

26. Johnson WT, Goodrich JL, James GA. Replantation of avulsed teeth with immature root development. Oral Surg Oral Med Oral Pathol 1985;60:420–7.

27. Windley W 3rd, Teixeira F, Levin L, et al. Disinfection of immature teeth with a triple antibiotic paste. J Endod 2005;31:439–43.

28. Trope M. Treatment of the immature tooth with a non-vital pulp and apical periodontitis. Dent Clin North Am 2010;54(2):313–24.

29. Kling M, Cvek M, Mejare I. Rate and predictability of pulp revascularization in therapeutically reimplanted permanent incisors. Endod Dent Traumatol 1986;2: 83–9.

30. Huang GT, Lin LM. Letter to the editor: comments on the use of the term "revascularization" to describe. J Endod 2008;34(5):511.

31. Trope M. Reply. Letter to the editor: comments on the use of the term "revascularization" to describe. J Endod 2008;34(5):511–2.

32. Wang X, Thibodeau B, Trope M, et al. Histologic characterization of regenerated tissues in canal space after the revitalization/revascularization procedure of immature dog teeth with apical periodontitis. J Endod 2010;36:56–63.

33. Hargreaves K, Geisler T, Henry M, et al. Regeneration potential of the young permanent tooth: what does the future hold? J Endod 2008;34:S51–6.

34. Huang GT. Dental pulp and dentin tissue engineering and regeneration: advancement and challenge. Front Biosci 2011;E3:788–800.

35. Nygaard-Ostby B, Hjortdal O. Tissue formation in the root canal following pulp removal. Scand J Dent Res 1971;79:333–49.
36. Thibodeau B, Teixeira F, Yamauchi M, et al. Pulp revascularization of immature dog teeth with apical periodontitis. J Endod 2007;33:680–9.
37. Nevins A, Finkelstein F, Borden B, et al. Revitalization of pulpless open apex teeth in rhesus monkeys, using collagen-calcium phosphate gel. J Endod 1967;2: 159–65.
38. Myers MC, Fountain SB. Dental pulp regeneration aided by blood and blood substitutes after experimentally induced periapical infection. Oral Surg Oral Med Oral Pathol 1974;37:441–50.
39. Hoshino E, Kurihara-Ando N, Sato I, et al. In-vitro antibacterial susceptibility of bacteria taken from infected root dentine to a mixture of ciprofloxacin, metronidazole and minocycline. Int Endod J 1996;29:125–30.
40. Sonoyama W, Liu Y, Yamaza T, et al. Characterization of the apical papilla and its residing stem cells from human immature permanent teeth: a pilot study. J Endod 2008;34:166–71.
41. Zinman E. Endodontic records and legal responsibilities. In: Cohen S, Hargreaves KM, Keiser K, editors. Pathways of the pulp. 9th edition. St Louis (MO): Mosby; 2006. p. 400–57.
42. Trevino EG, Henry MA, Patwardhan A, et al. The effect of different irrigation solutions on the survival of stem cells of the apical papilla (SCAP) in a PRP scaffold in human root tips (abstract). J Endod 2009;35:428.
43. Basrani BR, Manek S, Sodhi RN, et al. Interaction between sodium hypochlorite and chlorhexidine gluconate. J Endod 2007;33:966–9.
44. Essner MD, Javed A, Eleazer PD. Effect of sodium hypochlorite on human pulp cells: an in vitro study. Oral Surg Oral Med Oral Pathol Oral Radiol Endod 2011;112(5):662–6.
45. Bose R, Nummikoski P, Hargreaves K. A retrospective evaluation of radiographic outcomes in immature teeth with necrotic root canal systems treated with regenerative endodontic procedures. J Endod 2009;10:1343.
46. Ruparel NB, Ruparel FB, Hargreaves KM, et al. Effect of intracanal medicaments on stem cells from apical papilla. J Endod 2012;38:e13–57.
47. Galler KM, D'Souza RN, Federlin M, et al. Dentin conditioning codetermines cell fate in regenerative endodontics. J Endod 2011;37(11):1536–41.
48. Yamauchi N, Yamauchi S, Nagaoka H, et al. Tissue engineering strategies for immature teeth with apical periodontitis. J Endod 2011;37:390–7.
49. Smith A. Dentin formation and repair. In: Hargreaves KM, Goodis HE, editors. Seltzer and Bender's dental pulp. 3rd edition. Chicago: Quintessence Publishing; 2002. p. 41–62.
50. Lovelace TW, Henry MA, Hargreaves KM. Evaluation of clinically delivered SCAP cells in regenerative endodontic procedures. J Endod 2010;36:554.
51. Geisler TM. Mattscheck AAE Annual Session. 2009.
52. Geisler TM. Law. AAE Annual Session. 2010.
53. Geisler TM. Texeira. AAE Annual Session. 2011.
54. Anitua E, Sánchez M, Nurden AT, et al. New insights into and novel applications for platelet-rich fibrin therapies. Trends Biotechnol 2006;24(5):227–34.
55. Mullane EM, Dong Z, Sedgley CM, et al. Effects of VEGF and FGF2 on the revascularization of severed human dental pulps. J Dent Res 2008;87(12):1144–8.
56. Torabinejad M, Rastegar AF, Kettering JD, et al. Bacterial leakage of mineral trioxide aggregate as a root-end filling material. J Endod 1995;21:109–12.

57. Lawley GR, Schindler WG, Walker WA 3rd, et al. Evaluation of ultrasonically placed MTA and fracture resistance with intracanal composite resin in a model of apexification. J Endod 2004;30:167–72.
58. Watts JD, Holt DM, Beeson TJ, et al. Effects of pH and mixing agents on the temporal setting of tooth-colored and gray mineral trioxide aggregate. J Endod 2007;33:970–3.
59. Boutsioukis C, Noula G, Lambrianidis T. Ex vivo study of the efficiency of two techniques for the removal of mineral trioxide aggregate used as a root canal filling material. J Endod 2008;34:1239–42.

Outcomes of Regenerative Endodontic Procedures

Alan S. Law, DDS, PhD

KEYWORDS

- Revascularization • Outcome • Regeneration • Revitalization • Radiograph
- Histology

KEY POINTS

- Radiographic evidence of apical bone healing, increased root length, and increased root wall width has been shown after the use of regenerative endodontic techniques in human teeth with immature roots and necrotic pulp tissue.
- The histologic evidence from animal models using similar regenerative procedures has shown varied hard and soft tissues in the canal space.
- Future research should focus on demonstrating consistent bone healing and continued root development in humans, while developing techniques that increase the likelihood of achieving regeneration of the pulp-dentin complex.

INTRODUCTION

When pulp tissue becomes necrotic in immature teeth, the long-term prognosis is compromised. Treatment of these teeth presents many challenges, including difficulties in cleaning and shaping large canals with blunderbuss apices, obturation of canals with open apices, and potential root fractures caused by thin and/or weakened root walls.[1–3] The use of regenerative techniques holds the promise of recreating the pulp-dentin complex.

Therapeutic options for the immature tooth with a necrotic pulp include apexification and regeneration, revascularization, or revitalization. There has been a debate as to which term, revascularization, revitalization, or regeneration, is most appropriate to describe the outcome of procedures used to regenerate pulp tissue.[3–5] The debate continues because of the lack of definitive evidence of the outcomes of the procedures.[3,6,7] The term revascularization is more commonly associated with dental trauma literature and describes reestablishment of vascular supply to immature permanent teeth.[8] Revitalization describes ingrowth of vital tissue that does not resemble the original lost tissue.[9] Endodontic regeneration is the replacement of "damaged structures, including dentin and root structures, as well as cells of the pulp-dentin complex."[10] In this article, the term revitalization is used to encompass all potential outcomes.

Private Practice, The Dental Specialists, 8650 Hudson Boulevard, Lake Elmo, MN 55042, USA
E-mail address: endolaw@comcast.net

Dent Clin N Am 56 (2012) 627–637
doi:10.1016/j.cden.2012.05.012
0011-8532/12/$ – see front matter © 2012 Elsevier Inc. All rights reserved.

dental.theclinics.com

CLINICAL OUTCOMES
Early Outcomes

The attempt to revitalize teeth with necrotic pulp tissue is not new to endodontics. In 1961, Nygaard-Ostby and Hjortdal[11] demonstrated the ingrowth of fibrous connective tissue and cementum in mature teeth with necrotic pulp tissue after instrumentation, interappointment disinfection with sulfathiazole and 4% formaldehyde, overinstrumentation beyond the apex to evoke bleeding, and obturation short of the apex with Kloroperka paste and a gutta-percha.

In 1974, Myers and Fountain[12] reported that a majority of incisors with mature apices that were disinfected with NaOCl and then had the apical openings intentionally enlarged and filled with citrated whole blood or gel foam experienced "root resorption, which correlated with the presence of chronically inflamed granulation tissue." In the same experimental protocol, canines with immature apices (as opposed to incisors with mature apices) had evidence of increased root length and calcified material in the canals.

In 1976, Nevins and colleagues[13] showed "various forms of hard and soft connective tissue," including "cementum, bone, and reparative dentin" lining the walls of the root canal in immature necrotic incisors of monkeys after the placement of a gel (containing collagen, calcium chloride, and dipotassium hydrogen phosphate) and short obturation with gutta-percha. Thus, findings from early case series and studies demonstrated the possibility of obtaining revitalization of a previously infected canal space, albeit with varied histologic outcomes.

Recent Outcomes

In the past decade there has been increased interest in regenerative endodontic procedures following published case reports describing clinical procedures for revitalizing necrotic immature teeth.[14,15] Using the methods described in these case reports, many clinicians have demonstrated radiographic evidence of increased root length and root wall thickness. An example of this outcome is shown in **Fig. 1**. The techniques

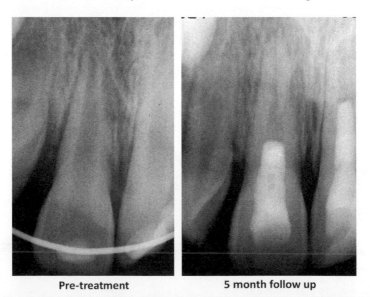

Pre-treatment   5 month follow up

Fig. 1. Pretreatment and follow-up radiographs from regenerative endodontic procedure. Note apparent increase in root length and root wall thickness.

(eg, single vs multiple appointment, type of irrigant, type of antibiotic paste, and type of pulp space barrier) and recall periods vary, but all follow the principles of canal disinfection, creation of an environment and scaffolding for stem cell ingrowth, and placement of a coronal seal.[14–32] A summary of the recall periods and outcome findings is shown in **Table 1**.

There are several challenges in interpreting the outcomes of case series and case report outcomes. These challenges include significant variability in technique and recall period, a potential bias of only successful cases being reported, and the lack of consistent radiographic angulation between pretreatment and follow-up radiographs. Case reports and case series do, however, demonstrate that regenerative endodontic techniques can result in healing apical pathosis and root development. The American Association of Endodontists maintains a database of revitalization cases with follow-up radiographs. Analysis of this data adds to the existing case reports/series and assists in the development of controlled clinical trials.

Two recent reports[30,33] have attempted to account for variability in radiographic angulation by using a geometric imaging program to minimize potential differences in angulation between the preoperative and recall images. The standardization of radiographic images enabled the calculation of continued development of root length and dentin wall thickness. Bose and colleagues[33] compared outcomes from teeth that were medicated with $Ca(OH)_2$ with triple antibiotic paste and with formocresol. Their results showed that teeth treated with triple antibiotic paste and $Ca(OH)_2$ had significantly greater increases in root length than the control teeth (apexification or NSRCT) and that triple antibiotic paste produced significantly greater differences in root wall thickness than either the $Ca(OH)_2$ or formocresol groups. The investigators also found that the percentage change in root length and root width increased over time (**Fig. 2**). Cehreli and colleagues[30] evaluated the changes in root length and width in 6 immature necrotic permanent first molars that were treated by a revitalization protocol using 2.5% NaOCl irrigation and medication and with calcium hydroxide. The investigators found, after 9 to 10 months follow-up, progressive thickening of dentinal walls (15%–38%) and increased root length (2%–18%) in all teeth.

These case reports and case series emphasize the importance of follow-up, including recording symptoms, radiographs, and clinical tests. Because of the variability in recall, it is difficult to establish time frames in which practitioners may expect to see radiographic changes. This information is important because it can help in assessing if and when alternative treatments (ie, apexification, traditional nonsurgical root canal therapy, or extraction) may be necessary. Chueh and colleagues[22] did attempt to determine the timing of radiographic changes. In this case series, 23 necrotic immature permanent teeth were irrigated with 2.6% NaOCl and treated with either short- (<3 months) or long-term treatment (<3 months) $Ca(OH)_2$ paste medication. The investigators found radiographic evidence of apical bone healing in 3 to 21 months (mean = 8 months), and radiographic evidence of root development in 10 to 29 months (mean = 16 months). These results suggest that if radiographic evidence of healing and root development has not occurred within approximately 2 years after the completion of treatment, alternative treatments may be necessary.

Radiographic assessment can be enhanced with the use of cone beam computed tomography (CBCT) because it reveals views of the tooth and surrounding bone not seen with periapical radiographs. This technique was demonstrated in a recent case report[31] of adjacent incisors, 1 of which was revitalized successfully and the other that had radiographic signs of failed treatment. An example of the additional radiographic information (eg, lateral view) that can be seen in CBCT images is shown in **Fig. 3**. Given the increased radiation exposure associated with CBCT, it is important

Table 1
Outcomes of revitalization/regeneration case reports/series

References	Recall Period	Apical Pathosis Healed? (# of Teeth)	Root Lengthened? (# of Teeth)	Root Wall Thickening? (# of Teeth)
Iwaya et al,[14] 2001	30 mo	Healed (1)	Yes (1)	Yes (1)
Banchs & Trope,[15] 2004	2 y	Healed (1)	Yes (1)	Yes (1)
Chueh & Huang,[16] 2006	7 mo–5 y	Healed (4)	Yes (4)	Yes (4)
Petrino,[17] 2307	8 mo	Healed (1)	Yes (1)	Yes (1)
Thibodeau & Trope,[18] 2007	12.5 mo	Healed (1)	Yes (1)	Yes (1)
Jung et al,[19] 2008	1–5 y	Healed (8) Reduced (1)	Yes (7) Questionable (2)	Yes (9)
Cotti et al,[20] 2008	30 mo	Healed (1)	Yes (1)	Yes (1)
Shah et al,[21] 2008	6 mo–3.5 y	Healed (4) Reduced (5)	Unable to determine (9)	Unable to determine (9)
Chueh et al[22] 2009	6–108 mo	Healed (23)	Continued root development (23)	Continued root development (23)
Ding et al,[23] 2009	≥1 y	Healed (3) Dropped out (6) Lost to recall (3)	Complete root development with closed apex (3)	Complete root cevelopment with closed apex (3)
Reynolds et al,[24] 2009	18 mo	Healed (2)	None (2)	Yes (2)
Shin et al,[25] 2009	19 mo	Healed	Yes (1)	Yes (1)
Thibodeau,[26] 2009	16 mo	Healed	Yes (1)	Yes (1)
Kim et al,[27] 2010	8 mo	Healed (1)	Yes (1)	Yes (1)
Petrino et al,[28] 2010	9–12 mo	Healed (1)	Yes (2) No (4)	Yes (2) No (4)
Cehrreli et a,[30] 2011	9–10 mo	Healed (6)	Yes (6)	Yes (6)
Nosrat et al[29] 2011	15–18 mo	Healed (2)	None (2)	Yes (2)
Torabinejad & Turman,[31] 2011	5.5 mo	Healed	Unable to determine (1)	Yes (1)
Lenzi & Trope,[32] 2012	21 mo	Healed (2)	Unable to determine (2)	Yes (1) No (1)

When available, recall radiographs were interpreted by the author of this article. If radiographs were not shown in the case report/series, the summary information provided in the article was included in the table.

Data from Hargreaves KM, Law AS. Regenerative endodontics. In: Hargreaves KM, Cohen S, editors. Pathways of the pulp. 10th edition. St Louis: Mosby/Elsevier; 2010.

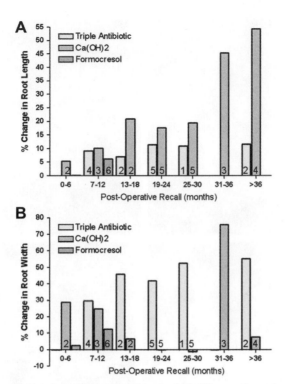

Fig. 2. Percentage change in root length (*A*) and width (*B*) over time, for teeth medicated with triple antibiotic paste, Ca(OH)$_2$, or formocresol. (*Data from* Bose R, Nummikoski P, Hargreaves K. A retrospective evaluation of radiographic outcomes in immature teeth with necrotic root canal systems treated with regenerative endodontic procedures. J Endod 2009;10:1343–9.)

to weigh the benefits of the increased visualization with the risks of radiation exposure and minimize the field of view as much a possible.[34] As with follow-up after other endodontic procedures, if there are persistent symptoms, recurrence of symptoms, increased apical radiolucency, and/or radiographic evidence of root resorption at any point, alternative treatment should be considered.

In addition to radiographic evidence of healing apical bone and continued root development, some case reports and case series have demonstrated positive responses to cold and/or electric pulp tests[14,23,28,30,31] in teeth that underwent revitalization procedures. The positive response to pulp tests may be an indication of regeneration of innervation in the canal space. The lack of a pulp response, however, does not necessarily indicate a lack of vitality. The case series in which there was no response to pulp testing,[30] there was radiographic evidence of continued root development, indicating the presence of vital tissue in the canal space. Future developments in assessing pulp vitality will allow for a more accurate assessment of treatment success.

The healing of the apical bone and resolution of symptoms, in the absence of continued root growth, may be an acceptable outcome for many patients and practitioners. Survival, or retention of the treated tooth, is an accepted outcome measure.[35,36] Given that loss of a permanent tooth before completion of alveolar bone development can lead to atrophy of the alveolar ridge,[37] thus potentially compromising future implant replacement, a reasonable goal of revitalization procedures should be retention of the treated tooth until completion of alveolar ridge development,

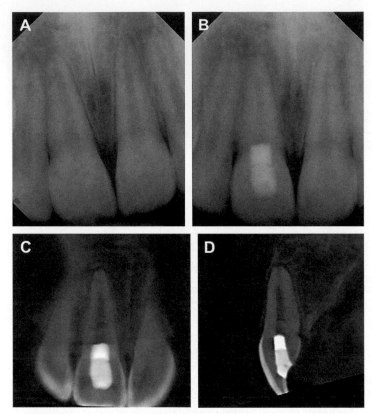

Fig. 3. Periapical radiographs at pretreatment (*A*) and 1 year after (*B*) a revitalization treatment. Cone beam computed tomography of the same tooth in coronal (*C*) and sagittal (*D*) views at 1 year after treatment. (*Courtesy of* Dr Jason Hales.)

even in the absence of continued root development. Examples of tooth retention without continued root development are shown in **Fig. 4**.

HISTOLOGY FROM ANIMAL STUDIES

The reported outcomes from case reports/series showing continued root development after revitalization/regeneration procedures, although encouraging, is not sufficient to demonstrate regeneration of pulp tissue. In a recent review by Andreasen and Bakland,[7] based on an analysis of more than 1200 traumatized teeth and 370 autotransplanted premolars, 4 types of healing outcomes following regeneration procedures have been discussed: (1) Revascularization of the pulp with accelerated dentin formation leading to pulp canal obliteration (PCO); (2) Ingrowth of cementum and PDL; (3) Ingrowth of cementum, PDL, and bone; and (4) Ingrowth of bone and bone marrow. There is a lack of histologic data on human teeth following intentional revitalization procedures, making it impossible to determine with any certainty the type of tissue occupying the canal space.

Results from animal studies may provide a glimpse into possible outcomes in human teeth following revitalization procedures. A recent study by Wang and colleagues[9] on immature necrotic teeth of dogs that underwent revitalization procedures demonstrated the presence of intracanal cementum on the dentinal walls and

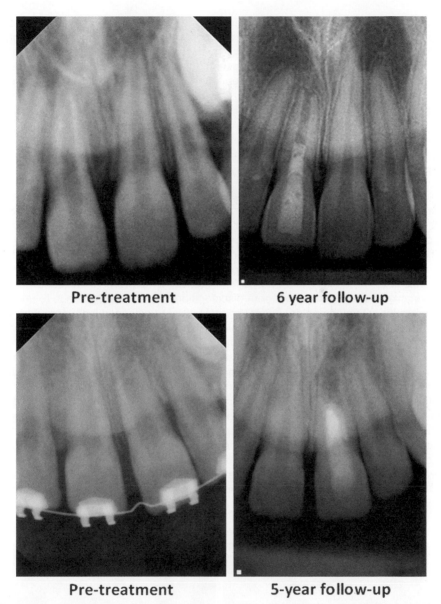

Pre-treatment   6 year follow-up

Pre-treatment   5-year follow-up

Fig. 4. Examples of bone healing and tooth retention, but lack of continued root development following revitalization. The procedure for both teeth consisted of rubber dam isolation, irrigation with NaOCl, medication with triple antibiotic paste. After 3 weeks, the apical tissues were lacerated to initiate blood clot formation, a mineral trioxide aggregate barrier was placed over the blood clot, and the teeth were restored with composite. The tooth in the top figures has an incisal edge fracture that gives it the appearance of being submerged, but the cervical height is similar to the adjacent central incisor.

cementum on the apical portion of the root. In addition, some of the teeth had evidence of intracanal bone or bone-like tissue and connective tissue similar to the periodontal ligament. The evidence from this study on dogs suggests that the tissue in the canal space may be closer to extracanal tissues than pulp tissue.

Another animal study demonstrated that it may be possible to obtain pulp-like tissue after a revitalization procedure. Huang and colleagues[38] subcutaneously implanted 6- to 7-mm long human tooth fragments containing dental stem cells seeded onto a poly-D,L,-lactide and glycolide (PLG) scaffold into immunodeficient mice. Three to 4 months after the transplantation, the tooth fragments were harvested. The histology revealed the formation of well-vascularized soft tissue in the root canal space, and a continuous layer of dentinlike tissue lined with odontoblast-like cells. Although subcutaneous tissue is much different than alveolar bone, these results suggest that it is possible to obtain pulp-like tissue after regeneration/revitalization procedures.

POTENTIAL COMPLICATIONS/UNDESIRED OUTCOMES

Although revitalization procedures are designed to heal bone and promote root development, potential complications and undesired outcomes must be addressed with patients and guardians before treatment. These complications include potential tooth discoloration, adverse reaction to intracanal antibiotics, and treatment failure.

Tooth discoloration after revitalization procedures has been demonstrated in several case reports/series.[24,27,28] The likely cause for bluish-gray discoloration reported in some cases is minocylcline from medicaments placed in the canal space; the removal of which eliminated tooth discoloration.[3,27] Another approach to prevent discoloration is to place a Root Canal Projector (CJM Engineering Inc, Santa Barbara, CA, USA) into the access, seal the coronal dentin with composite, and then remove the Projector and place the triple antibiotic paste in the canal.[24] Discoloration can also be avoided by using $Ca(OH)_2$ paste. If discoloration does occur after the placement of a minocycline-containing paste in the canal, sodium perborate bleach can be used in the tooth internally (**Fig. 5**).

Another potential source of discoloration resulting from revitalization procedures is the placement of mineral trioxide aggregate (MTA). Both gray and white MTA have been shown to discolor dentin following placement in the canal.[39,40] To avoid potential discoloration from MTA, the MTA could be placed apical to the esthetic zone, but this placement would necessarily decrease the potential for revitalization in the coronal portion of the canal, thus eliminating the potential for increased root wall thickness in the cervical area. Alternatively, a different pulp space barrier, such as glass ionomer, could be used.[14,21]

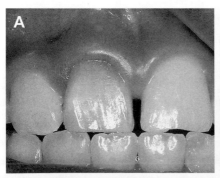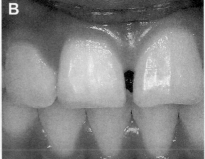

Fig. 5. Bluish discoloration caused by minocycline in triple antibiotic paste (*A*), and same tooth following internal bleaching with sodium perborate (*B*). (*From* Kim JH, Kim Y, Shin SJ, et al. Tooth discoloration of immature permanent incisor associated with triple antibiotic therapy: a case report. J Endod 2010;36:1086–91; with permission.)

A potentially more serious consequence of using antibiotics in the canal space is an allergic reaction. Allergic reactions have been reported after topical use of the antibiotics in the triple antibiotic paste.[41–45] There are no reports, however, of allergic reactions after the use of these antibiotics in root canals. Nonetheless, patients and guardians should be informed of the possibility of a reaction and asked about related allergies.

Another potential outcome of the revitalization procedure is the failure of the apical bone to heal and/or tissue to grow into the canal space, or apical bone to heal. This may be evidenced radiographically by a persistent or enlarging apical radiolucency, and/or the lack or root development. As discussed earlier in this article, one should expect to see apical bone healing at approximately 8 months after the completion of treatment, and root development at approximately 16 months. Additionally, a sign of treatment failure would be radiographic evidence of root resorption. Persistent pain, swelling, or sinus tract would also indicate failure of the treatment. If any of these signs or symptoms should occur, alternative treatments should be considered, including apexification, nonsurgical root canal treatment, or extraction.

SUMMARY

Radiographic evidence of apical bone healing, increased root length, and increased root wall width has been shown after the use of regenerative endodontic techniques in human teeth with immature roots and necrotic pulp tissue. Histologic evidence from animal models using similar revitalization procedures has shown varied hard and soft tissues in the canal space. Future research should focus on demonstrating histologic changes in human teeth, and developing techniques that increase the likelihood of achieving regeneration of the pulp-dentin complex.

REFERENCES

1. Cvek M. Prognosis of luxated non-vital maxillary incisors treated with calcium hydroxide and filled with gutta-percha. A retrospective clinical study. Endod Dent Traumatol 1992;8:45.
2. Andreasen JO, Farik B, Munksgaard EC. Long-term calcium hydroxide as a root canal dressing may increase risk of root fracture. Dent Traumatol 2002;18:134.
3. Trope M. Treatment of the immature tooth with a non-vital pulp and apical periodontitis. Dent Clin North Am 2010;54:313–24.
4. Huang GT, Lin LM. Letter to the editor: comments on the use of the term "revascularization" to describe root regeneration. J Endod 2008;34:511.
5. Trope M. Reply. J Endod 2008;34:511–2.
6. Thibodeau B, Teixeira F, Yamauchi M, et al. Pulp revascularization of immature dog teeth with apical periodontitis. J Endod 2007;33:680–9.
7. Andreasen JO, Bakland LK. Pulp regeneration after non-infected and infected necrosis, what type of tissue do we want? A review. Dent Traumatol 2011;28(1):13–8.
8. Andreasen JO, Andreasen FM. Textbook and color atlas of traumatic injuries to the teeth. Copenhagen (Denmark): Munksgaard; 1994.
9. Wang X, Thibodeau B, Trope M, et al. Histologic characterization of regenerated tissues in canal space after the revitalization/revascularization procedure of immature dog teeth with apical periodontitis. J Endod 2010;36:56–63.
10. Murray PE, Garcia-Godoy F, Hargreaves KM. Regenerative endodontics: a review of current status and a call for action. J Endod 2007;33:377–90.
11. Nygaard-Ostby B, Hjortdal O. Tissue formation in the root canal following pulp removal. Scand J Dent Res 1971;79:333–49.

12. Myers MC, Fountain SB. Dental pulp regeneration aided by blood and blood substitutes after experimentally induced periapical infection. Oral Surg Oral Med Oral Pathol 1974;37:441–50.
13. Nevins A, Finkelstein F, Borden B, et al. Revitalization of pulpless open apex teeth in rhesus monkeys, using collagen-calcium phosphate gel. J Endod 1976;2: 159–65.
14. Iwaya SI, Ikawa M, Kubota M. Revascularization of an immature permanent tooth with apical periodontitis and sinus tract. Dent Traumatol 2001;17:185–7.
15. Banchs F, Trope M. Revascularization of immature permanent teeth with apical periodontitis: new treatment protocol? J Endod 2004;30:196–200.
16. Chueh LH, Huang GT. Immature teeth with periradicular periodontitis or abscess undergoing apexogenesis: a paradigm shift. J Endod 2006;32:1205–13.
17. Petrino JA. Revascularization of necrotic pulp of immature teeth with apical periodontitis. Northwest Dent 2007;86:33–5.
18. Thibodeau B, Trope M. Pulp revascularization of a necrotic infected immature permanent tooth: case report and review of the literature. Pediatr Dent 2007; 29:47–50.
19. Jung IY, Lee SJ, Hargreaves KM. Biologically based treatment of immature permanent teeth with pulpal necrosis: a case series. J Endod 2008;34:876–87.
20. Cotti E, Mereu M, Lusso D. Regenerative treatment of an immature, traumatized tooth with apical periodontitis: report of a case. J Endod 2008;34:611–6.
21. Shah N, Logani A, Bhaskar U, et al. Efficacy of revascularization to induce apexification/apexogenesis in infected, nonvital, immature teeth: a pilot clinical study. J Endod 2008;34:919–25.
22. Chueh LH, Ho YC, Kuo TC, et al. Regenerative endodontic treatment for necrotic immature permanent teeth. J Endod 2009;35:160–4.
23. Ding RY, Cheung GS, Chen J, et al. Pulp revascularization of immature teeth with apical periodontitis: a clinical study. J Endod 2009;35:745–9.
24. Reynolds K, Johnson JD, Cohenca N. Pulp revascularization of necrotic bilateral bicuspids using a modified novel technique to eliminate potential coronal discolouration: a case report. Int Endod J 2009;42:84–92.
25. Shin SY, Albert JS, Mortman RE. One step pulp revascularization treatment of an immature permanent tooth with chronic apical abscess: a case report. Int Endod J 2009;42:1118–26.
26. Thibodeau B. Case report: pulp revascularization of a necrotic, infected, immature, permanent tooth. Pediatr Dent 2009;31:145–8.
27. Kim JH, Kim Y, Shin SJ, et al. Tooth discoloration of immature permanent incisor associated with triple antibiotic therapy: a case report. J Endod 2010;36: 1086–91.
28. Petrino JA, Boda KK, Shambarger S, et al. Challenges in regenerative endodontics: a case series. J Endod 2010;36:536–41.
29. Nosrat A, Seifi A, Asgary S. Regenerative endodontic treatment (revascularization) for necrotic immature permanent molars: a review and report of two cases with a new biomaterial. J Endod 2011;37:562–7.
30. Cehreli ZC, Isbitiren B, Sara S, et al. Regenerative endodontic treatment (revascularization) of immature necrotic molars medicated with calcium hydroxide: a case series. J Endod 2011;37:1327–30.
31. Torabinejad M, Turman M. Revitalization of tooth with necrotic pulp and open apex by using platelet-rich plasma: a case report. J Endod 2011;37:265–8.
32. Lenzi R, Trope M. Revitalization procedures in two traumatized incisors with different biological outcomes. J Endod 2012;38:411–4.

33. Bose R, Nummikoski P, Hargreaves K. A retrospective evaluation of radiographic outcomes in immature teeth with necrotic root canal systems treated with regenerative endodontic procedures. J Endod 2009;10:1343–9.

34. American Association of Endodontists, American Academy of Oral and Maxillofacial Radiology. Use of cone-beam computed tomography in endodontics Joint Position Statement of the American Association of Endodontists and the American Academy of Oral and Maxillofacial Radiology. Oral Surg Oral Med Oral Pathol Oral Radiol Endod 2011;111(2):234–7.

35. Lazarski MP, Walker WA III, Flores CM, et al. Epidemiological evaluation of the outcomes of nonsurgical root canal treatment in a large cohort of insured dental patients. J Endod 2001;27:791–6.

36. Salehrabi R, Rotstein I. Endodontic treatment outcomes in a large patient population in the USA: an epidemiological study. J Endod 2004;30(12):846–50.

37. Rodd HD, Malhotra R, O'Brien CH, et al. Change in supporting tissue following loss of a permanent maxillary incisor in children. Dent Traumatol 2007;23:328–32.

38. Huang GT, Yamaza T, Shea LD, et al. Stem/progenitor cell-mediated de novo regeneration of dental pulp with newly deposited continuous layer of dentin in an in vivo model. Tissue Eng 2010;16:605–15.

39. Watts JD, Holt DM, Beeson TJ, et al. Effects of pH and mixing agents on the temporal setting of tooth-colored and gray mineral trioxide aggregate. J Endod 2007;33:970–3.

40. Boutsioukis C, Noula G, Lambrianidis T. Ex vivo study of the efficiency of two Techniques for the removal of mineral trioxide aggregate used as a root canal filling material. J Endod 2008;34:1239–42.

41. de Paz S, Perez A, Gomez M, et al. Severe hypersensitivity reaction to minocycline. J Investig Allergol Clin Immunol 1999;9:403–4.

42. Hausermann P, Scherer K, Weber M, et al. Ciprofloxacin-induced acute generalized exanthematous pustulosis mimicking bullous drug eruption confirmed by a positive patch test. Dermatology 2005;211:277–80.

43. Jappe U, Schnuch A, Uter W. Rosacea and contact allergy to cosmetics and topical medicaments–retrospective analysis of multicentre surveillance data 1995–2002. Contact Dermatitis 2005;52:96–101.

44. Isik SR, Karakaya G, Erkin G, et al. Multidrug-induced erythema multiforme. J Investig Allergol Clin Immunol 2007;17:196–8.

45. Madsen JT, Thormann J, Kerre S, et al. Allergic contact dermatitis to topical metronidazole–3 cases. Contact Dermatitis 2007;56:364–6.

Regenerative Endodontics
Barriers and Strategies for Clinical Translation

Jeremy J. Mao, DDS, PhD[a],*, Sahng G. Kim, DDS, MS[a,b],
Jian Zhou, DDS, PhD[a], Ling Ye, DDS, PhD[c], Shoko Cho, MD, PhD[a],
Takahiro Suzuki, DDS, PhD[a], Susan Y. Fu, MD, PhD[a],
Rujing Yang, MD[a], Xuedong Zhou, DDS, PhD[c]

KEYWORDS

- Regenerative • Endodontics • Pulp • Dentin • Regeneration • Stem cells
- Tissue engineering

KEY POINTS

- Despite a great deal of enthusiasm and effort, regenerative endodontics has encountered substantial challenges toward clinical translation. The recent adoption by the American Dental Association of evoked pulp bleeding in immature permanent teeth is an important step for regenerative endodontics. However, there is no regenerative therapy for most endodontic diseases.
- Simple recapitulation of cell therapy and tissue engineering strategies that are under development for other organ systems have not led to clinical translation in regenerative endodontics. Dental pulp stem cells may seem to be a priori choice for dental pulp regeneration. However, dental pulp stem cells may not be available in patients who are in need of pulp regeneration.
- Even if dental pulp stem cells are available autologously or perhaps allogeneically, one must address a multitude of scientific, regulatory, and commercialization barriers; unless these issues are resolved, transplantation of dental pulp stem cells will remain a scientific exercise rather than a clinical reality.
- Recent work using novel biomaterial scaffolds and growth factors that orchestrate the homing of host endogenous cells represents a departure from traditional cell transplantation approaches and may accelerate clinical translation. Given the functions and scale of dental pulp and dentin, regenerative endodontics is poised to become one of the early biologic solutions in regenerative dental medicine.

The work for composition of this article is supported by NIH grants R01DE018248, R01EB009663, and RC2DE020767 (to J.J.M.) as well as NSFC grants 81070801 (to L.Y.) and 30973324 (to X.D.Z.).
Conflict of interest: Columbia University is the owner of patents for several regenerative endodontic agents and methods on behalf of Dr Jeremy Mao's laboratory.
[a] Center for Craniofacial Regeneration, Columbia University, 630 West 168 Street, PH7E, New York, NY 10032, USA; [b] Division of Endodontics, College of Dental Medicine, Columbia University, 630 West 168 Street, PH7Stem #128, New York, NY 10032, USA; [c] Department of Endodontics, West China School of Stomatology, Sichuan University, 14#, 3rd section of Ren Min Nan Lu, Chengdu, Sichuan, 610041, China
* Corresponding author. Center for Craniofacial Regeneration, Columbia University, 630 West 168 Street, PH7E, New York, NY 10032.
E-mail address: jmao@columbia.edu

Dent Clin N Am 56 (2012) 639–649
http://dx.doi.org/10.1016/j.cden.2012.05.005
0011-8532/12/$ – see front matter

INTRODUCTION

Endodontics is a dental specialty that treats trauma and infections involving the dental pulp, dentin, and periapical lesions. Each year, a total of approximately 16 million endodontic procedures are performed in the United States.[1] Root canal treatment (RCT) that involves the extirpation of the injured or infected dental pulp and filling of the root canal and pulp chamber with bioinert materials is the most common endodontic treatment.[2] Success rates for endodontic therapies vary, depending on case selection, practitioner skills, availability of instruments and materials, etc. In general, current endodontic treatments are effective to eliminate pain and control infections.[3,4] Therefore, why regenerative endodontics? Endodontic therapies, like many other dental treatments, are not without failure. Reinfections and tooth fractures are among some of the undesirable and frustrating complications for patients and practitioners, leading to additional lost work hours. **Table 1** demonstrates causes and incidences of failure of common endodontic treatments and how regenerative endodontics may address current endodontic failures.

In January 2011, the American Dental Association adopted a new procedure code to allow practitioners to induce apical bleeding into the root canal in immature permanent teeth with necrotic pulps that have been extirpated.[5] This is an important step by the endodontic community on its path to explore avenues of pulp and dentin regeneration. The endodontic treatment of immature permanent teeth with the root apex not yet fully developed presents a unique clinical challenge. The delivery of conventional RCT in an injured or infected immature permanent tooth, although effective in removing infections and in managing symptoms, has a tendency to cause the arrest of root development. As meritorious as it is, the clinical consistency of induced pulp bleeding technique is lacking at this time. The endodontic community has, for decades, been searching for vital pulp therapies.[6] Regenerative endodontics was proposed as an alternative to conventional endodontic therapies, including RCT and others.[7] In this review, the authors discuss the challenges for translating current concepts in regenerative endodontics and identify strategies to address existing barriers toward the development of clinical viable therapies.

CLINICAL STUDIES OF PULP REVASCULARIZATION

Regenerative endodontics benefit from previous studies of pulp revascularization. The clinical observation has been that pulp revascularization may be accomplished in immature teeth with apical foramen greater than 1 mm in diameter.[8,9] As early as 1966, Rule and Winter[10] presented a case of continued root formation with the apical

Table 1			
Causes and incidence of failure of nonsurgical endodontic treatments and benefits of regenerative endodontic therapy			
Therapy	Causes	Incidence of Failure	Regenerative Therapy
Primary root canal treatment	Pulp infections Trauma	15%–32%[3]	Immunologic defense Restored homeostasis Functional pulp-dentin complex
Secondary root canal treatment	Persistent infection Tooth/root fracture Restoration failure	23%[4]	Immunologic defense Restored vascular supply Option to deliver antibiotics

closure of a nonvital immature mandibular premolar following pulp bleeding. The root canal was mechanically instrumented and dressed with polyantibiotics, followed by absorbable iodoform placement. Nygaard-Ostby and colleagues[11] reported new connective tissue formation in root canals after complete pulpectomy and root filling short of the apical foramen. Nevin and colleagues[12] showed root maturation with a collagen-calcium phosphate gel introduced in an intruded maxillary lateral incisor with an immature root apex after root canal debridement. A case report by Iwaya and colleagues[13] showed revascularization with apical closure and thickening of the root canal wall in a 13-year-old patient with a necrotic, immature, mandibular premolar secondary to a fractured tooth. A similar case was reported by Banchs and Trope[14] in an 11-year-old patient with a necrotic, immature, mandibular premolar following a fractured dental tubercle. The canal was irrigated with 5.25% sodium hypochlorite and chlorhexidine gluconate (Peridex) without mechanical debridement. A triple antibiotic paste (minocycline, metronidazole, and ciprofloxacin) was placed into the canal for 1 month and removed before bleeding was induced into the root canal space with an endodontic explorer. Mineral trioxide aggregate (MTA) was placed over the blood clot approximately 3 mm below the cemento-enamel junction followed by a bonded restoration. The tooth was responsive to cold at a 2-year follow-up and showed continued root maturation.[14] There are additional case reports of pulp revascularization in necrotic immature teeth that show continuous root maturation with dentinal wall thickening and a positive response to vitality tests.[15–22] However, no randomized clinical trials have been performed on the efficacy of pulp revascularization and root development following induced pulp bleeding in immature permanent teeth.

Torabinejad and Turman[23] reported a case of pulp revascularization using platelet-rich plasma (PRP) in a replanted, immature, necrotic, maxillary premolar following accidental extraction. The necrotic pulp was removed with a barbed broach. The canal was irrigated with 5.25% sodium hypochlorite and medicated with a triple antibiotic paste for 22 days. PRP prepared from the patient's blood was injected into the canal space. The canal was sealed with Cavit and amalgam after MTA was placed over the PRP clot. At the 5- to 6-month follow-up, continued root maturation and root canal thickening was observed radiographically, along with a positive vitality test.

In summary, isolated clinical case reports have shown tangible results of pulp revascularization and some level of dentin/root development in immature permanent teeth following pulp bleeding or PRP delivery. As clinically meritorious as these attempts are, treatment outcomes are anticipated to be variable, depending on a multitude of factors, including the patients' intrinsic responses, the severity of the disease, case selection, and practitioner skills. There is a lack of randomized prospective clinical trials and, without them, it is virtually impossible to compare 2 or more therapies or even to achieve a consistent outcome for a single therapy. PRP suffers from the shortcoming of drawing blood from patients and the complexity of centrifuge and purification. Again, practitioner variation is expected to affect the clinical outcome of PRP as a regenerative endodontics therapy. A clinically meritorious trial is currently underway to compare a triple antibiotic paste and induced bleeding into the root canal system with the standard treatment of immature necrotic teeth (MTA apexification).[24]

Are there differences between pulp revascularization and pulp regeneration? In the endodontic literature, pulp revascularization is usually defined as the reintroduction of vascularity in the root canal system.[25] Pulp regeneration, on the other hand, has not been precisely defined. Given that rigid definitions tend to restrict the development of new drugs, devices, and therapies, it may be beneficial not to excessively debate the differences between pulp revascularization and pulp regeneration at this time.

Synopses from several recent review articles on regenerative endodontics seem to indicate that pulp regeneration is the restoration of the pulp-dentin complex, which is still somewhat vague.[7,26–28] The authors' view is that pulp regeneration cannot take place without revascularization or angiogenesis, but pulp revascularization seems to indicate the restoration of vascularity in the pulp but not necessarily the repopulation of odontoblasts that align on dentin surfaces. Although blood vessels are indispensable constituents of dental pulp, pulp regeneration is likely considered incomplete without an odontoblastic layer lining the dentin surface. Pulp regeneration may also be considered incomplete without nociceptive and sympathetic and parasympathetic nerve fibers, in addition to interstitial fibroblasts and, perhaps most importantly, stem/progenitor cells that serve to replenish all pulp cells in the regenerated pulp when they undergo apoptosis and turnover. Thus, it may be helpful to conceptualize:

- Pulp revascularization is the induction of angiogenesis in an endodontically treated root canal.
- Pulp regeneration is pulp revascularization plus the restoration of functional odontoblasts and/or nerve fibers.

REGENERATIVE ENDODONTICS: IS IT JUST A SCIENTIFIC EXERCISE OR CAN IT BECOME CLINICAL TREATMENTS?

The American Association of Endodontists deserves credit for its vision to enthusiastically endorse regenerative endodontics as one of the profession's future directions. However, approximately 16 years following the introduction of the concept of regenerative endodontics to the profession,[29] there is an element of palpable uncertainty and perhaps frustration that regenerative endodontics remains a scientific exercise rather than a clinical reality. This point is demonstrated vividly by an acute and yet collegial exchange of letters to the editor of *Oral Surgery, Oral Medicine, Oral Pathology, Oral Radiology, and Endodontology.* Professor Spångberg wrote the initial letter entitled, "The Emperor's new cloth,"[30] expressing concerns over the view that pulp revascularization, by evoked bleeding or triple antibiotic pastes, equates to pulp regeneration that is regarded as a paradigm shift in endodontics. The Spångberg letter was countered by a letter entitled, "The wrong emperor," from Professor Kenneth Hargreaves and Dr Alan Law, which stated that pulp revascularization, as in the classic endodontic literature, has not used the principles of tissue engineering, namely stem cells, scaffolds, and growth factors and differs from recent experimental studies of pulp regeneration.[31] The matter is perhaps not as clear-cut as we may all have wished for, as evidenced by the following challenges.

Challenge Number 1: What Cells Should Be Used for Pulp/Dentin Regeneration?

Several studies have shown that the transplantation of dental pulp or other stem cells can yield ectopic dental pulplike tissues in tooth slices or fragments in vivo.[32–36] Huang and colleagues[34] showed the formation of pulplike tissue with dentin deposition in root fragments in mice by implanting stem/progenitor cells from the apical papilla and dental pulp. Cordeiro and colleagues[37] demonstrated the formation of vascular pulplike tissue by the implantation of a tooth slice with a gel that was seeded with stem cells from human exfoliated deciduous teeth (SHED). Cell delivery has certain advantages, such as its ability to control the number of cells transplanted and the potential utility of subpopulation of stem/progenitor cells. For example, isolated stem/progenitor cells can be sorted to select the best subpopulations, which are yet to be identified, for pulp regeneration. Iohara and colleagues[35,38] showed that CD31⁻/CD146⁻ or CD105⁺ side population cells from dental pulp had higher self-renewal capacity and differentiation potential compared with the parent, heterogeneous cells. These fractionated cells have been shown to have a greater potential of inducing the formation of nerves, vasculature, and dentin in the root canal space.[33]

Why should there be a question as to what cells are to be used for dental pulp regeneration? Many would say: dental pulp stem cells. But consider this: what is the source of dental pulp stem cells for patients in need of regenerative RCT for a given tooth with the rest of the dentition completely healthy? tooth, if present, may be a theoretical source. However, the cost of the therapy is likely excessive by the time dental pulp stem cells are extracted from the tooth, processed ex vivo, and shipped back to the practitioner, not to mention the risks of contamination, the potential for acquisition of tumorigenesis during cell culture, the lack of expertise of practitioners to handle cells, the perceived poor consistency between patients, the difficulty with regulatory approval, and so forth. Cell therapy for medically incurable diseases, such as diabetes, Parkinson disease, or spinal cord injuries, may well be acceptable at a high cost and some risks but perhaps not for vital root canal therapy. Also, it is probable that the cost of ex vivo cell manipulation for the development of cell therapies of a medically incurable disease, such as spinal cord injuries, may be not that different from that of dental pulp regeneration. A recent study showed that stem/progenitor cells can be isolated from inflamed pulp tissues.[39] Inflammation is known to stimulate the recruitment or differentiation of stem/progenitor cells. However, the risks of contamination and inconsistency are likely associated with the delivery of stem/progenitor cells that are isolated from infected pulp tissues not to mention potential practitioner liabilities in case stem/progenitor cells from the patients' infected pulp tissue fail to regenerate the pulp. Other stem cells, including periodontal ligament, oral mucosa, dental follicle, apical papilla, bone marrow, and adipose stem cells, not only suffer from some of the same pitfalls as dental pulp stem cells as far as pulp regeneration is concerned but also face additional uncertainty whether they can regenerate multiple pulp tissues.

Despite its scientific validity, cell transplantation has encountered major difficulties in translation into a clinical therapy. The therapeutic use of stem cell products derived from nonhuman species will be limited because of the risk of immunorejection. Allogeneic cell transplantation has concerns of potential immunorejection and contamination. The cell cryopreservation/banking system suffers from the potential loss of cells and additional costs. Potential contamination during cell manipulation and the costs of shipping and storage are additional barriers of cell transplantation. Few practitioners today know how to handle a vial of cells. In case a few cells, among thousands or millions of cells that are transplanted, acquire oncogenes during ex vivo cell processing, a practitioner, company, or hospital would likely be held liable.

As an alternative to cell transplantation, Kim and colleagues[40] showed the regeneration of the pulp-dentin complex by cell homing. RCT was performed in clinically extracted human teeth, including pulp extirpation and instrumentation, with the only exception of root canal filling, followed by autoclaving of the teeth to remove any biologic or organic components. Instead of gutta percha, growth factors in a collagen scaffold were placed in surgically treated root canals of the human teeth. Following a 3- to 6-week in vivo implantation in the dorsum of rats, dental pulplike tissue formed in the length of root canals with vascular, odontoblastic, and neural components.[40] This study was the first to demonstrate the regeneration of dental pulplike tissues by the homing of host endogenous cells and without cell transplantation. Growth factors selected for pulp-dentin regeneration in this study include basic fibroblast growth factors (bFGFs), vascular endothelial growth factors (VEGFs), platelet-derived growth factors (PDGFs), nerve growth factors (NGFs), and bone morphogenetic protein-7

(BMP-7). bFGF was selected for chemotaxis and angiogenesis; VEGF was selected for chemotaxis, mitogenesis, and angiogenesis; PDGF was selected for angiogenesis; NGF was selected for survival and growth of nerve fibers; and BMP-7 was selected for mineralized tissue formation. Cell homing was originally defined as the migration of hematopoietic stem cells from bone marrow to the periphery and ultimately to stem cell niches. The authors extended this concept to describe the recruitment of host endogenous cells, likely including stem/progenitor cells, and subsequent tissue formation.[41] A major advantage of cell homing is to regenerate by host endogenous cells and the elimination of all ex vivo cell processing steps that are necessarily associated with cell transplantation.

Certain signaling molecules serve as bioactive cues that orchestrate the regenerative process. Signaling molecules include growth factors, cytokines, chemical compounds, or hormones. Among them, PDGF, VEGF, bFGF, BMPs, and NGF have been tested in dental pulp regeneration.[40] Their effects have been extensively discussed in "Effects of growth factors on dental stem/progenitor cells" by Kim and colleagues in this issue of the *Dental Clinics of North America*. The controlled release of signaling molecules may be necessary to address rapid diffusion and the enzymatic breakdown of peptides and proteins.[41,42] For example, control-released FGF-2 from gelatin hydrogels promoted the formation of dentin particles in amputated rat molar pulp, whereas the adsorption of FGF-2 in collagen sponges induced reparative dentin formation.[43] In an effort to develop scaffolds with controlled release of growth factors, poly ($_{D,L}$-lactide-co-glycolide) (PLGA)–based fibrous scaffolds have been developed to demonstrate the release of BMP-2 in a linear pattern over 4 weeks.[44,45] **Table 2** compares the pros and cons of cell transplantation and cell homing approaches in dental pulp regeneration.

Challenge Number 2: What Scaffolding Material Should Be Used in Pulp/Dentin Regeneration?

Scaffolds are likely indispensable for pulp/dentin regeneration and provide structural support for cells, either transplanted or endogenously homed while they synthesize tissues.[46] Scaffolds can be either native or synthetic materials.[46] An ideal scaffold should promote cell attachment and provide a conducive environment for pulp or dentin regeneration.

Table 2 Comparison of cell transplantation and cell homing approaches for regenerative endodontics		
	Cell Transplantation	**Cell Homing**
Benefits	Ability to control cell number Availability of a cell source in periapical defects Utility of subpopulations of stem/progenitor cells	No cell isolation No immunorejection No ex vivo cell processing steps
Barriers	Cell isolation from patients required Immunorejection Contamination during cell manipulation, transplantation, and storage Tumorigenesis High cost for commercialization and manufacturing stem cell products	Shortage of cells for regeneration in periapical defects?

Natural polymers include natural extracellular matrix components, such as collagen and fibronectin, which are typically biocompatible and biodegradable. Zhang and colleagues[47] used a collagen sponge, a porous ceramic, and a fibrous titanium mesh seeded with dental pulp stem cells. Mineralized deposits were observed with the expression of dentin sialoprotein after cells were cultured in an osteogenic medium for 4 weeks. On the implantation of cell-seeded scaffolds subcutaneously in nude mice for 6 or 12 weeks, dentin sialophosphoprotein was expressed in all scaffolds but mainly connective tissues were regenerated, except for in the ceramic group whereby some calcification was observed.[47]

The hyaluronic acid (HA) sponge as a natural polymer has been used in dental pulp regeneration. Inuyama and colleagues[48] investigated the effect of the HA sponge on odontoblastic cell lines (KN-3) in vitro and on the amputated dental pulp of a rat molar in vivo. In vitro, KN-3 cells attached to HA and collagen sponges. The expression of interleukin (IL)-6 and tumor necrosis factor α in a KN-3 cell-seeded HA sponge was almost equivalent to those in the collagen sponge, and the numbers of granulated leukocytes that migrated into the HA sponge were significantly lower than those that migrated into the collagen sponge.

Chitosan, chemically similar to cellulose, has been investigated for use as a scaffold for dental pulp regeneration.[49] Chitosan monomers (D-glucosamine hydrochloride) were tested to investigate the cell metabolism and wound healing in in vitro and in vivo experiments. The expression of alkaline phosphatase (ALP) activity increased significantly in 3 days of culture in the chitosan monomer group. Bone morphogenetic protein-2 activity also increased after 7 days of osteoblast culture. IL-8 synthesis was suppressed by the chitosan monomer in dental pulp cells. In vivo, direct pulp capping with chitosan monomer in rats showed that chitosan monomer induced minimal inflammatory cell infiltration after 1 day, promoted proliferation of pulp fibroblasts after 3 days, and induced mineralization by odontoblastic cells after 5 and 7 days.[49]

Several additional synthetic polymers, such as polylactic acid (PLA), poly(l-lactic) acid (PLLA), polyglycolic acid, poly($_{D,L}$-lactide-co-glycolide) (PLGA), and poly(ε-caprolactone) (PCL), have been suggested as potential scaffolds for pulp regeneration. The synthetic polymers are nontoxic; biodegradable; and allow precise manipulation of the physicochemical properties, such as mechanical stiffness, degradation rate, porosity, and microstructure.[50]

PLA and PLLA have been used as synthetic scaffolds in in vivo studies for pulp regeneration. Cordeiro and colleagues[37] used PLA scaffolds seeded with SHED in a tooth-slice implantation model. The subcutaneously implanted tooth slices with SHED-seeded PLA scaffolds into immunodeficient mice have been demonstrated to induce differentiation into odontoblastlike cells and endothelial-like cells in newly regenerated tissue based on the expression of dentin sialoprotein and B-galactosidase staining, respectively, and facilitate the regeneration of pulplike tissue. Similar experiments were performed by Sakai and colleagues,[51] which showed that SHED-seeded PLLA scaffolds promoted dental pulp cell differentiation into endothelial cells and odontoblasts.

PLGA has been widely used as a synthetic polymer scaffold in tissue engineering[44,52] and recently used in an in vivo pulp regeneration study. Huang and colleagues[34] used PLGA scaffolds seeded with stem/progenitor cells from apical papilla and dental pulp stem cells in a tooth-slice implantation model. It was demonstrated that dentinlike tissue along the wall of root canals and pulplike tissue could be regenerated after 3 to 4 months of subcutaneous implantation of teeth with cell-seeded PLGA scaffolds into immunocompromised mice.

A few studies have investigated the performance of nanofiber scaffolds for the regeneration of the dentin-pulp complex. In a study by Yang and colleagues,[53] electrospun nanofibers consisting of PCL/gelatin with or without nano-hydroxyapatite were seeded with rat dental pulp stem cells and tested in in vitro and in vivo experiments. Nanofiber scaffolds supported cell proliferation and odontoblastic differentiation by DNA content, ALP activity, and osteocalcin expression. Subcutaneous implantation of the cell-seeded nanoscaffolds showed mineralized tissue formation without inflammatory response, suggesting a potential use for pulp capping. Wang and colleagues[54,55] also showed that nanofibers fabricated from PLLA polymers could enhance attachment, proliferation, and odontoblastic differentiation of human dental pulp stem/progenitor cells in vivo and in vitro.

SUMMARY

Despite the initial promise, regenerative endodontics has encountered substantial barriers in clinical translation. Dental pulp stem cells may seem to be a priori choice for dental pulp regeneration. However, dental pulp stem cells may not be available in patients who are in need of pulp/dentin regeneration therapy. Even if dental pulp stem cells are available autologously or perhaps allogeneically, one must address a multitude of scientific, regulatory, and commercialization barriers; unless these issues are resolved, the transplantation of dental pulp stem cells for dental pulp regeneration will remain a scientific exercise rather than a clinical reality. These barriers include cell isolation; ex vivo manipulation with the potential for changing cell phenotype; and safety issues, including immunorejection, potential contamination, pathogen transmission, and potential tumorigenesis. Excessive costs associated with these issue in addition to shipping; storage; handling issues; and regulatory difficulties, including unclear pathway and the general inability to ensure batch-to-batch consistency in cell quality, cast multidimensional questions for the practicality of cell transplantation. Cell homing offers an alternative to cell transplantation for dental pulp/dentin regeneration. Biomaterial scaffolds are another area of innovation in regenerative endodontics. Several natural and synthetic polymers have shown positive results in vivo. Preclinical animal models and randomized clinical trials that test novel therapies are indispensable for translating regenerative technologies into clinical therapies.

ACKNOWLEDGMENTS

The authors thank Dr Charles Solomon for critiques, and H. Keyes, F. Guo and J. Melendez for technical and administrative assistance.

REFERENCES

1. Available at: http://www.aae.org/rootcanalspecialists/dentalprofessionalsandstudents/factsheet/. Accessed April 2, 2012.
2. Ingle JI, Slavkin HC. Modern endodontic therapy: past, present and future. In: Ingle JI, Bakland LK, Baumgartner JC, editors. Ingle's endodontics. 6th edition. Hamilton (Canada): BC Decker Inc; 2008. p. 1–35.
3. Ng YL, Mann V, Rahbaran S, et al. Outcome of primary root canal treatment: systematic review of the literature - part 1. Effects of study characteristics on probability of success. Int Endod J 2007;40(12):921–39.
4. Ng YL, Mann V, Gulabivala K. Outcome of secondary root canal treatment: a systematic review of the literature. Int Endod J 2008;41(12):1026–46.
5. American Dental Association. CDT 2011-2012: the ADA practical guide to dental procedure codes. Chicago: American Dental Association; 2010.

6. Aguilar P, Linsuwanont P. Vital pulp therapy in vital permanent teeth with cariously exposed pulp: a systematic review. J Endod 2011;37(5):581–7.
7. Murray PE, Garcia-Godoy F, Hargreaves KM. Regenerative endodontics: a review of current status and a call for action. J Endod 2007;33(4):377–90.
8. Andreasen JO, Paulsen HU, Yu Z, et al. A long-term study of 370 autotrans-planted premolars. Part II. Tooth survival and pulp healing subsequent to trans-plantation. Eur J Orthod 1990;12(1):14–24.
9. Kling M, Cvek M, Mejare I. Rate and predictability of pulp revascularization in thera-peutically reimplanted permanent incisors. Endod Dent Traumatol 1986;2(3):83–9.
10. Rule DC, Winter GB. Root growth and apical repair subsequent to pulpal necrosis in children. Br Dent J 1966;120(12):586–90.
11. Nygaard-Ostby B, Hjortdal O. Tissue formation in the root canal following pulp removal. Scand J Dent Res 1971;79(5):333–49.
12. Nevins A, Wrobel W, Valachovic R, et al. Hard tissue induction into pulpless open-apex teeth using collagen-calcium phosphate gel. J Endod 1977;3(11):431–3.
13. Iwaya SI, Ikawa M, Kubota M. Revascularization of an immature permanent tooth with apical periodontitis and sinus tract. Dent Traumatol 2001;17(4):185–7.
14. Banchs F, Trope M. Revascularization of immature permanent teeth with apical periodontitis: new treatment protocol? J Endod 2004;30(4):196–200.
15. Jung IY, Lee SJ, Hargreaves KM. Biologically based treatment of immature permanent teeth with pulpal necrosis: a case series. J Endod 2008;34(7):876–87.
16. Chueh LH, Ho YC, Kuo TC, et al. Regenerative endodontic treatment for necrotic immature permanent teeth. J Endod 2009;35(2):160–4.
17. Ding RY, Cheung GS, Chen J, et al. Pulp revascularization of immature teeth with apical periodontitis: a clinical study. J Endod 2009;35(5):745–9.
18. Bose R, Nummikoski P, Hargreaves K. A retrospective evaluation of radiographic outcomes in immature teeth with necrotic root canal systems treated with regen-erative endodontic procedures. J Endod 2009;35(10):1343–9.
19. Reynolds K, Johnson JD, Cohenca N. Pulp revascularization of necrotic bilateral bicuspids using a modified novel technique to eliminate potential coronal disco-louration: a case report. Int Endod J 2009;42(1):84–92.
20. Shin SY, Albert JS, Mortman RE. One step pulp revascularization treatment of an immature permanent tooth with chronic apical abscess: a case report. Int Endod J 2009;42(12):1118–26.
21. Petrino JA, Boda KK, Shambarger S, et al. Challenges in regenerative endodon-tics: a case series. J Endod 2010;36(3):536–41.
22. Nosrat A, Seifi A, Asgary S. Regenerative endodontic treatment (revasculariza-tion) for necrotic immature permanent molars: a review and report of two cases with a new biomaterial. J Endod 2011;37(4):562–7.
23. Torabinejad M, Turman M. Revitalization of tooth with necrotic pulp and open apex by using platelet-rich plasma: a case report. J Endod 2011;37(2):265–8.
24. Available at: http://projectreporter.nih.gov/project_info_description.cfm?aid=7876114&icde=11743516&ddparam=&ddvalue=&ddsub=&cr=2&csb=default&cs=ASC. Accessed April 2, 2012.
25. Hargreaves KM, Law AS. Regenerative endodontics. In: Hargreaves KM, Cohen S, editors. Cohen's pathways of the pulp. 10th edition. St Louis (MO): Mos-by Elsevier; 2011. p. 602–19.
26. Sun HH, Jin T, Yu Q, et al. Biological approaches toward dental pulp regeneration by tissue engineering. J Tissue Eng Regen Med 2011;5(4):e1–16.
27. Bansal R, Bansal R. Regenerative endodontics: a state of the art. Indian J Dent Res 2011;22(1):122–31.

28. Demarco FF, Conde MC, Cavalcanti BN, et al. Dental pulp tissue engineering. Braz Dent J 2011;22(1):3–13.
29. Garcia-Godoy F, Murray PE. Recommendations for using regenerative endodontic procedures in permanent immature traumatized teeth. Dent Traumatol 2012;28(1):33–41.
30. Spångberg LS. The emperor's new cloth. Oral Surg Oral Med Oral Pathol Oral Radiol Endod 2009;108(5):643–4.
31. Hargreaves KM, Law A. The wrong emperor. Oral Surg Oral Med Oral Pathol Oral Radiol Endod 2010;109(3):327–8.
32. Ishizaka R, Iohara K, Murakami M, et al. Regeneration of dental pulp following pulpectomy by fractionated stem/progenitor cells from bone marrow and adipose tissue. Biomaterials 2012;33(7):2109–18.
33. Iohara K, Imabayashi K, Ishizaka R, et al. Complete pulp regeneration after pulpectomy by transplantation of CD105+ stem cells with stromal cell-derived factor-1. Tissue Eng Part A 2011;17(15–16):1911–20.
34. Huang GT, Yamaza T, Shea LD, et al. Stem/progenitor cell-mediated de novo regeneration of dental pulp with newly deposited continuous layer of dentin in an in vivo model. Tissue Eng Part A 2010;16(2):605–15.
35. Iohara K, Zheng L, Ito M, et al. Regeneration of dental pulp after pulpotomy by transplantation of CD31(-)/CD146(-) side population cells from a canine tooth. Regen Med 2009;4(3):377–85.
36. Kuo TF, Huang AT, Chang HH, et al. Regeneration of dentin-pulp complex with cementum and periodontal ligament formation using dental bud cells in gelatin-chondroitin-hyaluronan tri-copolymer scaffold in swine. J Biomed Mater Res A 2008;86(4):1062–8.
37. Cordeiro MM, Dong Z, Kaneko T, et al. Dental pulp tissue engineering with stem cells from exfoliated deciduous teeth. J Endod 2008;34(8):962–9.
38. Iohara K, Zheng L, Ito M, et al. Side population cells isolated from porcine dental pulp tissue with self-renewal and multipotency for dentinogenesis, chondrogenesis, adipogenesis, and neurogenesis. Stem Cells 2006;24(11):2493–503.
39. Alongi DJ, Yamaza T, Song Y, et al. Stem/progenitor cells from inflamed human dental pulp retain tissue regeneration potential. Regen Med 2010;5(4):617–31.
40. Kim JY, Xin X, Moioli EK, et al. Regeneration of dental-pulp-like tissue by chemotaxis-induced cell homing. Tissue Eng Part A 2010;16(10):3023–31.
41. Lee CH, Cook JL, Mendelson A, et al. Regeneration of the articular surface of the rabbit synovial joint by cell homing: a proof of concept study. Lancet 2010;376(9739):440–8.
42. Stosich MS, Moioli EK, Wu JK, et al. Bioengineering strategies to generate vascularized soft tissue grafts with sustained shape. Methods 2009;47(2):116–21.
43. Kikuchi N, Kitamura C, Morotomi T, et al. Formation of dentin-like particles in dentin defects above exposed pulp by controlled release of fibroblast growth factor 2 from gelatin hydrogels. J Endod 2007;33(10):1198–202.
44. Fu YC, Nie H, Ho ML, et al. Optimized bone regeneration based on sustained release from three-dimensional fibrous PLGA/HAp composite scaffolds loaded with BMP-2. Biotechnol Bioeng 2008;99(4):996–1006.
45. Nie H, Soh BW, Fu YC, et al. Three-dimensional fibrous PLGA/HAp composite scaffold for BMP-2 delivery. Biotechnol Bioeng 2008;99(1):223–34.
46. Yuan Z, Nie H, Wang S, et al. Biomaterial selection for tooth regeneration. Tissue Eng Part B Rev 2011;17(5):373–88.

47. Zhang W, Walboomers XF, van Kuppevelt TH, et al. The performance of human dental pulp stem cells on different three-dimensional scaffold materials. Biomaterials 2006;27(33):5658–68.
48. Inuyama Y, Kitamura C, Nishihara T, et al. Effects of hyaluronic acid sponge as a scaffold on odontoblastic cell line and amputated dental pulp. J Biomed Mater Res B Appl Biomater 2010;92(1):120–8.
49. Matsunaga T, Yanagiguchi K, Yamada S, et al. Chitosan monomer promotes tissue regeneration on dental pulp wounds. J Biomed Mater Res A 2006;76(4): 711–20.
50. Sharma B, Elisseeff JH. Engineering structurally organized cartilage and bone tissues. Ann Biomed Eng 2004;32(1):148–59.
51. Sakai VT, Zhang Z, Dong Z, et al. SHED differentiate into functional odontoblasts and endothelium. J Dent Res 2010;89(8):791–6.
52. Agrawal CM, Ray RB. Biodegradable polymeric scaffolds for musculoskeletal tissue engineering. J Biomed Mater Res 2001;55(2):141–50.
53. Yang X, Yang F, Walboomers XF, et al. The performance of dental pulp stem cells on nanofibrous PCL/gelatin/nHA scaffolds. J Biomed Mater Res A 2010;93(1): 247–57.
54. Wang J, Liu X, Jin X, et al. The odontogenic differentiation of human dental pulp stem cells on nanofibrous poly(L-lactic acid) scaffolds in vitro and in vivo. Acta Biomater 2010;6(10):3856–63.
55. Wang J, Ma H, Jin X, et al. The effect of scaffold architecture on odontogenic differentiation of human dental pulp stem cells. Biomaterials 2011;32(31): 7822–30.

Therapeutic Potential of Mesenchymal Stem Cells for Oral and Systemic Diseases

Reuben H. Kim, DDS, PhD[a,b], Shebli Mehrazarin, DDS[b],
Mo K. Kang, DDS, PhD[c,*]

(categorization)

KEYWORDS

- Mesenchymal stem cells • Tissue engineering • Immunosuppression
- Epithelial–mesenchymal transition • Pulp capping • Pulp revitalization

KEY POINTS

- Mesenchymal stem cells (MSCs) are adult stem cells whose self-renewal, multipotency, and immunosuppressive functions have been investigated for therapeutic applications.
- Although initially isolated from systemic tissue sources, MSCs have also been isolated from dental and orofacial tissues yielding odontoblastic and cementoblastic differentiation capacities. These unique features facilitate their application for pulpal, periradicular, and mineralized dental tissue regeneration.
- MSCs have used for various systemic organ regenerative therapies, allowing rescue of tissue function in damaged or failing organs. MSCs also possess immunosuppressive functions that allow improved management and treatment of chronic inflammatory disorders. However, their propensity to undergo cellular senescence, as well as host immune response-mediated loss of potency of allogenically transplanted MSCs, may limit their use in clinical settings.

INTRODUCTION

Interest in mesenchymal stem cells (MSCs) for tissue regenerative and other medical applications has stemmed from their multilineage and self-renewal capacity and ease of isolation.[1] Since their initial discovery in the early 1960s,[2] MSCs have been extensively characterized, and their tissue origin, morphology, self-renewal capacity, and

Financial Disclosure: The current study was supported by grants DE18295 and DE18959 from NIDCR/NIH and by the Jack Weichman Endowed fund.
[a] Division of Restorative Dentistry, University of California Los Angeles School of Dentistry, 10833 Le Conte Avenue, Los Angeles, CA 90095, USA; [b] Section of Oral Biology & Medicine, University of California Los Angeles School of Dentistry, 10833 Le Conte Avenue, Los Angeles, CA 90095, USA; [c] Section of Endodontics, Division of Associated Clinical Specialty, University of California Los Angeles School of Dentistry, 10833 Le Conte Avenue, Los Angeles, CA 90095, USA
* Corresponding author.
E-mail address: mkang@dentistry.ucla.edu

Dent Clin N Am 56 (2012) 651–675
http://dx.doi.org/10.1016/j.cden.2012.05.006
dental.theclinics.com
0011-8532/12/$ – see front matter © 2012 Elsevier Inc. All rights reserved.

multipotency have been well documented. Recently, new types of MSCs originating from dental and oral tissues have been identified and characterized.[3] Although similar in morphology and replicative capacity, these dental MSCs (dMSCs) have been shown to possess distinct tissue and cell type-specific lineage paths, as well as immunosuppressive capacities, which have sparked interest in their application in dental and systemic tissue regeneration.

The first characterized MSCs were identified in bone marrow tissues.[2] Although bone marrow stem cells (BMMSCs) are among the most widely characterized, MSCs have been derived from many tissues, including umbilical cord,[4] adipose tissue,[5] and hair follicle.[6] Within the last decade and a half, a new type of MSC derived from dental and orofacial tissues has been identified. Among these MSC are dental pulp stem cells (DPSCs),[3] stem cells from apical papilla (SCAPs),[7] and periodontal ligament stem cells (PDLSCs),[8] as well as stem cells from exfoliated deciduous teeth (SHEDs),[9] and the more recently discovered dental follicle progenitor cells (DFPC).[10] In contrast to BMMSCs, dMSCs primarily follow odontogenic (DPSC, SCAP, and SHED) or cementoblastic (PDLSC) rather than osteogenic development and are responsible for developing and repairing mineralized dental tissues during development and in response to disease.[11] In addition, the authors' laboratory recently reported generation of induced MSCs (iMSCs) from epithelial cells through retroviral transduction of gene ΔNp63α through process called epithelial–mesenchymal transition (EMT).[12] These cells have demonstrated odontogenic and adipocytic differentiation properties under appropriate induction conditions. Since iMSCs can be derived from widely available tissues (eg, skin or mucosal keratinocytes), these cells may represent alternative source of MSCs, and further research will elucidate their therapeutic potential in oral and systemic conditions.

Morphologically, MSCs possess a spindle shape similar to that of fibroblasts. Upon serial subculture in vitro, dMSCs have been shown to develop morphologic changes consistent with cellular senescence, losing their spindle shape and exhibiting flattened, enlarged morphology.[13] Although they exhibit a universal morphology, MSCs originate from different tissue sources, and not all cells collected from these tissues are MSCs. Several distinct cell surface markers have been identified for each class of MSCs that have been used to isolate MSCs from non-MSCs during tissue primary culture. CD44, CD73, and CD105 are expressed consistently across all BMMSCs and dMSCs, and selection of STRO-1 by flow cytometry has become the gold standard of MSC selection and isolation.[14]

In addition to cell surface immunotype markers used to selectively isolate MSCs, several lineage-specific markers have also been identified. The osteogenic/odontoblastic lineage is among the most well characterized found in MSCs, and BMMSCs and dMSCs have been found to express common osteogenic/odontoblastic markers, such as collagen type 1, alkaline phosphatase, and bone sialoprotein.[11] Altered gene expression of these markers has been used to investigate adverse effects of senescence in MSCs.[13]

Unlike embryonic stem cells (ESCs), MSCs are adult stem cells possessing a committed lineage and lacking an indefinite self-renewal and totipotent capacity. MSCs have been shown to possess limited lifespan and ultimately undergo replicative senescence or aging in vitro.[11,13] Self-renewal has been documented as ranging from 30 to 50 population doublings (PDs) in BMMSCs to more than 120 PDs in DPSC.[11] Although self-renewal capacity of MSCs is more extensive than many somatic cells, studies have shown that, upon replicative senescence, dMSCs undergo morphologic and functional changes, in turn losing their multipotency and differentiative capacity.[13,15] The limited self-renewal capacity and senescence-associated loss of function in MSCs subcultured in vitro may present an obstacle for therapeutic application.

Although MSCs may possess comparable phenotype and replicative capacities, their multipotency and differentiation capacity differ widely and are tissue specific. BMMSCs primarily possess osteogenic differentiation capacity and express osteogenic markers, whereas DPSC and SCAP follow odontoblastic lineages, and PDLSCs possess cementoblastic differentiation.[11]

The committed lineage difference between these MSC is believed to be tissue directed. When transplanted, DPSC and SCAP form dentin–pulp-like complexes. For DPSC, this odontoblastic commitment facilitates the deposition of reparative dentin near pulp chamber in response to trauma or bacterial insult. In SCAP, this odontoblastic commitment facilitates tooth root formation during development. PDLSCs do not form dentin–pulp complexes and instead possess osteoblastic and cementoblastic lineages to regenerate periodontal tissue and maintain PDL integrity.[11] Thus, the distinct lineages adopted by MSCs are believed to be tissue-specific to address the needs of the tissue of origin. Other than osteoblastic, odontoblastic, and cementoblastic lineages, MSCs have also been induced toward adipogenic, chrondogenic, and neurogenic lineages in vitro (**Tables 1** and **2**). Alternate lineage commitment has been achieved in MSCs cultured in lineage-specific medium in vitro and evaluated by lineage-specific assays.

Despite their limited replicative potential, MSCs continue to be investigated due to their immunomodulatory and immunosuppressive properties. MSCs have been shown

Table 1				
Phenotypic comparison of MSC types				
MSCs	**Tissue Origin**	**Stem Cell Gene/Markers**	**Differentiation Markers**	**Multipotent Lineages**
BMMSC	Bone marrow	STRO-1, Oct4, Nanog	Col I, Col III, ALP, BSP, OCN, OSX	Osteogenic Adipogenic Neurogenic Chrondogenic
DPSC	Dental pulp	STRO-1, Oct 4, TGFβR Endostatin, bFGF, FGFR3	Col I, Col III, ALP, BSP, DSP, OSX, Runx2	Odontoblastic Osteogenic Adipogenic Neurogenic Chrondogenic
SCAP	Immature, developing apical papilla	STRO-1, Survivin, TGFβR, GFGR3, Endostatin, bFGF	ALP, BSP, DSP, Runx2	Odontoblastic Osteogenic Adipogenic Neurogenic
PDLSC	Periodontal ligament	STRO-1, MUC18, TGFβR	ALP, BSP, OCN	Cementogenic Osteogenic Neurogenic Chrondogenic
iMSC	Skin (keratinocytes)	Nanog, Lin28	ALP, BSP, DSP, DMP-1, OCN, ON	Osteogenic Adipogenic

Summary of MSC in vivo locations, gene expression, multipotency, and markers as known in the literature.[3,8,11,12,140]

Abbreviations: ALP, alkaline phosphatase; BSP, bone sialoprotein; BMMSC, bone marrow mesenchymal stem cells; Col I, collagen type I; Col III, collagen type III; DMP, dentin matrix protein; DPSC, dental pulp stem cells; DSP, dentin sialoprotein; iMSC, induced mesenchymal stem cell; OCN, osteocalcin; OSX, osterix; PDLSC, periodontal ligament stem cells; SCAP, stem cells of apical papillae.

Table 2
In vitro induction of MSC toward different cell lineages

Lineage	Induction Condition	Phenotypic Marker	References
Osteogenic/odontoblastic	α-MEM, 10% FBS, ascorbic acid, β-GP, dexamethasone	Alizarin red staining Von Kossa staining	3
Adipogenic	α-MEM, 20% FBS, dexamethasone	Oil Red - O staining	141
Neurogenic	DMEM, 20% FBS, FGF-2, BHA, forskolin, valproic acid, KCl, K252a, N2 supplement	Immunostaining (NSE, NeuN, Tau)	142
Chondrogenic	DMEM, insulin, transferin, selenious acid, BSA, linoleic acid, ascorbic acid	Alcian blue staining Safranin-O Staining	143,144

Abbreviations: β-GP, β-glycerophosphate; BHA, butylated hydroxyanisole; BSA, bovine serum albumin; DMEM, Dulbecco modified eagle medium; FBS, fetal bovine serum; K252a, tyrosine kinase inhibitor; MEM, minimum essential medium; N2 supplement, neuron growth supplement; NeuN, neuronal nuclear antigen; NSE, neuron-specific enolase.

to abrogate B cell antibody production, Th2 cell activation, and inflammatory cytokine production.[1,16] Studies by Pevsner-Fischer and colleagues[17] and Tomchuck and colleagues[18] have shown Toll-like receptors 3 and 4 (TLR3, TLR4) to serve a critical role in MSC immunomodulation by regulation MSC inhibition of T lymphocytes. MSCs' immunosuppressive capacity has also been shown to be regulated by proinflammatory cytokines (interferon [IFN]-γ, tumor necrosis factor [TNF]α, interleukin [IL]-1α, and IL-1β) that result in recruitment of MSCs and T cell mobilization.[1] Spaggiari and colleagues[19] demonstrated that MSCs possess the capacity to inhibit IL-2 mediated natural killer cell proliferation and cytokine production. MSCs have also been shown to lack functional MHC 2, which may further explain their immunosuppressive capacity. dMSC-specific immunosuppression has been demonstrated but not fully characterized.[11,20,21]

Although complex, multifactorial, and highly regulated, MSCs' immunosuppressive capacity has been of great interest due to therapeutic potential. Immunosuppression exhibited by MSCs may be manipulated to allow allogeneic tissue regeneration and host rejection-free transplantation. It may also facilitate treatment of degenerative conditions such as graft versus host disease and autoimmune diseases. This article will discuss the regenerative and immunomodulatory properties of MSCs and their applications in oral and systemic tissue regeneration and treatment of inflammatory disorders. It will also discuss challenges to MSC-mediated therapeutics that arise from aging of MSC donors and immunogenicity of allogeneic MSCs, and alternative sources of MSC aimed at overcoming these limitations.

TISSUE ENGINEERING OF DENTAL STRUCTURES AND PERIODONTIUM USING dMSCs

Relevance of dMSCs for dentistry lies in their potential use in tissue regeneration of dental and dentofacial structures. The authors present 4 distinct categories of tissue regeneration for dental and periodontal structures, the underlying rationale, and current status of clinical translation (**Fig. 1**). The first and simplest means of dental tissue regeneration is reparative dentine formation in dental pulp following direct pulp capping (DPC). Second, pulp revitalization allows for disinfection of necrotic, immature root canals and restoration of pulp-like tissues and pulp vitality. Third, pulp tissue engineering is aimed at regeneration of the pulp–dentin complex using

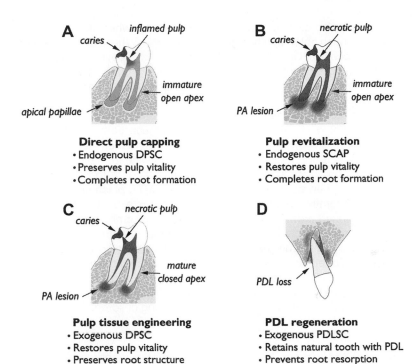

Fig. 1. Dental tissue regeneration using dMSCs. (*A*) Direct pulp capping is performed for immature tooth with open apices to preserve the pulp vitality and allow complete root formation. (*B*) Pulp revitalization aids in restoration of pulp vitality in necrotic teeth with immature root formation. This procedure also enhances root stability by continued formation of root structure. (*C*) Pulp tissue engineering restores pulp vitality in necrotic, mature teeth. This procedure would be an alternative to conventional root canal therapy (RCT) yet would preclude the need to remove tooth structure for shaping purposes for root canal obturation. In doing so, excessive removal of root structure is not necessary, leading to longer and stable dentition. (*D*) PDL regeneration would allow management of avulsed teeth for delayed replantation. Other applications would be to regenerate PDL in extracted teeth for autotransplantation and around metal implants.

exogenous dMSCs, biocompatible scaffolds, and growth factors. This approach might be considered an alternative to conventional root canal therapy (RCT) for mature permanent teeth with necrotic pulp and closed root apex. Finally, investigations are underway for tissue engineering of PDL for avulsed or extracted natural teeth and dental implants. The first 2 categories are using endogenous dMSCs, namely DPSC and SCAP, respectively, while the latter 2 categories rely on exogenous dMSCs for tissue engineering.

Direct Pulp Capping

Concept and practice of DPC goes back more than half century after the original publication by Castagnola and Orlay.[22] Since then, DPC has been regarded as a viable alternative to RCT to preserve vital pulp following pulp exposure to caries or trauma. Examination of 359 DPC cases with follow-up ranging from 1 to 8 years demonstrated overall success of 61% when $Ca(OH)_2$ was used as the capping material.[23] Several studies have demonstrated higher success with mineral trioxide aggregate (MTA) over those capped with $Ca(OH)_2$. Mente and colleagues[24] have shown 78% success with MTA pulp capping and 60% success with Ca(OH)$_2$, while higher success rates (93%–98%) have been noted in other studies.[25,26] Many of these studies demonstrate that long-term success of DPC depends, in part, on tooth type, capping material, incidence related to pulp exposure (eg, trauma vs caries), and patient's age. For instance, Auschill and colleagues[23] noted that the most successful DPC was seen with central incisors and in young (age 10–19 years) patients.

In many cases, DPC induces regenerative dentin formation, presumably from the resident DPSCs that were recruited to the site of defect. Earlier studies by Cvek[27] demonstrated formation of hard dentin structure in permanent teeth with complex crown fracture. This report indicated that initial hard tissue formation was noted in 3 to 12 weeks, and complete bridge formation was noted in 3 to 6 months following partial pulpotomy. Likewise, in a routine DPC case, MTA placement led to notable formation of regenerative dentin in 6 months time in a young (9 years) patient (**Fig. 2**). As mentioned earlier, DPC with Ca(OH)$_2$ is generally less successful than DPC capped with MTA. This may be attributed to the structural defects, known as tunnel defects, in hard tissue formed under Ca(OH)$_2$, causing bacterial leakage.[28] As such, dental pulp retains robust healing capacity through differentiation of DPSCs into odontoblasts, and DPC has been shown to be highly successful with newer materials like MTA. Clinically, DPC should be considered as a viable alternative to RCT, especially for immature teeth with open apices in young children.

Pulp Revitalization

Recent studies demonstrate the feasibility of revitalizing chronically abscessed necrotic teeth through regenerative endodontics procedures.[29–32] This approach

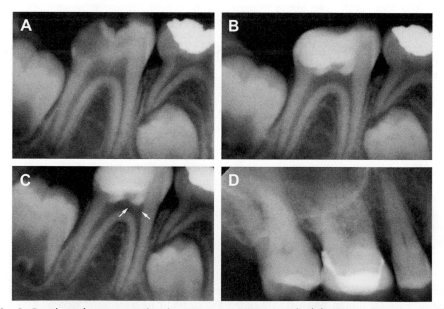

Fig. 2. Dentin–pulp regeneration in young permanent tooth. (*A*) Carious lesion on tooth #30 of a 9-year-old patient was excavated and the defect repaired by direct pulp capping using MTA. (*B*) Immediately after treatment, pulp exposure was covered with MTA. (*C*) There is radiographically visible reparative dentin formation underneath MTA after 6 months postoperatively, demonstrating robust regenerative potential (*arrows*). (*D*) Tooth #3 from a 50-year-old patient demonstrates heavily calcified pulp and root canal.

would be greatly beneficial for immature teeth with divergent apices, because revitalization of such teeth would allow for continued root development and apical closure. On the contrary, conventional treatment would involve apexification, which permanently arrests root development, leaving the tooth more susceptible to fracture. A study by Bose and colleagues[33] demonstrated significantly increased root length and thickness in teeth after revitalization when compared with those that had received apexification. Thus, there is clear justification for this new approach for immature, necrotic teeth.

While varied clinical protocols are reported, the unifying theme of pulp revitalization procedures is to disinfect the root canals using either $Ca(OH)_2$ or triple antibiotic paste, induce intracanal bleeding through the apical foramen, and allow endogenous MSCs to resume odontogenic differentiation and complete the root formation. Underlying assumptions are that there is residual pool of SCAPs surviving the chronic infection and that these cells are reactivated once the source of inflammation is resolved. A recent study showed enriched population of CD73+ and CD105+ MSCs in intracanal blood during revitalization procedure.[34] Thus, evidence suggests recruitment of MSCs during revitalization into the root canal, although the source of these cells and their role in pulp–dentin reconstitution remain completely unknown.

Validity of pulp revitalization as routine endodontic therapy requires understanding of long-term outcome and predictability. So far, this information is generally limited to several case reports, with follow-up periods ranging from a few months to 2 to 3 years postoperatively. However, preliminary results shown in the case reports are striking. Chueh and colleagues[30] report successful resolution of apical lesions and root development in 23 necrotic immature permanent teeth after the revitalization procedure using $Ca(OH)_2$. In another study, revitalization was performed using platelet-rich plasma (PRP) on a necrotic maxillary second premolar that had regained sensitivity to cold and electric pulp testing.[32] Clearly, growing evidence is in favor of revitalization as a viable alternative to apexification, although systematic evaluation of treatment outcomes with larger numbers of cases and longer follow-up periods is needed.

Pulp Tissue Engineering

Both DPC and revitalization discussed previously harness the regeneration capacities of endogenous dMSCs, either representing DPSCs or SCAPs, respectively. Revitalization of necrotic mature teeth with closed apex may necessitate pulp tissue engineering, which may require biodegradable scaffolds, addition of exogenous dMSCs, and growth factors (eg, TGF-β, BMP-7, and bFGF).[35–37] Pulp tissue engineering is far more complicated than revitalization using endogenous dMSCs and is being developed as an alternative to conventional RCT. Although literature supports high success rates upwards of 90%,[38,39] structural defects are the leading cause of tooth extraction among endodontically treated teeth. Vire[40] reported that 59.4% of endodontically treated teeth were extracted due to prosthetic failure (eg, crown fracture, root fracture, and recurrent decay), whereas 8.6% were extracted due to endodontic failure. Such structural failure may simply be due to removal of dentinal matter during cleaning and shaping, rather than any substantive changes to dentin by lack of vitality. Sedgley and Messer[41] showed no significant difference in dentinal shear strength, toughness, or fracture resistance between vital dentin and those treated endodontically. Thus, structural imperfections associated with conventional RCT may be avoided by devising regenerative therapies, which may reinforce dentinal structure.

Recent studies demonstrated proof-of-concept for pulp tissue engineering using extracted root model transplanted onto immunocompromised animals. Huang and colleagues[42] used a hollowed root filled with polylactide/glicolide (PLG) scaffolds and DPSCs, and showed pulp regeneration and dentin formation inside the root canal wall. Subsequently, the tooth slice model developed by Sakai and colleagues[43] showed de novo dentinogenesis in artificial pulp regenerated with poly-L-lactic acid (PLLA) and DPSCs. Pulp regeneration therefore allowed for new hard tissue formation in dental pulp that may aid in reinforcing structural stability. Other advantages of pulp tissue engineering may include reinstating immune defense mechanisms and innervation for environmental stimuli, including temperature changes, excessive load, and bacterial invasion. These functions of dental pulp are critical for protecting the tooth structure from potential fractures and recurrent decay. Conventional RCT offers no functional restoration of pulp, and such deficiencies may account for the need to extract endodontically treated teeth. At present, there is no clinical study demonstrating successful restoration of functional pulp through tissue engineering, although preclinical studies using dMSC and the scaffolds have yielded promising results.

PDL Regeneration

PDLSCs have been isolated from extracted human teeth and have shown ability to form cementum- and PDL-like structures when transplanted in vivo.[8] These cells opened the possibility of PDL regeneration on root surfaces of extracted or avulsed teeth. Traditionally, tooth avulsion and replantation have had poor long-term survival resulting from root resorption and ankylosis. Donaldson and Kinirons[44] showed that 68% of all replanted teeth undergo root resorption and that resorption is enhanced by extended dry-time (ie, duration of tooth being out of socket) and presence of contamination. PDL regeneration may prevent root resorption in avulsion–replantation cases or intentional tooth replantation or transplantation. Like pulp tissue engineering, PDL regeneration would require an exogenous source of dMSCs. A preclinical animal study was recently published by Dangaria and colleagues[45] to demonstrate feasibility of PDL regeneration. This study used the extraction–replantation model using rat maxillary molars with or without PDLSC coating on the root surface; when evaluated 6 months after replantation, almost complete resorption occurred on the denuded root surface. However, those teeth with PDLSC coating revealed newly formed PDL structure and absence of root resorption. Thus, PDLSCs are able to regenerate PDL tissue on a replanted tooth. Further development of this technology will allow better management of avulsion–replantation cases and possibly extraoral manipulation of teeth for routine dental work. In addition, PDL regeneration is a possibility on titanium implant surfaces, as recently demonstrated in an animal model.[46] One clinical study demonstrated cell-coated dental implant placement in the mandible and PDL formation around the implant surface.[47] This is the proof-of-concept study for ligament-anchored implants or ligaplant for clinical use in people. Among many, 1 obvious benefit for ligaplant would be the possibility to mobilize dental implants using orthodontic appliances.

REGENERATIVE THERAPIES USING MSCs FOR SYSTEMIC DISEASES

Recent advances in the use of MSC-mediated therapies hold great promises to potentially managing and treating systemic diseases. Systemic applications of MSC therapies are grossly divided into 2 categories, regenerative and immunomodulatory therapies. Regenerative therapy refers to a therapeutic modality in which structures and functions of an organ are regenerated to the clinically acceptable level with MSCs. Immunomodulatory therapy uses immunomodulatory characteristics of MSCs capable of intervening both innate and adaptive immunity. This section will discuss about use of MSCs for both therapeutic purposes.

The main goals of using MSCs for regenerative therapies for systemic diseases include restoration of forms or functions of cells, tissues, and organs that are missing or malfunctioning. MSCs have been shown to differentiate into different types of cells in vitro (**Table 3**). In addition, preclinical animal studies provided rationales to push the use of MSCs at the clinical trial levels to regenerate functionally failed organs. In this section, the authors will discuss potential role of MSCs for functional restoration of critical organ systems, such as skin, cardiac muscle, pancreas, and liver.

Skin Wound Closure

Currently, the standard of care for skin defects is split-thickness autograft,[48] but its practice is limited to availability and sizes of wounds. For large skin defects such as traumatic, burned, or nonhealing wounds, regenerative therapies are promising therapeutic modalities. The primary goals of skin regenerative therapies are to restore physical barriers to prevent infection and the loss of body fluid and to provide esthetically acceptable appearance. Skin regenerative therapies are largely divided into 3 categories: (1) artificially bioengineered skin substitutes, (2) cell-based therapies, and (3) combination of skin substitutes and cell-base therapies. Integra is a bilayer artificial skin substitute with silicone in the external layer and bovine collagen/chondroitin sulfate matrix in the inner layer. Integra serves as a temporary matrix, which allows for ingrowth of cells including fibroblasts, and it has been used and widely accepted as the prototypical biomaterials for restoration of skin defects. Cultured epithelial autografts (CEAs) are cell-based therapies in which keratinocytes and fibroblasts are integrated onto a collagen sheet to reconstitute skin-like constructs. CEA is advantageous, because of its autologous tissue constructs; however, its use is limited due to high cost, the fragility of the graft materials, and increased total costs including hospital care for the follow-ups. Studies have shown that combination of CEA and Integra allows for rapid healing and complete restoration of the skin at the wound site[49]; however, complete skin regeneration is not achievable because (1) cultured keratinocytes and fibroblasts contain minimal, if not all, amounts of multipotent stem cells required to reconstitute fully functional skin, and (2) stem cells are most likely needed to reconstitute different functional components of skin including hair follicles and sweat glands.

Recent studies demonstrate that skin-regenerative therapies using MSCs are potentially promising. Several groups reported complete closure of chronic wounds when freshly prepared or in vitro-cultured bone marrow-derived cells were topically applied to the wounded sites.[50–52] Bone marrow MSC impregnated onto collagen matrix has been shown to be effective in closure of chronic wounds.[53,54] MSC derived from adipose tissues were also used with or without fibrin glue to expedite closure of perianal fistula, and the long-term follow-ups revealed that 17 out of 24 patients treated with MSCs had the fistula remained closed, whereas 3 out of 25 patients treated without MSCs had the open fistula.[55,56] Therefore, use of MSCs to enhance cutaneous wound healing in the clinical settings is a promising therapeutic modality in skin regeneration.

Despite the promising clinical outcomes of MSC-mediated therapy on chronic wound healing, direct conversion of MSCs to the skin epithelial cells (eg, keratinocytes) as a underlying mechanisms has only been recently suggested. Fujita and colleagues[57] showed that hematopoietic-derived MSCs exhibited keratinocyte-specific markers when either co-cultured with keratinocytes or cultured in keratinocyte-conditioned medium. However, because expedited cutaneous wound healing mediated by MSCs is most likely associated with enhanced reepithelialization, cellularity, and angiogenesis,[58] whether such results are associated with de novo conversion of

Table 3
In vitro transdifferentiation potential of MSCs into different cell types

Organ/Cells	MSC Sources	Induction Conditions	Differentiation Markers	References
Skin/keratinocytes	Hematopoietic	Keratinocyte-conditioned medium	↑KRT14 ↑TGM1	57
Heart/cardiomyocytes	Bone marrow	5-azacytidine	↑ action potential ↑ Nkx2.5/Csx, GATA4 ↑ MEF-2A, MEF-2D	61
	Bone marrow	Insulin, dexamethasone, ascorbic acid	↑ Nkx2.5/Csx, GATA4 ↑ MEF-2A, MEF-2D	62
Pancreas/β-cells	Bone marrow	1. High glucose (for expansion) 2. Nicotinamide, exendin4, glucose (for differentiation)	↑ insulin 1 and 2 ↑Glut2, PDX-1, Pax6	70
	Bone marrow	Rat pancreatic extract (RPE)	↑ insulin 1 and 2 ↑glucagon ↑pancreatic polypeptide ↑somatostatin	71
	Bone marrow	1. Ectopic expression of IPF1, HLXB9, and FOXA2 2. Islet-conditioned medium	↑FOXA2, PAX4, and ISL1 ↑ insulin 1 and 2 ↑glucagon	72
Liver/hepatocytes	Bone marrow	1. ITS, FGF, EGF (for expansion) 2. HGF, NTA, Dexamethazone (for differentiation)	↑albumin, HepPar-1, α-fetoprotein, KRT18, KRT19, nestin	79
	Bone marrow	1. IGF-I, HGF, dexamethasone (for expansion) 2. Oncostatin M (for differentiation)	↑albumin, α-fetoprotein	81

Upward arrow indicates increased level.

Abbreviations: EGF, epidermal growth factor; FOXA2, forkhead box transcription factor; FGF, fibroblast growth factor; Glut, glucose transporter; HGF, hepatocyte growth factor; HLXB9, homeobox gene encoding Hb9; IGF, insulin-like growth factor; IPF, insulin promoter factor; ISL, insulin gene enhancer protein; KRT, keratin; MEF, myocyte enhancer factor; Nkx,2.5, NK2 homeobox 5; NTA, nicotinamide; Pax, paired box protein; PDX, pancreatic and duodenal homeobox; TGM, transglutaminase.

MSCs into functional keratinocytes (eg, formation of epithelial barriers) and play an important role in wound healing of the skin in vivo requires further examination.

Cardiac Muscle

Progressive functional failure of heart muscle after a myocardial infarction is among the major heart problems in elderly population worldwide.[59] Because the cardiac muscle has long been considered as a postmitotic organ without regenerative potential, the infarcted heart fails to regenerate contractile cardiac tissues but is replaced by noncontractile fibrous tissues. Therefore, the goal of cardiac muscle regeneration is to rejuvenate the cardiac muscles and to restore the contractile forces.

Recent in vitro studies suggest that MSCs can be induced to differentiate into contractile cardiomyocytes. Fukuda[60] and Makino and colleagues[61] showed that MSC treated with 5-aza-cyidine became cardiomyocytes as demonstrated by increased expression of cardiac-specific transcription factors such as GATA4 and Nkx2.5. MSCs cultured in medium containing insulin, dexamethasone, and ascorbic acid also differentiated into cardiomyocytes,[62] suggesting that MSC may serve as an adequate source for cardiac muscle regeneration therapy.

Preclinical animal studies demonstrated that MSCs improve cardiac function after myocardial infarction, although the mechanisms behind such improvement are incompletely understood. Miyahara and colleagues[63] showed that a sheet of MSCs transplanted onto the scarred myocardium after myocardial infarction in mice grew to form a thick stratum and improved cardiac function. MSCs directly injected into the infarcted cardiac muscle in mice also showed improved cardiac function.[64,65]

As of 2011, there were total of 19 clinical trials for MSC-mediated heart therapy for heart diseases.[66,67] Recent phase 1 clinical study showed significant improvement in cardiac contractility as determined by left ventricular ejection fraction.[68] Nonetheless, there are still unsolved challenges such as transient enhancement of cardiac contractility without structural repair, lack of evidence in long-term survival, and efficient delivery of the MSCs to the donor sites.

Pancreatic β-Cells

The pancreas is an important organ that produces insulin, a critical factor that regulates the blood glucose levels. Insulin is produced by β-cells within the pancreatic islets of Langerhans, and destruction of β-cells leads to hypoglycemia and type 1 diabetes mellitus. Patients with type 1 diabetes mellitus are susceptible to vascular damages, and, over period of time, develop chronic complications such as retinopathy, neuropathy, nephropathy, and cardiovascular diseases.

Current treatment of type 1 diabetes mellitus is exogenous insulin administration. Whole-organ transplantation has been performed on those who are nonresponsive to exogenous insulin-based treatment[69]; however, it is limited by systemic infection and lifelong immunosuppression secondary to organ transplantation, and relapse due to incomplete achievement for insulin independence.

Because type 1 diabetes mellitus is primarily due to the functional loss of a single cell type, β-cells within the pancreatic islets of Langerhans, MSC-mediated therapy is a plausible treatment modality. In vitro, MSCs have been demonstrated to be reprogrammed to insulin-producing cells. Several groups demonstrated that MSCs derived from human or rodent bone marrow can be differentiated into insulin-producing cells.[70–73] MSCs derived from different anatomic sources have also also been shown to be differentiated into insulin-producing cells.[74,75] It additionally has been demonstrated that these insulin-producing cells are responsive to glucose stimulation,[75] suggesting MSCs are the promising alternative cell population that can functionally replace damaged pancreatic β-cells.

Preclinical studies using animal models demonstrated that MSCs can functionally and structurally replace pancreatic β-cells in vivo. Ianus and colleagues[76] genetically engineered MSCs that produce enhanced green fluorescent protein (EGFP) when the insulin gene is actively transcribed. These MSCs were transplanted onto the immune-suppressed mice, and EGFP-positive cells were detected in the pancreatic islets. When these cells were explanted and grown in vitro, they produced glucose-dependent and incretin-enhanced insulin secretion, suggesting MSCs can be differentiated into pancreatic β-cells to produce insulin in vivo. However, subsequent studies by other groups showed different results; transplanted MSCs became pancreatic β-cells, but no insulin was secreted from these cells.[77] Nonetheless, MSC transplantation resulted in endogenous pancreatic tissue repair,[78] suggesting that MSC-mediated therapy is a viable therapeutic modality for nonfunctional or damaged pancreas such as in type 1 diabetes mellitus.

Liver

The liver is a vital organ that detoxifies toxic substances. Damages to the liver by portal hypertension, chronic liver failure, or viral- or nonviral-mediated cancer lead to fibrosis. The end-stage fibrosis or cirrhosis requires liver transplantation. However, similar to pancreas transplantation, the limitations to liver transplantation are availability of the liver donors, immune rejection, surgical intervention, and high costs. Cell-based therapy can be beneficial as an alternative to transplantation.

Several groups reported successful differentiation of MSCs into the hepatocytes in vitro. Chivu and colleagues[79] used a 2-stage method to differentiate MSCs to hepatocytes. Histone deacetylase, valproic acid, and cytokines such as hepatocyte growth factor (HGF) and insulin-like growth factor 1 (IGF-1) were also used for hepatogenic differentiation.[80,81]

Preclinical animal studies also demonstrated the potential use of MSCs to manage liver fibrosis. In a D-galatosamine induced rat model of acute liver injury, MSC-mediated therapy caused a reduction of apoptotic hepatocellular death and enhancement of hepatocyte proliferation.[82] The improvement of liver functions by MSCs has been demonstrated in other liver injury models.[83–85] Similarly, recent clinical trials demonstrated efficacy and safety of MSC-mediated liver generation therapy,[86,87] suggesting that MSC-mediated therapy for liver failures is promising therapeutic modality.

IMMUNOMODULATORY THERAPIES USING MSCs FOR SYSTEMIC DISEASES

In addition to pluripotency of MSCs that can differentiate into different types of cells such as keratinocytes, cardiomyocytes, hepatocytes, and pancreatic cells, MSCs have immunomodulatory functions. MSCs modulate both innate and adaptive immunity (Fig. 3), and such properties are promising in direct use to clinical applications. In particular, MSCs are involved in innate immunity by inhibiting the functions of IL-2-stimulated natural killer (NK) cells[88] and maturation of monocytes into the dendritic cells.[89] MSCs also interfere with the adaptive immune functions by inhibiting B cell and CD4+ T proliferation, gaining resistance to cytotoxic T lymphocytes (CTL)-mediated lysis, and inducing Treg cells.[90–92] These studies suggest that MSCs generally assert immunosuppressive functions and that immune-associated disorders may be intervened with MSC-mediated therapy.

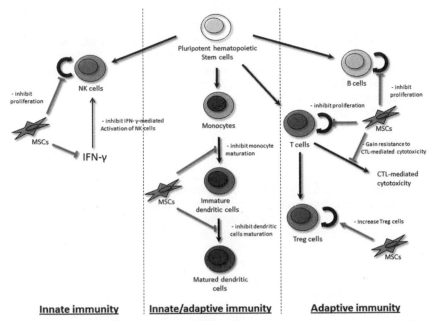

Fig. 3. Immunomodulatory functions of MSCs. MSCs modulate both innate and adaptive immunity by inhibition proliferation of NK cells, B cells, and T cells. MSCs interfere with monocyte differentiation by inhibiting dendritic cell maturation. In contrast, MSCs induce Treg cells, maintaining tolerance to self-antigens.

Systemic Lupus Erythematosus

Systemic lupus erythematosus (SLE) is an autoimmune inflammatory disease with involvement of multiple organs, destruction of which may lead to life-threatening situations. As such, lifelong immune suppression may be required for severe SLE. To date, there are no cures for SLE; however, recent studies have suggested potential therapeutic effects of MSCs for SLE. It was initially thought that SLE is associated with MSC deficiency and that allogeneic transplantation of MSC to lupus patients may be effective. It was then experimentally proven that MSCs in SLE were defective in phenotype.[93,94] Using an SLE mouse model, MSCs from healthy a mouse were transplanted onto a mouse with SLE at the early as well as matured stages of the SLE disorder. Regardless of the SLE stages, allogenetically transplanted MSC significantly improved SLE conditions including significant reduction in anti-dsDNA antibodies immunoglobulin (Ig)G and IgM, antinuclear antibody (ANA), and immunoglubulins.[95,96] MSC transplantation also reduced renal disorders, 1 of the common organ sites affected by SLE. The same group demonstrated that MSCs derived from bone marrow and umbilical cords were safe and effective in treating SLE patients,[97,98] suggesting that the immunomodulatory role of MSC potentially holds promise to treating autoimmune diseases. It would be interesting to see further validations of MSC-mediated therapy in SLE patients by other groups.

Rheumatoid Arthritis

Rheumatoid arthritis (RA) is also a type of immune diseases with chronic inflammation specific to the joints and the surrounding tissues mediated by immune cells including T cells.[99] Because MSCs modulate and interfere with T cells' proliferation and function, MSCs were used in preclinical animal models to examine effects of MSC-mediated therapy on RA. In a collagen-induced arthritis (CIA) mouse model, MSCs derived from adipose tissues ameliorated CIA as demonstrated by inhibition of various inflammatory cytokines and a decrease in antigen-specific Th1/Th17 cell expansion.[100] Similarly, umbilical cord-derived MSCs showed similar results.[101] Genetically modified MSCs have been also used. For example, CIA-induced mice received intraperitoneal administration of TGF-β-transduced MSCs, and these mice showed suppression of arthritis development and improvement in joint inflammation.[102] On the other hand, allogeneic MSC transplantation in refractory RA patients revealed unclear effectiveness,[103] suggesting that effects of MSC-mediated therapy for RA need further investigation.

Multiple Sclerosis

Multiple sclerosis (MS) is another type of autoimmune diseases that affect the central nervous system including brain and spinal cores, leading to gradual and progressive deterioration of neurologic functions. Although the pathophysiology of MS is still unclear, it is believed to be an autoimmune disorder associated with uncontrolled T cells and other immune cells such that the body's own immune system damages the myelin,[104] healing of which leaves multiple scars (hence multiple sclerosis), particularly in the white matter. There is no complete cure for MS, but it is currently managed by suppressing the immune systems.

The preclinical studies of MS were well characterized and performed in an experimental allergic encephalomyelitis (EAE) model in which animals were immunized with myelin proteins or peptides to cause damages to myelin.[105] Early studies showed that bone marrow-derived MSCs injected intravenously into the EAE mouse ameliorated EAE as demonstrated by decreased inflammatory infiltrates and demyelination.[106] Subsequent studies consistently revealed that MSCs improved neurologic functions and suppressed immune responses.[107–110] Allogeneic MSCs were also used and showed a significant decrease in disease score in the EAE mouse model.[111]

Recent clinical studies have shown that MSCs improved clinical outcomes in MS patients. Mohyeddin Bonab and colleagues[112] showed that 6 out of 10 patients who underwent MSC-mediated therapy showed some degree of improvement in clinical functional tests, although magnetic resonance imaging (MRI) assessment revealed only 1 patient with a decrease in the number of plaques. Similarly, other groups reported that MSC-mediated therapy for MS patients showed improved clinical outcomes without radiological efficacy.[113] Clearly, randomized and well-controlled clinical studies with larger samples are needed.

CHALLENGES AND FUTURE DIRECTIONS OF MSC THERAPIES

As mentioned previously, many of the degenerative diseases that may have therapeutic benefit from MSCs, whether systemic or dental, are associated with chronologic aging of patients. For instance, indisputably, the greatest risk factor for myocardial infarct is aging.[114] Numerous other disease conditions, (eg, neurodegenerative diseases, liver cirrhosis, and diabetes) have great propensity to occur in aged individuals. The aged population is retaining more teeth, presumably due to the advancement of dental care and enhanced patient education.

Nonetheless, earlier studies showed progressive changes in demographics of endodontic therapies such that conventional RCTs have been performed in aged patients in more recent years than before.[115] This would indicate that the pulp tissue engineering approach for mature teeth should be made available to the aged population in the future. With these considerations, there are 3 main remaining questions: (1)

what are the effects of aging on the tissue sources and regenerative capacities of MSCs; (2) whether allogeneic MSCs can be used for regenerative therapies just as efficaciously as autologous MSCs; and (3) if there is any alternative source of MSCs.

Effects of Aging on MSC Function

Aging in general causes tissue deterioration and loss of regenerative capacity in part due to age-associated tissue changes and accumulation of environmental factors.[116] When the bone marrow content in cadaver femoral heads was compared against age, a young (22 years) cadaver showed mostly red marrow, indicative of active hematopoietic regeneration.[117] On the contrary, those from an 86 year-old cadaver showed complete fatty transformation of bone marrow, suggesting absence of tissue regeneration. Comparison of periapical radiographs of young patients versus middle-aged patients demonstrates drastic loss of pulp tissue space with aging (see **Fig. 2**). Changes in dental pulp with aging are well characterized by the article by Morse.[118] Based on this review, aging dental pulp progressively accumulates secondary dentin and undergoes fatty degeneration, loss of cellularity, and fibrous degeneration in pulp proper. Secondary dentin formation at the apical foramen leads to closure of blood and nerve supplies to the pulp, compromising the pulp vitality in aged patients. Clearly, there is a rather drastic loss of tissue sources from which MSCs may be derived from the aged population, whether it is bone marrow or dental pulp.

At the cellular level, several studies indicate diminution of regenerative capacity of MSCs with aging of the host/donor. Global gene expression profiling of bone marrow MSCs demonstrated aging-associated decline in markers (eg, osteogenic and homeobox markers and adipogenic markers), representing tissue regenerative capacity.[119] Similarly, BMMSCs of rhesus monkeys showed notable diminution of differentiation potential as a function of age.[120] This same study also elucidated that such decline occurs by accumulation of senescent cells in aged bone marrow compared with younger bone marrow. Cellular senescence is a phenomenon whereby the cells spontaneously arrest their replication after finite number of cell doublings.[121] In their recent study, the authors showed that DPSCs lose their odontogenic differentiation potential after extended in vitro culture due to onset of senescence.[13] The authors also revealed the underlying mechanism that involves progressive loss of expression level of Bmi-1, which is associated with stemness,[122] in DPSC approaching senescence. These studies present fundamental limitations of MSC therapies for which primary MSCs have to be isolated from tissues and expanded in vitro to acquire sufficient number of regenerative cells. This becomes a more limiting fact for systemic infusion of MSCs, which requires in the range of 150 to 300 million cells per infusion.[123] Furthermore, even if MSCs isolated from aged donors could be used, despite their limited tissue source, they would present with reduced regenerative potential, possibly associated with cellular senescence. For these reasons, allogeneic MSCs have been used in place of autologous MSCs for stem cell therapies. Many reports indicate promising results using allogeneic MSCs; other studies also raise possibilities that allogeneic MSCs are rapidly degraded by immune cells in the host, suggesting reduced efficacy.

Allogeneic Versus Autologous MSCs

In part due to the limitations of MSC therapies with aging, allogeneic MSCs, such as those from newborn umbilical cord bloods,[124] have been thought to be attractive alternatives to autologous MSCs. Furthermore, allogeneic MSCs are much more feasible as a commercial product than autologous MSCs, because these cells can be prepared in large quantities from various donors and be ready for use off the shelf for all patients. On the contrary, autologous MSCs must be isolated, expanded, and prepared for the patient who will be the donor and the beneficiary of the particular MSC therapy. Many studies have demonstrated treatment of inflammatory or degenerative conditions using allogeneic MSCs without adverse effects.[123] For instance, allogeneic MSCs from bone marrow infused into patients who suffered from acute myocardial infarct showed improved cardiac function compared with placebo controls.[125] These studies demonstrate safety of allogeneic MSCs, which may be attributed to the immune suppressive function of MSCs[126] or to the fact that most (99%) MSCs are rapidly cleared from the systemic circulation within 5 minutes after infusion.[127] Despite initial success using MSCs, several studies raised questions as to the long-term benefit of using MSC infusion therapy.[128] Meyer[128] reported that a single dose of intracoronary infusion of MSCs (bone marrow-derived) in myocardial infarction patients showed no significant effect 18 months after initial therapy, although there was some benefit initially after 6 months.

The article by Griffin and colleagues[129] summarized studies that compared the therapeutic efficacy between allogeneic MSC versus autologous MSC infusion. The authors concluded that allogeneic MSCs are immunogenic despite prior findings that MSCs are in general immunosuppressive and therefore immune-privileged. Eliopoulos and colleagues[130] reported increase of host-derived CD8+ and NK cells after allogeneic MSC infusion, resulting in alloimmunization, while syngeneic MSCs showed no such effects in a mouse model. A recent study showed that intravenous injection of allogeneic MSCs triggers donor-specific antibody production in the recipient host and triggers complement-mediated lysis of allogeneic MSCs.[131] Such immunogenic response by primary allogeneic MSC injection led to significantly reduced survival of subsequently injected allogeneic MSCs. Solid evidence is found in the literature supporting immunogenicity of allogeneic MSCs, although therapeutic benefit of allogeneic MSCs has been demonstrated in several disease models. In summary, allogeneic MSCs are a valuable tool in regenerative medicine and have potential for commercialization that may benefit a wide patient pool. Further research is needed to investigate the long-term therapeutic benefit of allogeneic MSCs.

Induced Stemness By Epithelial–Mesenchymal Transition

Earlier studies demonstrated potential regenerative therapies using ESCs, which have the capability to differentiate into any cell type in the body.[132] This ESC concept was soon challenged by ethical concerns over destruction of life and the fact that the studies involve short-term culture of human embryos.[128] Subsequently, induced pluripotent stem cells (iPSCs) were generated from adult somatic cells by introduction of defined reprogramming factors (ie, Oct3/4, Sox2, c-Myc, and Klf4).[133] iPSCs circumvent the ethical issues over ESC but present with safety concerns due to genetic instability and possibility of tumorigenic conversion of cells after long-term engraftment.[134,135] Use of MSCs isolated from adult tissues may bypass these ethical and safety issues that hamper clinical application of regenerative therapies using ESC/iPSCs. However, for reasons discussed previously, MSCs may have limitations for clinical use, and there is need to seek alternative sources of MSCs for regenerative therapies.

Recently, the authors' laboratory reported the possibility of induced stemness in primary human keratinocytes through epithelial–mesenchymal transition (EMT).[12] EMT is a process by which epithelial cells gain mesenchymal phenotype, and it plays a normal physiologic role in embryogenesis and wound healing.[136,137] Introduction of ΔNp63α into primary human keratinocytes led to EMT and acquisition of characteristics resembling MSCs, such as spindle-shaped morphology, increased cell migration, and differentiation ability into other lineages, such as osteogenic and adipocytic cell types (**Fig. 4**).[136] In addition, the transformed cells have lost the expression of

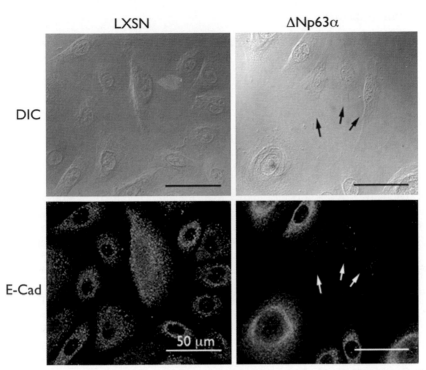

Fig. 4. Epithelial–mesenchymal transition induced by transduction of ΔNp63α. Rapidly proliferating normal human epidermal keratinocytes were retrovirally transduced with ΔNp63α. As a control, empty vector (LXSN) was used as mock viral infection. Arrow indicates emerging mesenchymal cells that have lost the expression of E-Cadherin (E-Cad), which is shown as green staining. Blue nuclear staining was performed with DAPI. DIC, differential interference contrast.

E-Cadherin and cytokeratin 14, which are epithelial cell markers, and gained expression of fibronectin, like other mesenchymal cells. Based on this altered phenotype, the authors coined the term induced MSC (iMSC) to indicate that MSC-like phenotype was induced in epithelial (nonmesenchymal) cells by gene modulation. Importantly, iMSCs are generated in skin or oral mucosa, which are readily available and often discarded tissues, and the authors' recent studies demonstrate that transient modulation of p63 protein level in primary keratinocytes can also trigger EMT and iMSC formation without the use of viral vectors (Jun-Eun Oh, personal communication, 2011). It is possible that iMSCs may retain longer lifespan than endogenous MSCs (eg, those from bone marrow or dental tissues) and may retain the regenerative capacity even when derived from aged donors. In the authors' previous study, they showed that donor age has very little effect on the replicative lifespan of primary culture of human oral keratinocytes.[121] This may be due to the fact that the oral mucosa is undergoing constant tissue turnover through its lifespan.[138] An earlier study demonstrated that the number of cells undergoing DNA synthesis at the basal layer of oral epithelium is increased during postmaturational aging,[139] supporting mucosal tissue regeneration throughout chronologic aging. Further research is needed to elucidate the regenerative capacity of iMSCs derived from oral mucosa or skin, and to validate the potential use of these cells for oral and systemic tissue regenerative therapies.

ACKNOWLEDGMENTS

The authors thank Dr Ju-Eun Oh and Ms Zi Xiao Lau for assistance with EMT experiment.

REFERENCES

1. Kode JA, Mukherjee S, Joglekar MV, et al. Mesenchymal stem cells: immunobiology and role in immunomodulation and tissue regeneration. Cytotherapy 2009; 11:377–91.
2. Friedenstein AJ, Piatetzky-Shapiro I, Petrakova KV. Osteogenesis in transplants of bone marrow cells. J Embryol Exp Morphol 1966;16:381–90.
3. Gronthos S, Mankani M, Brahim J, et al. Postnatal human dental pulp stem cells (DPSCs). Proc Natl Acad Sci U S A 2000;97:13625–30.
4. Yang S, Huang S, Feng C, et al. Umbilical cord-derived mesenchymal stem cells: strategies, challenges, and potential for cutaneous regeneration. Front Med 2012;6:41–7.
5. Gonzalez RE, Gonzalez MA, Varela N, et al. Human adipose-derived mesenchymal stem cells reduce inflammatory and T cell responses and induce regulatory T cells in vitro in rheumatoid arthritis. Ann Rheum Dis 2010;69:241–8.
6. Nowak JA, Polak L, Pasolli HA, et al. Hair follicle stem cells are specified and function in early skin morphogenesis. Cell Stem Cell 2008;3:33–43.
7. Sonoyama W, Liu Y, Fang D, et al. Mesenchymal stem cell mediated functional tooth regeneration in swine. PLoS One 2006;1:e79.
8. Seo BM, Miura M, Gronthos S, et al. Investigation of multipotent postnatal stem cells from human periodontal ligament. Lancet 2004;364:149–55.
9. Miura M, Gronthos S, Zhao M, et al. SHED: stem cells from human exfoliated teeth. Proc Natl Acad Sci U S A 2003;100:5807–12.
10. Yao S, Pan F, Pripic V, et al. Differentiation of stem cells in the dental follicle. J Dent Res 2008;87:767–71.
11. Huang GT, Gronthos S, Shi S. Mesenchymal stem cells derived from dental tissues vs. those derived from other sources: their biology and role in regenerative medicine. J Dent Res 2009;88:792–806.
12. Oh JE, Kim RH, Shin KH, et al. DeltaNp63α protein triggers epithelial–mesenchymal transition and confers stem cell properties in normal human keratinocytes. J Biol Chem 2011;286:38757–67.
13. Mehrazarin S, Oh JE, Chung CL, et al. Impaired odontogenic differentiation of senescent dental mesenchymal stem cells is associated with loss of Bmi-1 expression. J Endod 2011;37:662–6.
14. Gronthos S, Graves SE, Ohta S, et al. The STRO-1 fraction of adult human bone marrow contains osteogenic precursors. Blood 1994;84:4164–73.
15. Wagner W, Horn P, Castoldi M, et al. Replicative senescence of mesenchymal stem cells: a continuous and organized process. PLoS One 2008;3:e2213.
16. Hoogduijn MJ, Popp F, Verbeek R, et al. The immunomodulatory properties of mesenchymal stem cells and their use for immunotherapy. Int Immunopharmacol 2010;10:1496–500.
17. Pevsner-Fischer M, Morad V, Cohen-Sfady M, et al. Toll-like receptors and their ligands control mesenchymal stem cell functions. Blood 2007;109:1422–32.
18. Tomchuck SL, Zwezdaryk KJ, Coffelt SB, et al. Toll-like receptors on human mesenchymal stem cells drive their migration and immunomodulating responses. Stem Cells 2008;26:99–107.

19. Spaggiari GM, Capobianco A, Abdelrazik H, et al. Mesenchymal stem cells inhibit natural killer-cell proliferation, cytotoxicity, and cytokine production: role of indoleamine 2,3-dioxygenase and prostaglandin E2. Blood 2008;111:1327–33.

20. Pierdomenico L, Bonsi L, Calvitti M, et al. Multipotent mesenchymal stem cells with immunosuppressive activity can be easily isolated from dental pulp. Transplantation 2005;80:836–42.

21. Tomic S, Djokic J, Vasilijic S, et al. Immunomodulatory properties of mesenchymal stem cells derived from dental pulp and dental follicle are susceptible to activation by Toll-like receptor agonists. Stem Cells Dev 2011;20: 695–708.

22. Castagnola L, Orlay HG. Direct capping of the pulp and vital amputation. Br Dent J 1950;88:324–30.

23. Auschill TM, Arweiler NB, Hellwig E, et al. Success rate of direct pulp capping with calcium hydroxide. Schweiz Monatsschr Zahnmed 2003;113:946–52.

24. Mente J, Geletneky B, Ohle M, et al. Mineral trioxide aggregate or calcium hydroxide direct pulp capping: an analysis of the clinical treatment outcome. J Endod 2010;36:806–13.

25. Farsi N, Alamoudi N, Balto K, et al. Clinical assessment of mineral trioxide aggregate (MTA) as direct pulp capping in young permanent teeth. J Clin Pediatr Dent 2006;31:72–6.

26. Bogen G, Kim JS, Bakland LK. Direct pulp capping with mineral trioxide aggregate: an observational study. J Am Dent Assoc 2008;139:305–15.

27. Cvek M. Treatment of non-vital permanent incisors with calcium hydroxide. IV. Periodontal healing and closure of the root canal in the coronal fragment of teeth with intra-alveolar fracture and vital apical fragment. A follow-up. Odontol Revy 1974;25:239–46.

28. Cox CF, Subay RK, Ostro E, et al. Tunnel defects in dentin bridges: their formation following direct pulp capping. Oper Dent 1996;21:4–11.

29. Banchs F, Trope M. Revascularization of immature permanent teeth with apical periodontitis: new treatment protocol? J Endod 2004;30:196–200.

30. Chueh LH, Ho YC, Kuo TC, et al. Regenerative endodontic treatment for necrotic immature permanent teeth. J Endod 2009;35:160–4.

31. Cehreli ZC, Isbitiren B, Sara S, et al. Regenerative endodontic treatment (revascularization) of immature necrotic molars medicated with calcium hydroxide: a case series. J Endod 2011;37:1327–30.

32. Torabinejad M, Turman M. Revitalization of tooth with necrotic pulp and open apex by using platelet-rich plasma: a case report. J Endod 2011;37: 265–8.

33. Bose R, Nummikoski R, Hargreaves KM. A retrospective evaluation of radiographic outcomes in immature teeth with necrotic root canal systems treated with regenerative endodontic procedures. J Endod 2009;35:1343–9.

34. Lovelace TW, Henry MA, Hargreaves KM, et al. Evaluation of the delivery of mesenchymal stem cells into the root canal space of necrotic immature teeth after clinical regenerative endodontic procedure. J Endod 2011;37:133–8.

35. Li Y, Lu X, Sun X, et al. Odontoblast-like cell differentiation and dentin formation induced with TGF-β1. Arch Oral Biol 2011;56:1221–9.

36. Suzuki T, Lee CH, Chen M, et al. Induced migration of dental pulp stem cells for *in vivo* pulp regeneration. J Dent Res 2011;90:1013–8.

37. Yang X, Han G, Fan M. Chitosan/collagen scaffold containing bone morphogenetic protein-7 DNA supports dental pulp stem cell differentiation in vitro and in vivo. J Biomed Mater Res 2012. [Epub ahead of print].

38. Imura N, Pinheiro ET, Gomes BP, et al. The outcome of endodontic treatment: a retrospective study of 2000 cases performed by a specialist. J Endod 2007; 33:1278–82.
39. Hannahan JP, Eleazer PD. Comparison of success of implants versus endodontically treated teeth. J Endod 2008;34:1302–5.
40. Vire DE. Failure of endodontically treated teeth: classification and evaluation. J Endod 1991;17:338–42.
41. Sedgley CM, Messer HH. Are endodontically treated teeth more brittle? J Endod 1992;18:332–5.
42. Huang GTJ, Yamaza T, Shea LD, et al. Stem/progenitor cell-mediated de novo regeneration of dental pulp with newly deposited continuous layer of dentin in an in vivo model. Tissue Eng 2010;16:605–15.
43. Sakai VT, Cordeiro MM, Dong Z, et al. Tooth slice/scaffold model of dental pulp tissue engineering. Adv Dent Res 2011;23:325–32.
44. Donaldson M, Kinirons MJ. Factors affecting the time of onset of resorption in avulsed and replanted incisor teeth in children. Dent Traumatol 2001;17: 205–9.
45. Dangaria SJ, Ito Y, Luan X, et al. Successful periodontal ligament regeneration by periodontal progenitor preceding on natural tooth root surfaces. Stem Cells Dev 2011;20:1659–68.
46. Lin Y, Gallucci GO, Buser D, et al. Bioengineered periodontal tissue formed on titanium dental implants. J Dent Res 2011;90:251–6.
47. Gault P, Black A, Romette JL, et al. Tissue-engineered ligament: implant constructs for tooth replacement. J Clin Periodontol 2010;37:750–8.
48. Lineen E, Namias N. Biologic dressing in burns. J Craniofac Surg 2008;19: 923–8.
49. Heimbach DM, Warden GD, Luterman A, et al. Multicenter postapproval clinical trial of Integra dermal regeneration template for burn treatment. J Burn Care Rehabil 2003;24:42–8.
50. Badiavas EV, Falanga V. Treatment of chronic wounds with bone marrow-derived cells. Arch Dermatol 2003;139:510–6.
51. Badiavas EV, Ford D, Liu P, et al. Long-term bone marrow culture and its clinical potential in chronic wound healing. Wound Repair Regen 2007;15: 856–65.
52. Lataillade JJ, Doucet C, Bey E, et al. New approach to radiation burn treatment by dosimetry-guided surgery combined with autologous mesenchymal stem cell therapy. Regen Med 2007;2:785–94.
53. Ichioka S, Kouraba S, Sekiya N, et al. Bone marrow-impregnated collagen matrix for wound healing: experimental evaluation in a microcirculatory model of angiogenesis, and clinical experience. Br J Plast Surg 2005;58:1124–30.
54. Yoshikawa T, Mitsuno H, Nonaka I, et al. Wound therapy by marrow mesenchymal cell transplantation. Plast Reconstr Surg 2008;121:860–77.
55. Garcia-Olmo D, Herreros D, Pascual I, et al. Expanded adipose-derived stem cells for the treatment of complex perianal fistula: a phase II clinical trial. Dis Colon Rectum 2009;52:79–86.
56. Guadalajara H, Herreros D, De-La-Quintana P, et al. Long-term follow-up of patients undergoing adipose-derived adult stem cell administration to treat complex perianal fistulas. Int J Colorectal Dis 2012;27(5):595–600.
57. Fujita Y, Inokuma D, Abe R, et al. Conversion from human haematopoietic stem cells to keratinocytes requires keratinocyte secretory factors. Clin Exp Dermatol 2012. [Epub ahead of print].

58. Wu Y, Chen L, Scott PG, et al. Mesenchymal stem cells enhance wound healing through differentiation and angiogenesis. Stem Cells 2007;25:2648–59.
59. Sun Y, Weber KT. Infarct scar: a dynamic tissue. Cardiovasc Res 2000;46: 250–6.
60. Fukuda K. Molecular characterization of regenerated cardiomyocytes derived from adult mesenchymal stem cells. Congenit Anom 2002;42:1–9.
61. Makino S, Fukuda K, Miyoshi S, et al. Cardiomyocytes can be generated from marrow stromal cells in vitro. J Clin Invest 1999;103:697–705.
62. Shim WS, Jiang S, Wong P, et al. Ex vivo differentiation of human adult bone marrow stem cells into cardiomyocyte-like cells. Biochem Biophys Res Commun 2004;324:481–8.
63. Miyahara Y, Nagaya N, Kataoka M, et al. Monolayered mesenchymal stem cells repair scarred myocardium after myocardial infarction. Nat Med 2006;12:459–65.
64. Amado LC, Saliaris AP, Schuleri KH, et al. Cardiac repair with intramyocardial injection of allogeneic mesenchymal stem cells after myocardial infarction. Proc Natl Acad Sci U S A 2005;102:11474–9.
65. Fazel S, Chen L, Weisel RD, et al. Cell transplantation preserves cardiac function after infarction by infarct stabilization: augmentation by stem cell factor. J Thorac Cardiovasc Surg 2005;130:1310.
66. Sun L, Zhang T, Lan X, et al. Effects of stem cell therapy on left ventricular remodeling after acute myocardial infarction: a meta-analysis. Clin Cardiol 2010; 33:296–302.
67. Trounson A, Thakar RG, Lomax G, et al. Clinical trials for stem cell therapies. BMC Med 2011;9:52.
68. Lasala GP, Silva JA, Kusnick BA, et al. Combination stem cell therapy for the treatment of medically refractory coronary ischemia: a phase I study. Cardiovasc Revasc Med 2011;12:29–34.
69. Robertson RP, Sutherland DE, Kendall DM, et al. Metabolic characterization of long-term successful pancreas transplants in type I diabetes. J Investig Med 1996;44:549–55.
70. Tang DQ, Cao LZ, Burkhardt BR, et al. In vivo and in vitro characterization of insulin-producing cells obtained from murine bone marrow. Diabetes 2004;53:1721–32.
71. Choi KS, Shin JS, Lee JJ, et al. In vitro trans-differentiation of rat mesenchymal cells into insulin-producing cells by rat pancreatic extract. Biochem Biophys Res Commun 2005;330:1299–305.
72. Moriscot C, de Fraipont F, Richard MJ, et al. Human bone marrow mesenchymal stem cells can express insulin and key transcription factors of the endocrine pancreas developmental pathway upon genetic and/or microenvironmental manipulation in vitro. Stem Cells 2005;23:594–603.
73. Karnieli O, Izhar-Prato Y, Bulvik S, et al. Generation of insulin-producing cells from human bone marrow mesenchymal stem cells by genetic manipulation. Stem Cells 2007;25:2837–44.
74. Sun Y, Chen L, Hou XG. Differentiation of bone marrow-derived mesenchymal stem cells from diabetic patients into insulin-producing cells in vitro. Chin Med J 2007;120:771–6.
75. Kim SJ, Choi YS, Ko ES, et al. Glucose-stimulated insulin secretion of various mesenchymal stem cells after insulin-producing cell differentiation. J Biosci Bioeng 2012;113(6):771–7.
76. Ianus A, Holz GG, Theise ND, et al. In vivo derivation of glucose-competent pancreatic endocrine cells from bone marrow without evidence of cell fusion. J Clin Invest 2003;111:843–50.

77. Choi JB, Uchino H, Azuma K, et al. Little evidence of transdifferentiation of bone marrow-derived cells into pancreatic beta cells. Diabetologia 2003;46: 1366–74.
78. Hess D, Li L, Martin M, et al. Bone marrow-derived stem cells initiate pancreatic regeneration. Nat Biotechnol 2003;21:763–70.
79. Chivu M, Dima SO, Stancu CI, et al. In vitro hepatic differentiation of human bone marrow mesenchymal stem cells under differential exposure to liver-specific factors. Transl Res 2009;154:122–32.
80. Dong XJ, Zhang GR, Zhou QJ, et al. Direct hepatic differentiation of mouse embryonic stem cells induced by valproic acid and cytokines. World J Gastroenterol 2009;15:5165–75.
81. Ayatollahi M, Soleimani M, Tabei SZ, et al. Hepatogenic differentiation of mesenchymal stem cells induced by insulin like growth factor-I. World J Stem Cells 2011;3:113–21.
82. van Poll D, Parekkadan B, Cho CH, et al. Mesenchymal stem cell-derived molecules directly modulate hepatocellular death and regeneration in vitro and in vivo. Hepatology 2008;47:1634–43.
83. Kuo TK, Hung SP, Chuang CH, et al. Stem cell therapy for liver disease: parameters governing the success of using bone marrow mesenchymal stem cells. Gastroenterology 2008;134:2111–21.
84. Sun CK, Chang CL, Lin YC, et al. Systemic administration of autologous adipose-derived mesenchymal stem cells alleviates hepatic ischemia-reperfusion injury in rats. Crit Care Med 2012;40:1279–90.
85. Zhao W, Li JJ, Cao DY, et al. Intravenous injection of mesenchymal stem cells is effective in treating liver fibrosis. World J Gastroenterol 2012;18: 1048–58.
86. Saito T, Okumoto K, Haga H, et al. Potential therapeutic application of intravenous autologous bone marrow infusion in patients with alcoholic liver cirrhosis. Stem Cells Dev 2011;20:1503–10.
87. Lyra AC, Soares MB, da Silva LF, et al. Infusion of autologous bone marrow mononuclear cells through hepatic artery results in a short-term improvement of liver function in patients with chronic liver disease: a pilot randomized controlled study. Eur J Gastroenterol Hepatol 2010;22:33–42.
88. Uccelli A, Moretta L, Pistoia V. Mesenchymal stem cells in health and disease. Nat Rev Immunol 2008;8:726–36.
89. English K, French A, Wood KJ. Mesenchymal stromal cells: facilitators of successful transplantation? Cell Stem Cell 2010;7:431–42.
90. Glennie S, Soeiro I, Dyson PJ, et al. Bone marrow mesenchymal stem cells induce division arrest anergy of activated T cells. Blood 2005;105:2821–7.
91. Morandi F, Raffaghello L, Bianchi G, et al. Immunogenicity of human mesenchymal stem cells in HLA-class I-restricted T-cell responses against viral or tumor-associated antigens. Stem Cells 2008;26:1275–8.
92. Tasso R, Ilengo C, Quarto R, et al. Mesenchymal stem cells induce functionally active T-regulatory lymphocytes in a paracrine fashion and ameliorate experimental autoimmune uveitis. Invest Ophthalmol Vis Sci 2012;53: 786–93.
93. Nie Y, Lau CS, Lie AK, et al. Defective phenotype of mesenchymal stem cells in patients with systemic lupus erythematosus. Lupus 2010;19:850–9.
94. Sun LY, Zhang HY, Feng XB, et al. Abnormality of bone marrow-derived mesenchymal stem cells in patients with systemic lupus erythematosus. Lupus 2007; 16:121–8.

95. Zhou K, Zhang H, Jin O, et al. Transplantation of human bone marrow mesenchymal stem cell ameliorates the autoimmune pathogenesis in MRL/lpr mice. Cell Mol Immunol 2008;5:417–24.

96. Sun L, Akiyama K, Zhang H, et al. Mesenchymal stem cell transplantation reverses multiorgan dysfunction in systemic lupus erythematosus mice and humans. Stem Cells 2009;27:1421–32.

97. Liang J, Zhang H, Hua B, et al. Allogenic mesenchymal stem cells transplantation in refractory systemic lupus erythematosus: a pilot clinical study. Ann Rheum Dis 2010;69:1423–9.

98. Shi D, Wang D, Li X, et al. Allogeneic transplantation of umbilical cord-derived mesenchymal stem cells for diffuse alveolar hemorrhage in systemic lupus erythematosus. Clin Rheumatol 2012;31:841–6.

99. Firestein GS. Immunologic mechanisms in the pathogenesis of rheumatoid arthritis. J Clin Rheumatol 2005;11:S39–44.

100. Zhou B, Yuan J, Zhou Y, et al. Administering human adipose-derived mesenchymal stem cells to prevent and treat experimental arthritis. Clin Immunol 2011;141:328–37.

101. Liu Y, Mu R, Wang S, et al. Therapeutic potential of human umbilical cord mesenchymal stem cells in the treatment of rheumatoid arthritis. Arthritis Res Ther 2010;12:R210.

102. Park MJ, Park HS, Cho ML, et al. Transforming growth factor β-transduced mesenchymal stem cells ameliorate experimental autoimmune arthritis through reciprocal regulation of Treg/Th17 cells and osteoclastogenesis. Arthritis Rheum 2011;63:1668–80.

103. Liang J, Li X, Zhang H, et al. Allogeneic mesenchymal stem cells transplantation in patients with refractory RA. Clin Rheumatol 2012;31:157–61.

104. Sospedra M, Martin R. Immunology of multiple sclerosis. Annu Rev Immunol 2005;23:683–747.

105. Martin R, McFarland HF, McFarlin DE. Immunological aspects of demyelinating diseases. Annu Rev Immunol 1992;10:153–87.

106. Zappia E, Casazza S, Pedemonte E, et al. Mesenchymal stem cells ameliorate experimental autoimmune encephalomyelitis inducing T-cell anergy. Blood 2005;106:1755–61.

107. Zhang J, Li Y, Chen J, et al. Human bone marrow stromal cell treatment improves neurological functional recovery in EAE mice. Exp Neurol 2005;195:16–26.

108. Gerdoni E, Gallo B, Casazza S, et al. Mesenchymal stem cells effectively modulate pathogenic immune response in experimental autoimmune encephalomyelitis. Ann Neurol 2007;61:219–27.

109. Gordon D, Pavlovska G, Glover CP, et al. Human mesenchymal stem cells abrogate experimental allergic encephalomyelitis after intraperitoneal injection, and with sparse CNS infiltration. Neurosci Lett 2008;448:71–3.

110. Bai L, Lennon DP, Eaton V, et al. Human bone marrow-derived mesenchymal stem cells induce Th2-polarized immune response and promote endogenous repair in animal models of multiple sclerosis. Glia 2009;57:1192–203.

111. Rafei M, Birman E, Forner K, et al. Allogeneic mesenchymal stem cells for treatment of experimental autoimmune encephalomyelitis. Mol Ther 2009;17:1799–803.

112. Mohyeddin Bonab M, Yazdanbakhsh S, Lotfi J, et al. Does mesenchymal stem cell therapy help multiple sclerosis patients? Report of a pilot study. Iran J Immunol 2007;4:50–7.

113. Yamout B, Hourani R, Salti H, et al. Bone marrow mesenchymal stem cell transplantation in patients with multiple sclerosis: a pilot study. J Neuroimmunol 2010; 227:185–9.

114. Wojtovich AP, Nadtochiy SM, Brookes PS, et al. Ischemic preconditioning: the role of mitochondria and aging. Exp Gerontol 2012;47:1–7.

115. Manogue M, Martin DM. Changes in patient age and tooth distribution for root canal treatment in a teaching hospital over a 15-year period. Int Endod J 1994;27:148–53.

116. Conboy IM, Rando TA. Aging, stem cells and tissue regeneration. Cell Cycle 2005;4:407–10.

117. Tuljapurkar SR, McGuire TR, Brusnahan SK, et al. Changes in human bone marrow fat content associated with changes in hematopoietic stem cell numbers and cytokine levels with aging. J Anat 2011;219:574–81.

118. Morse D. Age-related changes of the dental pulp complex and their relationship to systemic aging. Oral Surg Oral Med Oral Pathol 1991;72:721–45.

119. Wilson A, Shehadeh LA, Yu H, et al. Age-related molecular genetic changes of murine bone marrow mesenchymal stem cells. BMC Genomics 2010;11:229.

120. Yu JM, Wu X, Gimble JM, et al. Age-related changes in mesenchymal stem cells derived from rhesus macaque bone marrow. Aging Cell 2011;10:66–79.

121. Kang MK, Bibb C, Baluda MA, et al. In vitro replication and differentiation of normal human oral keratinocytes. Exp Cell Res 2000;258:288–97.

122. Park IK, Morrison SJ, Clarke MF. Bmi1, stem cells, and senescence regulation. J Clin Invest 2004;113:175–9.

123. Ankrum J, Karp JM. Mesenchymal stem cell therapy: two steps forward, one step back. Trends Mol Med 2010;16:203–9.

124. Hussain I, Magd SA, Eremin O, et al. New approach for isolation of mesenchymal stem cells (MSCs) from human umbilical cord blood. Cell Biol Int 2012;36:595–600.

125. Hare JM, Traverse JH, Henry TD, et al. Randomized, double-blind, placebo-controlled, dose-escalation study of intravenous adult human mesenchumal stem cells (Prochymal) after acute myocardial infarction. J Am Coll Cardiol 2009;54:2277–86.

126. Barry FP, Murphy JM, English K, et al. Immunogencity of adult mesenchymal stem cells: lessons from the fetal allograft. Stem Cells Dev 2005;14:252–65.

127. Lee RH, Pulin AA, Seo MJ, et al. Intravenous hMSCs improve myocardial infarction in mice because cells embolized in lung are activated to secrete the anti-inflammatory protein TSG-6. Cell Stem Cell 2009;5:54–63.

128. Meyer JR. Human embryonic stem cells and respect for life. J Med Ethics 2000; 26:166–70.

129. Griffin MD, Ritter T, Mahon BP. Immunological aspects of allogeneic mesenchymal stem cell therapies. Hum Gene Ther 2010;21:1641–55.

130. Eliopoulos N, Stagg J, Lejeune L, et al. Allogeneic marrow stromal cells are immune rejected by MHC class I- and class II-mismatched recipient mice. Blood 2005;106:4057–65.

131. Schu S, Nosov M, O'Flynn L, et al. Immunogenicity of allogeneic mesenchymal stem cells. J Cell Mol Med 2011. [Epub ahead of print].

132. He Q, Li J, Bettiol E, et al. Embryonic stem cells: new possible therapy for degenerative diseases that affect elderly people. J Gerontol A Biol Sci Med Sci 2003;58:279–87.

133. Takahashi K, Yamanaka S. Induction of pluripotent stem cells from mouse embryonic and adult fibroblast culture by defined factors. Cell 2006;126:663–76.

134. Yamashita T, Kawai H, Tian F, et al. Tumorigenic development of induced pluripotent stem cells in ischemic mouse brain. Cell Transplant 2011;20:883–91.
135. Griscelli F, Feraud O, Oudrhiri N, et al. Malignant germ cell-like tumors, expressing Ki-1 antigen (CD30), are revealed during in vivo differentiation of partially reprogrammed human-induced pluripotent stem cells. Am J Pathol 2012;180: 2084–96.
136. Nakamura M, Tokura Y. Epithelial–mesenchymal transition in skin. J Dermatol Sci 2011;61:7–13.
137. Kalluri R, Weinberg RA. The basics of epithelial–mesenchymal transition. J Clin Invest 2009;119:1420–8.
138. Squier CA, Kremer MJ. Biology of oral mucosa and esophagus. J Natl Cancer Inst Monogr 2001;29:7–15.
139. Sharav Y, Massler M. Age changes in oral epithelia. Progenitor population, synthesis index and tissue turnover. Exp Cell Res 1967;47:132–8.
140. Shi S, Bartold PM, Miura M, et al. The efficacy of mesenchymal stem cells to regenerate and repair dental structures. Orthod Craniofac Res 2005;8:191–9.
141. Sekiya I, Larson BL, Vuoristo JT, et al. Adipogenic differentiation of human adult stem cells from bone marrow stroma (MSCs). J Bone Miner Res 2004;19: 256–64.
142. Bertani N, Malatesta P, Volpi G, et al. Neurogenic potential of mesenchymal stem cells revisited: analysis by immunostaining, time-lapse video and microarray. J Cell Sci 2005;118:3925–36.
143. Bosnakovski D, Mizuno M, Kim G, et al. Chondrogenic differentiation of bovine bone marrow mesenchymal stem cells in pellet cultural system. Exp Hematol 2004;32:502–9.
144. Shih DT, Lee DC, Chen SC, et al. Isolation and characterization of neurogenic mesenchymal stem cells in human scalp tissue. Stem Cells 2005;23:1012–20.

Regenerative Endodontics and Tissue Engineering
What the Future Holds?

Harold E. Goodis, DDS[a,b,c,*], Bassam Michael Kinaia, DDS, MS[d,e,f], Atheel M. Kinaia, DDS[g], Sami M.A. Chogle, BDS, DMD, MSD[b,h,i]

KEYWORDS

- Stem cells • Repair • Regeneration • Progenitor cells • Cell signaling
- Growth factors • Dental pulp • Dentin

KEY POINTS

- The work performed by researchers in regenerative endodontics and tissue engineering over the last decades has been superb; however, many questions remain to be answered. The basic biologic mechanisms must be elucidated that will allow the development of the dental pulp and dentin in situ.
- Development of stem cell lines are needed that are easily cultured, grown, maintained, and ready to be placed in a tooth together with a proper scaffold and the introduction of growth factors that allow "-like-tissue" formation.
- The need for controlled odontogenesis (dentin, pulp) that will continue to protect the tooth, now somewhat successful in animals, must become a normal and usual clinical therapy. Stress must be placed on the many questions that will lead to the design of effective, safe treatment options and therapies.

Conflict of Interest: The authors declare that there are no conflicts of if interest related to this paper.
[a] The Boston University Institute for Dental Research and Education, PO Box 505097, Dubai Healthcare City, Dubai, United Arab Emirates; [b] Department of Endodontics, The Goldman School of Dental Medicine, Boston, MA, USA; [c] Department of Endodontics, The University of California School of Dentistry, San Francisco, CA, USA; [d] Postgraduate Periodontology Program, Periodontology Department, The Boston University Institute for Dental Research and Education, PO Box 505097, Dubai Healthcare City, Dubai, United Arab Emirates; [e] Department of Periodontology and Oral Biology, The Goldman School of Dental Medicine, Boston, MA, USA; [f] University of Detroit Mercy – School of Dentistry, Detroit, MI, USA; [g] Advanced Education in General Dentistry Program, The European University, PO Box 505097, Dubai Healthcare City, Dubai, United Arab Emirates; [h] Postgraduate Program in Endodontics, Endodontics Department, The Boston University Institute for Dental Research and Education, PO Box 505097, Dubai Healthcare City, Dubai, United Arab Emirates; [i] Department of Endodontics, Case School of Dental Medicine, Cleveland, OH, USA
* Corresponding author. 6065 Palermo Way, El Dorado Hills, CA 95762.
E-mail address: harold.goodis@ucsf.edu

Dent Clin N Am 56 (2012) 677–689
http://dx.doi.org/10.1016/j.cden.2012.05.007
0011-8532/12/$ – see front matter © 2012 Elsevier Inc. All rights reserved.

INTRODUCTION

Regenerative endodontics is concerned with the development of biologically based treatment modalities that are used to replace diseased portions of the dental pulp or to allow complete formation of a dental pulp–like tissue that will act as the original dental pulp.[1] Today, the major effort in regenerative endodontics appears to use several types of stem cells placed on a scaffold inside the diseased root canal system of a tooth. With the addition of growth factors, externally or from dentin and/or remaining dental pulp, a pulplike tissue forms.[2] (Please see a review of tooth formation from embryonic tissues to a fully formed tooth by Tziatas and Kodonas.[3]) A form of regenerative endodontics began many years ago with the development of direct and indirect pulp-capping procedures. The need for a scaffold, vascular supply, growth factors, signaling mechanisms, migration of cells, and differentiation were not well known, nor were the actual events that occurred during the formation and regenerative processes known. Today's placement of a direct calcium hydroxide pulp cap leads to growth factor activation from surrounding hard tissues, inclusion of native stem cells from the remaining pulp tissue, and hard tissue formation (dentinlike hard tissue) that may also act as a scaffold and as a source for growth factors. The body of work in regenerative endodontics has grown exponentially, therefore this article is concerned with the future possibilities of an understanding of the processes and mechanisms to restore a vital, healthy tissue within a tooth in situ and include a review of the progress of laboratory studies that may lead to greater knowledge of the interactions at the cellular and molecular levels of tissue engineering.[4]

In a healthy tooth, the pulp/dentin complex undergoes dentin matrix formation with eventual mineralization. The dentin formed is in a physiologic process. The dentin formed is very similar to primary dentin, with a tubular structure that covers primary dentin with the dentin tubules being continuous between both primary and secondary dentin formations. In teeth that have been injured in some manner (caries, restorations, trauma), another type of dentin forms called tertiary dentin. This is a unique type of dentin that is not tubular in its formation but rather occurs as an atubular structure. There are 2 types of tertiary dentin: reactive and reparative.[5] Reactive dentin is formed by the remaining, original odontoblasts forming a matrix that becomes almost completely solid with no tubules; however, tunneling has been seen to occur in this form of dentin.[6] Reparative dentin is a matrix formed by new odontoblastlike cells that form precursor and stem cells found in the remaining vital pulp tissue. It also is formed without tubules.

Regenerative endodontic procedures use biologically based treatment modalities and pulpal cells.[7–9] The information available in regenerative studies to date, however, indicate that more must be learned about the interactions that occur between all cells, growth factors, proliferation and differentiation of cells, and the ability to use materials that will result in a well-formed, functioning tooth.[7,8]

PULP REPAIR AND REGENERATION

An excellent review by Goldberg[10] suggests that there are more questions than answers in the ability to effect pulp repair and pulp regeneration. The following is a summary of the questions he poses as to the future of pulp repair, pulp regeneration, and tissue engineering.

A distinction between endodontic repair and regeneration must be understood before one can understand the processes that occur in repair and regeneration. Repair indicates that healing occurs because the remaining damaged tissue is vital, original odontoblasts survive, and the pulp tissue can be restored to a normal-like form and function. In the dental pulp, odontoblasts are reactivated, a dentin matrix is formed that becomes mineralized (reactionary dentin), and the pulp retains, for the most part, its biologic functions.

Regeneration indicates that the pulp is completely necrotic (complete degradation) and a tissue (pulplike) must be formed that may function as the original tissue. Questions arise as to how the resultant cells and tissue react in relation to the original tissue. Studies have demonstrated that a completely necrotic pulp, combined with a periapical lesion and incomplete root formation, is the usual clinical finding. Initial treatment is undertaken to remove the infection and heal the lesion. This is followed by formation of the tooth root, creation of new odontoblastlike cells functioning as a pulplike tissue.[1,11–15] In these cases, the new pulplike tissue continues to form a hard dentinlike tissue, generally without tubules closing the root canal space in what appears to be an event that occurs rapidly.[11] The events occurring in these teeth may cause the need for further therapeutic interventions, including root canal or surgical root end therapy. The mechanisms for these events are not fully understood, hence the term "-like tissue." Can the processes be controlled to produce a more natural tissue reaction that occurs over many years without closing down the root canal space? Ideally, the process should mimic the development of secondary dentin formation, which is physiologic in nature and occurs in an uninvolved pulp as a natural part of the aging process.

The future of repair and regeneration depends on answers to the questions posed in the Goldberg[10] article. What is the nature of the stem cells that should be used to regenerate pulp tissue? This is of great importance, as researchers appear to have isolated several different stem cell lines, which, in itself generates several other questions. Greater attention to the analysis of the biologic properties of dental tissue–derived mesenchymal stem cells using both in vitro and in vivo systems is necessary. A recent study concluded that both dental pulp stem cells (DPSCs) and stem cells from the apical papilla (SCAPs) could differentiate into odontoblastlike cells with the potential to migrate and mineralize leading to 3-dimensional dentinlike structures; however, SCAPs had a higher population capacity and proliferation rate compared with DPSCs. This may be an advantage for dental tissue repair and regeneration from the standpoint of cryopreservation of the cells in large quantities and a high mineralization rate may shorten the process.[15]

STEM CELLS

All stem cells in odontogenesis, with the exception of ameloblast progenitor cells, originate in the mesenchyme and are said to be of ectomesenchymal origin. DPSCs are isolated from the dental pulp and can regenerate into new stem cell lines that can differentiate into other cell lines. As the developmental ability of these cells in vitro is limited, they are more useful in in vivo studies, as more complex tissues arise. For example, dentin/pulplike tissues arise from DPSCs, such as dentinlike and pulplike tissues.[15–19]

SHEDS are stem cells from exfoliated, human, deciduous teeth, which are a readily accessible source of adult stem cells from impacted third molars. In vivo, removal of these teeth led to collection of multipotent stem cells having the potential to differentiate into odontoblastlike cells,[20] neurons,[21] and osteoinductive cells.[22–25] Periodontal ligament stem cells (PDLSCs) can form cementum and periodontal ligament and, when transplanted into mice, bone and cementum structures were seen.[26–29] Dental follicle stem cells (DFSCs) are collected from the follicles that surround developing third molars. These cells have a major role in the genesis of cementum and cementoblastlike cells.[30]

SCAPs are harvested from the apex of a developing tooth. The papilla is a precursor of the dental pulp. As in other stem cells, SCAPs express early mesenchymal surface markers.[16,31–34] A reading of the quoted articles will show that the previously listed references demonstrate that, in many instances, the studies compare one type of stem cell to another or several others. These stem cells are proliferative with characteristic markers such as Stro-1, CD146/MUC18, and CD44 (see articles by Sedgley and colleagues and Law and colleagues elsewhere in this issue). This leads to questions as to which markers should be recognized that will allow collection and development of a cell line that can be maintained and colonized and introduced into a tooth as an in vivo treatment option. A primary question must be asked as to what type of pulp-like tissue should be the result of implantation?

Is it possible to obtain a functional, nonmineralized pulp that is vascularized and innervated as the original tissue would be? Or is the aim to develop a pulp tissue that would induce an increased amount of mineralization that could serve as a substitute for root canal therapy? Cell differentiation can lead to either adult progenitor or an odontoblastlike/osteoblastlike cell, which is divergent from other results obtained.

The question of using multipotent stem cells remains unsettled, especially when attempting to regenerate pulpal tissue. The cells necessary are present in the pulp and can be associated with odontoblast and osteoblast cells, endothelial cells, and, later, formation of neurons. Therefore, is the use of multipotent progenitors or nonpotent cells, the cells of choice?[15,19]

In the future, it may be possible to minimally invade and isolate suitable stem cells, have them undergo differentiation in vitro, and combine and develop them into tooth structures.[35] Pulp cells differentiate in vitro into odontoblastlike stem cells. The dentin formed, as previously mentioned, is atubular. Is there a possibility of dental pulp cells producing tubular dentin?[36] A recent study mixed pulp cells with a hydroxyapatite (tricalcium phosphate powder) and generated a dentin-pulplike tissue.[17] Bartouli and coworkers[37] transplanted tubular dentin on the surface of dentin-pulp slices and generated increased amounts of tubular dentin; however, the origin of the progenitor cells giving rise to new odontoblasts (tubular dentin) and the signaling pathways in cell differentiation have not been clearly identified and remain a matter of debate.[36]

Greater knowledge related to the location and identity of odontogenic precursor cells that participate in reparative dentin formation is required. Implant experiments have begun to identify genuine progenitor cell markers and molecular signal pathways that allow stem cell recruitment. Implantation experiments using pulp-derived precursor cell lines have started to provide evidence that, in the absence of carriers or biomolecules, exogenous stem cells have the capacity to promote efficient tooth repair.[38]

Because repair and regeneration have different targets, the expectations of a particular therapy must be clear. Is regeneration of a nonmineralizing pulp the proper goal or is generation of a tissue that may become a completely mineralized root canal system the proper treatment option? Each aim uses specific tools that are valid for bioengineering treatment modalities.[10]

Caries may be the most common and dangerous of all types of injury, provoking adverse stimuli to the dental pulp. Understanding caries management (see article by Chogle and colleagues elsewhere in this issue for a review of the pulpal response to caries) has led to improved understanding of mineralization of teeth, further leading to therapies necessary to restore the biologic behavior of the entire pulp-dentin complex.[30]

The pulp-dentin complex is protective in nature, as its main roles are to manufacture dentin matrices and to restart dentinogenesis to protect the new pulplike tissue from injury or insult. Many of the processes involved are thought to be the same as the initial pulp developmental processes occurring embryonically.[40] Because the onset of injury in the dental pulp may be a result of caries, markers of inflammation are different, depending on the depth of the inflammatory process of the lesion.[41]

Still somewhat unclear is how inflammation may overwhelm and cause degeneration in the pulp, as opposed to its role in the regeneration of that tissue. To understand the treatment prognosis, understanding the balance between infection and inflammation is necessary, together with an understanding of proinflammatory and anti-inflammatory mediators and how they relate to the innate and adaptive immune systems.

Many studies have reported that several populations of stem cells in and around the tooth pulp are able to be used to repair or regenerate the pulp/dentin complex. These populations of cells include DPSCs,[17,18,20] SCAPs,[19,32,34] PDLSCs,[27,29] and mesenchymal stem cells.[33,42] SHEDs are human pulp cells of the dental follicle collected from impacted third molars.[20,43] These cells may have the dual ability to repair (heal), regenerate a particular tissue, or differentiate in a manner that causes a change in the ability of these cells to form original tissue. As previously mentioned, odontoblasts normally secrete a tubular dentin (both primary and secondary) as a normal physiologic function throughout life that maintains the tubular structure in both dentins. However, insults to the pulp may cause newly formed odontoblastlike cells to form an atubular (tertiary) dentin that is not tubular and not physiologic. Rather it is formed as a result of the pulplike tissue reacting as a defender of that tissue. To be able to use these cell lines clinically, translational research in the future will require both researchers and skilled clinicians who can develop new and novel therapies that can eventually be tested and used in clinical environments to answer these questions.

SCAFFOLDS

A scaffold is thought of as a 3-dimensional construct or support substance used for several tissue engineering applications. When stem cells are seeded on scaffolds, they are expected to attach, proliferate, and differentiate into new tissues that will eventually replace the scaffold. Scaffolds should be biocompatible, not elicit an inflammatory response or be cytotoxic, support cell organization and vascularization, allow new regenerated tissue to form, be sterilizable, and be stable while maintaining mechanical form and strength. They should have an inductive ability with added growth factors and morphogens for a more rapid cell attachment, proliferation, migration, and differentiation into a specific tissue.[44]

The choice of a scaffold is critical in tissue regeneration. Most scaffolds are organic in nature and used to provide surfaces on which cells may adhere, grow, and organize.[44] Scaffolds chosen for laboratory studies are diverse, including natural or synthetic polymers, extracellular matrices (EMCs), self-assembling systems, hydrogels, and bioactive ceramics. Recently, a synthetic polymer polycaprolactone was successful in growing increasing numbers of SCAP stem cells with apparent identification of NOTCH signaling expression.[44]

Although the number of scaffolds has increased (see the excellent review by Sakai and colleagues[45]), questions remain that must be addressed. For example, are scaffolds able to support various kinds of stem cells or are they stem cell–specific? Are stem cells able to be seeded with like results on more than one scaffold? What are the limitations of the use of one or another scaffold that may be natural or synthetic scaffolds? The use of a self-assembling peptide system that allows a "bottom-up" approach of generating EMC materials, offering high control at the molecular level, will be a major step forward in constructing future scaffolds.[44] The peptide system is referred to as a tunable matrix with several features that possibly allow scaffolds to be designed, as different requirements are needed to regenerate a tissue.[4]

NICHES

Today, the ability of stem cell–based tissue engineering of teeth faces dilemmas of methods from development owing to several differing conceptual issues. For example, where is the location and identity of odontogenic precursor cells that participate in reparative dentin formation?[38,46,47]

Stem cells appear to have the ability for tissue repair and regeneration throughout life. They may react by their ability to cause the self-renewal repair of a particular tissue by *differentiation* of the cells into other tissues and are influenced by a microenvironment called the stem cell niche. A niche determines how dental pulp cells regulate and participate in tissue maintenance, repair, and regeneration. Niches are located around the body in various tissues. The niches exist in specific anatomic locations where they house stem cells (few in number) where the cells can be renewed. These niches in their specific locations within the dental pulp and dentin regulate how stem cells participate in tissue repair and regeneration. Specific signals from precise areas (see section on NOTCH proteins) in the niche permit stem cells to maintain vitality and to change their ultimate fate and number.[48,49] When signaled to do so, they travel to the site of injury.[50] The signaling proteins functioning in these processes have been studied but more research is needed to determine the mechanisms that allow stem cells from a particular niche to increase in number and migrate to the area of injury. The stem cell niche may be thought of as an interactive structural unit that facilitates cell-fate decisions. Molecular cross-talk events, together with the signaling of specific molecules, occur in the right place at the right time. In other words, anatomic organization coordinates stem cell function in time and space. Both positive and negative signals are integrated with intercellular pathways that share the process with other signaling proteins and growth factors.[51]

Questions arise as to the environment of the niche surrounding the stem cells. Does that environment maintain stem cell lineage specificity? Are postnatal stem cells capable of converting from one type of cell into another, as they may do naturally in the body?[52] A stem cell niche is a group of cells in special tissue locations that maintain stem cells. Niches are variable, containing different cell types depending on the need of its environment. The niche may be thought of as an anchor for a particular stem cell that generates extrinsic factors that control stem cell numbers and their fate. Signaling molecules, such as bone morphogenic proteins (BMPs) and NOTCH molecules, regulate stem cell behavior, such as self-renewal and fate of that group of stem cells.[53]

NOTCH SIGNALING PROTEINS

NOTCH proteins are important regulators of stem cells in the cell's ability to function properly. They have the capacity to induce proliferation or differentiation in stem cells. For example, injuries to the dental pulp may lead to death of odontoblasts (apoptosis). This triggers the activation of pulp stem cells, leading to their proliferation, migration to the area of injury, and differentiation into another type of odontoblastlike cell to replace the apoptotic odontoblasts.[54]

When injury occurs to the dental pulp stem cells, large numbers leave their niche and travel to the areas of the injuries. NOTCH signaling proteins initiate migration of DPSCs through signaling mechanisms to the site of injury leading to proliferation and differentiation into odontoblastlike cells. This results in the formation of a reparativelike dentin matrix with eventual mineralization. The question still unanswered is that, although the niches contain only a few cells, what signaling molecules are responsible for the almost immediate increase in numbers of cells that are activated, proliferate and differentiate, and migrate to aid the pulp in its ability to be repaired?

The NOTCH proteins (1–4) are large, transmembrane receptors controlling cell fate decisions and the formation of cell compartments during embryonic development.[55,56] Ligands bind to the NOTCH receptors, triggering enzymatic activities. A complex is formed that activates the transcription of target genes that maintain cells in a proliferative/undifferentiated state. The expression of NOTCH receptors and ligands have been detected in developing dental pulp and teeth during injury and repair.[57] NOTCH proteins are involved in cell-cell signaling through direct cell-to-cell contact where one cell possesses a transmembrane receptor and the other cell possesses a membrane-bound ligand.[57]

The NOTCH family of signaling proteins causes an asymmetric stem cell division in the stem cells that ensures stem cell renewal. This allows the daughter cells to differentiate, leading to repair and regeneration of tissues. Signaling from NOTCH proteins plays a key role in the fate of the cell in determination and maintenance of stem cells. Its activation or inhibition can regulate the cell's fate.

In sum, when dental pulp is injured, stem cells are recruited from the niches where they reside to the areas of the injury. Odontoblasts survive, leading to repair, or die and are replaced by new odontoblastlike cells causing regeneration of the pulplike tissue.[43] Other molecules (BMPs, submembers of the transforming growth factor beta [TGF-β] family of growth factors) are released from dentin and play an important role in pulp healing.[58,59] Increased amounts of TGF-β are released during the death of the original cells, which leads to reparative dentin formation. When viewed microscopically, however, the areas thought to be niches appear as normal pulp tissue. More studies are needed to answer the previously mentioned questions, which will lead to the exact growth factor or combinations of growth factors that will mimic the reaction of repair mechanisms and allow the tooth to develop normally.

The above indicates that NOTCH signaling in their role of regulating stem cell behavior may be important for tooth repair. NOTCH receptors are absent in adult rat pulp tissue; their expression was found to occur after pulp tissue injury.[23,60] These studies also suggest that NOTCH signaling may act as a negative molecule in stem cell differentiation. The future of the full extent of NOTCH signaling abilities plus other signaling proteins that may be present are not fully known, which indicates that their ability in repair processing and participation in healing is not fully understood. Finally, it has not been demonstrated that NOTCH-positive stem cells participate in the repair process and leading to differentiation into odontoblastlike pulp cells.[10]

VASCULARIZATION

The understanding of the mechanisms that underlie dental pulp angiogenic responses still are not completely understood. Revascularization is critical for the development of new therapies necessary to regulate the dental pulp. New therapeutic methodology could be used for the regulation and expression of angiogenic factors, such as vascular endothelial growth factor and fibroblast growth factor 2 to revascularize the pulp tissue of avulsed or other traumatized teeth.[61] In cases of anterior tooth avulsion or intrusion and extrusion in a young child, displacement of the tooth may lead to apical blood vessel and nerve rupture. In these cases, the teeth remain with open apices and large pulp chambers favoring repair and regenerative treatment modalities occur that may involve stem cell therapy.[62,63]

GROWTH FACTORS AND SIGNALING PATHWAYS

Growth factors are peptide molecules that transmit signals to control cell behavior and activity. They act through interaction with specific receptors located on the surfaces of cells. A variety of growth factors have been identified and grouped into several classes. They include the following: TGF-α and TGF-β,[64] BMPs, fibroblast growth factors, Hedgehog proteins, and tumor necrosis factors.[65] Growth factors are responsible for signaling many of the events in tooth morphogenesis and response of the dental pulp to caries, microorganisms, and other noxious stimuli. Several studies have found that growth factors are present in the matrix of tooth dentin.[5,11,64,66]

Although studies have been performed, the results have yet to be used in a manner that allows regeneration and repair while not decreasing the volume of pulp tissue. Because the formation of secondary dentin is thought to be physiologic and occurs throughout life, the growth factors must be used in a manner that allows normal processes to continue as would occur in a virgin tooth with no restoration or caries or other stimuli that would increase the chance of narrowing and limiting natural processes in the dental pulp.

INFLAMMATION-REGENERATION

Although much is known about the mechanisms of both inflammation and regeneration, a failing in most studies occurs because there is a tendency to consider these entities separately rather than together.[67] Future studies should concentrate on both at the same time as they both occur, one step at a time (continuous until repair occurs). Inflammatory processes are seen as being antagonistic to these same processes that indicate that regeneration is occurring. Direct data have now emerged indicating that there is a relationship between the 2 processes.[41] The first (inflammation) results in tissue breakdown, whereas the latter develops regenerative (new tissue formation) actions. No doubt, increased inflammation may impede regeneration; however, if the inflammatory response is low grade, it may promote regenerative mechanisms that may include angiogenic stem cell processes. The data, however, are somewhat ambivalent, as greater levels of inflammation are studied alone without comparing the data that occur with regenerative effects. Therefore, it is necessary in the future not to separate the processes but attempt to study both at the same time. In the future, proper animal studies are necessary to demonstrate that these processes are fully described before clinical studies are undertaken. The limiting factor in both processes is the location of the dental pulp. Dentin surrounds the dental pulp and, although an inflammatory response to incipient caries may either regenerate or become a scar, the pulp tissue will be reduced in volume and other forms of dentin will occur that narrow the pulp tissue space. Studies need to be performed that develop suitable materials that will be able to reach the dental pulp through dentin tubules to regenerate original tissue without limiting the root canal system space.

SUMMARY

Tissue regeneration and engineering is the most challenging part of a tissue repair/regeneration program. The dental pulp is very small in relation to other human body tissues. Therefore, the idea of regenerated dental pulp tissue in a tooth has become a common thought among dental researchers. The regenerated tissue must contain the following attributes: it should be vascularized, contain similar cell density and architecture of the EMC, give rise to new odontoblasts lining dentin surfaces, and produce new dentin matrices that become mineralized and be innervated.[42,66]

The aspect of dentin-pulp tissue engineering is of great interest, with a large number of studies performed over the past several years. However, the science is still not able to allow clinical procedures to be performed routinely in animals or in humans. There are no clinical studies that can be routinely performed in an effort that will lead to dentin-pulp repair and regeneration.[50] Manufacturers must be able to produce materials, both biologic and synthetic, that are reliable and safe. Expanded cell populations must consider the possibility of genetic instability. The hope of research to date rests on the ability that the use of naturally occurring cells at the site of injury may lessen side-effect risks. Better understanding of the dentin-pulp complex biology will lead to an exciting era of the development of cell-based approaches.[50]

Other challenges have become apparent as a result of the large number of studies involving stem cells, growth factors, and so forth in repair and regeneration and tissue engineering. An interesting aspect of these challenges involves the necessity of revascularization, which, although not ignored, has not been overly stressed in the science needed to repair/regenerate dental pulp tissue. Most procedures concerned with revascularization are conducted using a young group of individuals, 12 to 15 years old, with fully developed teeth whose pulp tissue contains high stem cell populations. The various components, stem cells, scaffolds, and growth factors, together with establishing an adequate vascular supply, can become optimized and integrated to produce, repair, and regenerate the dentin-pulp complex on a regular basis; however, there have been few, if any studies on adults. A survey of endodontists in 2009 found 96% of respondents believed that regenerative treatment modalities would become a normal, therapeutic option for teeth that otherwise would be removed.[69] Although supportive of research, endodontists foresaw the need for increased funding, increased clinical trials, and development of new therapies.

Many teeth are not treated because of the fear that they cannot be restored. Endodontics now has a better than 90% or higher rate of success.[70–74] Many endodontic specialists report success of 95% or better, especially when survival is considered with success and failure. More patients are treated by placement of Implant-restored crowns rather than treated with root canal procedures on teeth that lend themselves to successful endodontic therapy. Therefore, there is a need for clinical specialties in dentistry to agree to a formula or creation of definitive standards that allow endodontists to successfully treat teeth or re-treat failures, allow prosthodontists to develop materials that prevent microleakage, and allow periodontists the ability to place implants when necessary. The development of regenerative endodontics may make those other procedures not needed (extraction and implant replacement), especially with the expectation that both hard (dentin, enamel) and soft (innervated and vascularized dental pulp) tissues would become a normal and successful procedure.

REFERENCES

1. Bose R, Nummikoski P, Hargreaves K. A retrospective evaluation of radiographic root canal systems treated with regenerative endodontic procedures. J Endod 2009;35(10):1343-9.
2. Kadar K, Kiraly M, Porcsalmy B, et al. Differentiation potential of stem cells from human dental origin—promise of tissue engineering. J Physiol Pharmacol 2009; 60(Suppl 7):167-75.
3. Tziafas D, Kodonas K. Differentiation potential of dental papilla, dental pulp and apical papilla progenitor cells. J Endod 2010;36(5):781-9.
4. Galler KM, D'Souza RN. Tissue engineering approaches for regenerative dentistry. Regen Med 2011;6(1):111-24.
5. Smith AJ, Tobias RS, Plant CG, et al. In vivo morphogenetic activity of dentin matrix proteins. J Biol Buccale 1990;18(2):123-9.
6. Cox CF, Subay RK, Ostro E, et al. Tunnel defects in dentin bridges: their formation following direct pulp capping. Oper Dent 1996;21(1):4-11.

7. Murray PE, About I, Lumley P, et al. Odontoblast morphology and dental repair. J Dent 2003;31(1):75–82.

8. Murray PE, Garcia-Godoy F, Hargreaves KM. Regenerative endodontics: a review of current status and a call for action. J Endod 2007;33(4):377–90.

9. About I, Mitsiadis TA. Molecular aspect of tooth pathogenesis and repair: in vivo and in vitro models. Adv Dent Res 2001;15(14):59–62.

10. Goldberg M. Pulp healing and regeneration: more questions than answers. Adv Dent Res 2011;23(3):270–4.

11. Smith AJ, Tobias RS, Cassidy N, et al. Odontoblast stimulation in ferrets by dentine matrix components. Arch Oral Biol 1994;39(1):13–22.

12. Trope M. Regenerative potential of dental pulp. J Endod 2008;34(Suppl 7):S13–7.

13. Ding RY, Cheung GS, Chen J, et al. Pulp revascularization of immature teeth with apical periodontitis: a clinical study. J Endod 2009;35(5):745–9.

14. Kusgoz A, Yildrim T, Er K, et al. Retreatment of a resected tooth associated with a large periradicular lesion by using a triple antibiotic paste and mineral trioxide aggregate: a case report with a thirty-month follow-up. J Endod 2009;35(11): 1603–6.

15. Mrozik KM, Zump S, Bagley CJ, et al. Protomic characterization of mesenchymal stem-cell like populations derived from ovine periodontal ligament, dental pulp, and bone marrow: analysis of differentially expressed proteins. Stem Cell Dev 2009;19(10):1485–99.

16. Gronthos S, Mankani M, Brahim J, et al. Postnatal human dental pulp stem cells (DPSCs) in vitro and in vivo. Proc Natl Acad Sci U S A 2000;97(25):13625–30.

17. Gronthos S, Brahim J, Li W, et al. Stem cell properties of human dental pulp stem cells. J Dent Res 2002;81(8):531–5.

18. Young-Min J, Jeon SH, Park JY, et al. Dental stem cell therapy with calcium hydroxide in dental pulp capping. Tissue Eng Part A 2009;16(6):1823–33.

19. Bakopoulou A, Leyhausen G, Volk J, et al. Assessment of the impact of two different isolation methods on the osteo/odontogenic differentiation potential of human stem cells derived from deciduous teeth. Calcif Tissue Int 2011;88(2): 130–41.

20. Miura M, Gronthos S, Zhao M, et al. SHED: stem cells from human exfoliated deciduous teeth. Proc Natl Acad Sci U S A 2003;100(10):5807–12.

21. Cordeiro MM, Dong Z, Kaneko T, et al. Dental pulp tissue engineering with stem cells from exfoliated deciduous teeth. J Endod 2008;34(8):962–9.

22. Seo BM, Sonoyama W, Yamaza T, et al. SHED repair critical calvarial defects in mice. Oral Dis 2008;14(5):428–34.

23. Zhang C, Chang J, Sonoyama W, et al. Inhibition of human dental pulp stem cell differentiation by NOTCH signaling. J Dent Res 2008;87(3):250–5.

24. Dissanayaka WL, Zhan X, Zhang C, et al. Coculture of dental pulp stem cells with endothelial cells enhances osteo-/odontogenic and angiogenic potential in vitro. J Endod 2012;38(4):454–63.

25. Pivoriuunas A, Surovas A, Borutinskaite Y, et al. Proteomic analysis of stromal cells derived from the dental pulp of human exfoliated deciduous teeth. Stem Cells Dev 2010;19(7):1081–93.

26. Sonoyama W, Liu Y, Fang D, et al. Mesenchymal stem cell-mediated functional tooth regeneration in swine. PLoS One 2006;1(1):e79.

27. Peng L, Ye L, Zhou XD. Mesenchymal stem cells and tooth engineering. Int J Oral Sci 2009;1(1):6–12.

28. Menicanin D, Bartold PM, Zannettino AC, et al. Identification of a common gene expression signature associated with immature clonal mesenchymal cell

populations derived from bone marrow and dental tissues. Stem Cells Dev 2010; 19(10):1501–10.

29. Estrela C, Alencar AH, Kitten GT, et al. Mesenchymal stem cells in the dental tissues: perspectives for tissue regeneration. Braz Dent J 2011;22(2):1–8.

30. Morsczek C, Gotz W, Schierholz J, et al. Isolation of precursor cells (PCs) from human dental follicle of wisdom teeth. Matrix Biol 2005;24:155–65.

31. Gronthos S, Mrozik K, Shi S, et al. Ovine periodontal ligament stem cells: isolation, characterization, and differentiation potential. Calcif Tissue Int 2006;79(5):310–7.

32. Huang GT, Sonoyama W, Liu Y, et al. The hidden treasure in apical papilla: the potential role in pulp/dentin regeneration and bio-root engineering. J Endod 2008;34(2):645–51.

33. Huang GT, Gronthos S, Shi S. Mesenchymal stem cells derived from dental tissues vs. those from other sources: their biology and role in regenerative medicine. J Dent Res 2009;88(9):792–806.

34. Sonoyama W, Liu Y, Yamaza T, et al. Characterization of apical papilla and its residing stem cells from human immature permanent teeth: a pilot study. J Endod 2008;34(1):166–71.

35. Ulmer FL, Winkel A, Kohorst P, et al. Stem cells—prospects in dentistry. Schweiz Monatsschr Zahnmed 2010;120(10):860–72 [in English, German].

36. About I. Dentin regeneration in vitro: the pivotal role of supportive cells. Adv Dent Res 2011;23(3):320–4.

37. Bartouli S, Miura M, Brahim J, et al. Comparison of stem-cell-mediated osteogenesis and dentinogenesis. J Dent Res 2003;82:976–81.

38. Harichane Y, Hirata A, Dimitrova-Nakov S, et al. Pulpal progenitors and dentin repair. Adv Dent Res 2011;23(3):307–12.

39. Simon SR, Berdal A, Cooper PR, et al. Dentin-pulp complex regeneration: from lab to clinic. Adv Dent Res 2011;23(3):340–5.

40. Smith AJ, Lesof H. Introduction and regulation of crown dentino-genesis: embryonic events as a template for dental tissue repair? Crit Rev Oral Biol Med 2001; 12(12):425–37.

41. Cooper PR, Takahasi Y, Graham LW, et al. Inflammation-regeneration interplay in the dentine-pulp complex. J Dent 2010;38(9):687–97.

42. Huang GT, Yamaza T, Shea LD, et al. Stem/progenitor cell medicated de novo regeneration of dental pulp with newly deposited continuous layer of dentin in an in vivo model. Tissue Eng Part A 2010;16(2):605–15.

43. Shi S, Gronthos S. Perivascular niche of postnatal mesenchymal stem cells in human bone marrow and dental pulp. J Bone Miner Res 2003;18(4):696–704.

44. Galler KM, D'Souza RN, Hartgerink JD, et al. Scaffolds for dental pulp tissue engineering. Adv Dent Res 2011;23(3):333–9.

45. Sakai VT, Corderio MM, Dong Z, et al. Tooth slice/scaffold model of dental pulp tissue engineering. Adv Dent Res 2011;23(3):325–32.

46. Mitsiadis TA, Fried K, Goridis C, et al. Reactivation of Delta-Notch signaling: complementary expression patterns of ligand and receptor in dental pulp. Exp Cell Res 1999;246(2):312–8.

47. Lovshall H, Mitsidias TA, Poulsen K, et al. Co-expression of Notch3 and Rgs5 in the pericyte-vascular smooth muscle cell axis in response to pulp injury. Int J Dev Biol 2007;51(8):715–21.

48. Scadden DL. The stem cell niche as an entity of action. Nature 2006;441(7097): 1075–9.

49. Djouad F, Ghannam S, Noel D, et al. Mesenchymal stem cells: innovative therapeutic tools for rheumatic diseases. Nat Rev Rheumatol 2009;5:392–9.

50. Mitsiadis TA, Feki A, Papaccio G, et al. Dental pulp stem cells, niches, and NOTCH signaling in tooth injury. Adv Dent Res 2011;23(3):275–9.
51. Moore KA, Lemischka IR. Stem cells and their niches. Science 2006;311(5769): 1880–5.
52. Kindler V. Postnatal stem cell survival: does the niche, a rare harbor where to resist the ebb tide of differentiation, also provide lineage-specific instructions? J Leukoc Biol 2005;78(4):836–44.
53. Li L, Xie T. Stem cell niche: structure and function. Annu Rev Cell Dev Biol 2005; 21:605–31.
54. Ahmed MJ. The ability of stem cells of the apical papilla to grow, proliferate and differentiate on polycaprolactone based scaffolds. Dubai (United Arab Emirates): Boston University Institute for Dental Research and Education; 2011.
55. Artavanis-Tsakonas S, Rand MD, Lake RJ. Notch signaling: cell fate control and signal integration in development. Science 1999;284(5415):770–6.
56. Artavanis-Tsakonas S. Notch: the past, the present and the future. Curr Top Dev Biol 2010;92:1–29.
57. Mitsiadis TA, Regaudiat L, Gridley T. Role of Notch signalling pathway in tooth morphogenesis. Arch Oral Biol 2005;50(2):137–40.
58. Tziafas D, Smith AJ, Lesot H. Designing new treatment strategies in vital pulp therapy. J Dent 2000;28(2):77–82.
59. Mitsiadis TA, Rahiotis C. Parallels between tooth development and repair: conserved molecular mechanisms following carious and dental injury. J Dent Res 2004;83(12):896–902.
60. Lovschall H, Tummers M, Thesleff I, et al. Activation of the Notch signaling pathways in response to pulp capping of rat molars. Eur J Oral Sci 2005;113(4): 312–7.
61. Mullane EM, Dong Z, Sedgley CM, et al. Effects of VEGF And FGF2 on the revasculature of severed human dental pulps. J Dent Res 2008;87(12):1144–8.
62. Rosa V, Tatiana MB, Botero M. Regenerative endodontics in light of stem cell paradigms. Int Dent J 2011;61(Suppl 1):23–8.
63. Gebhardt M, Murray PE, Namerow KN. Cell survival within pulp and periodontal constructs. J Endod 2009;35(1):63–6.
64. Smith AJ, Cassidy N, Perry H. Reactionary dentinogenesis. Int J Dev Biol 1995; 39(1):273–80.
65. Thesleff I, Mikkola M. The role of growth factors in tooth development. Int Rev Cytol 2002;217:93–135.
66. Jamal M, Chogle S, Goodis H, et al. Dental stem cells and their potential role in regenerative medicine. J Med Sci 2011;4(2):53–61.
67. Cooper PR, McLachlan JL, Simon S, et al. Mediators of inflammation and regeneration. Adv Dent Res 2011;23(3):290–5.
68. Huang GT. Dental pulp and dentin tissue engineering and regeneration: advances and challenges. Front Bio Science (Elite Ed) 2011;3:788–800.
69. Eppleman I, Murray PE, Garciua-Godoy F. A practitioner survey of opinions toward regenerative endodontics. J Endod 2009;35(9):1204–10.
70. Friedman S, Mor C. Success of endodontic therapy-healing and functionality. J Calif Dent Assoc 2004;32(6):493–503.
71. Farzaneh M, Abitbol S, Friedman S. Treatment outcome in endodontics: the Toronto Study. Phases I and II: Orthograde retreatment. J Endod 2004;30(9): 627–33.
72. Farzaneh M, Abitbol S, Lawrence HP, et al. Treatment outcome in endodontics; the Toronto Study. Phase II: initial treatment. J Endod 2004;30(5):302–9.

73. Wang N, Knight K, Dao T, et al. Treatment outcome in endodontics: the Toronto Study. Phase I and II: apical surgery. J Endod 2004;30(11):751–61.
74. Ikeda E, Morita R, Nakao K, et al. Fully functional bioengineering tooth replacement as an organ replacement therapy. Proc Natl Acad Sci U S A 2009; 106(32):13475–80.

Index

Note: Page numbers of article titles are in **boldface** type.

Dent Clin N Am 56 (2012) 691–697
doi:10.1016/S0011-8532(12)00053-5
0011-8532/12/$ – see front matter © 2012 Elsevier Inc. All rights reserved.

dental.theclinics.com

T

Moving?

Make sure your subscription moves with you!

To notify us of your new address, find your **Clinics Account Number** (located on your mailing label above your name), and contact customer service at:

Email: **journalscustomerservice-usa@elsevier.com**

800-654-2452 (subscribers in the U.S. & Canada)
314-447-8871 (subscribers outside of the U.S. & Canada)

Fax number: **314-447-8029**

Elsevier Health Sciences Division
Subscription Customer Service
3251 Riverport Lane
Maryland Heights, MO 63043

*To ensure uninterrupted delivery of your subscription, please notify us at least 4 weeks in advance of move.

Announcing
Dental Advance

The new, online home just for dentistry professionals

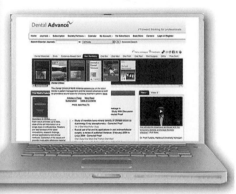

DentalAdvance.org is the gateway offering high-quality **research, news, jobs** and more for the **global community** of dental professionals.

What you'll find at DentalAdvance.org

* Journal profiles with quick links to **Tables of Contents, author submission** information, and subscription details
* Important information and valuable resources on how to submit a journal article
* Dentistry **Articles in Press** from participating journals
* Quick links to the leading dentistry societies worldwide
* **Dentistry News** from Elsevier Global Medical News (formerly IMNG)
* **Dentistry Jobs** powered by ElsevierHealthCareers.com

Bookmark us!
Visit DentalAdvance.org today.

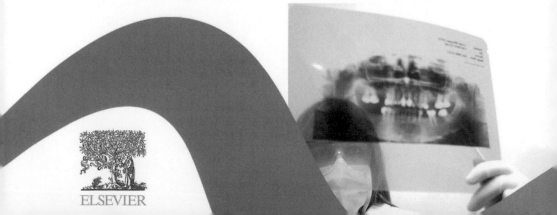

ELSEVIER